Environment and Breast Cancer

Jose Russo
Editor

Environment and Breast Cancer

Springer

Editor
Jose Russo MD, FACP
Breast Cancer Research Laboratory
Breast Cancer and the Environment Research Center
Fox Chase Cancer Center
Philadelphia, PA 19111
USA
jose.russo@fccc.edu

ISBN 978-1-4419-9895-8 e-ISBN 978-1-4419-9896-5
DOI 10.1007/978-1-4419-9896-5
Springer New York Dordrecht Heidelberg London

Library of Congress Control Number: 2011934046

Printed on acid-free paper

Springer is part of Springer Science+Business Media (www.springer.com)

This book is dedicated to
Dr. Kenneth Olden
That through his efforts and vision
the concept of Environment
and Breast Cancer was established

Prologue

Breast cancer is a complex disease caused by multiple environmental and lifestyle factors interacting with genetic susceptibility across the life span. Therefore, environmental factors are of intense interest to both researchers and community members, including women with breast cancer. There is not adequate literature that addresses this issue comprehensively from epidemiological, experimental, and translational research perspective. This book fills this gap in 11 chapters written by the most recognized expert in the field of breast biology and cancers with special interests in environmental issues.

Philadelphia, PA, USA

Jose Russo, MD

Acknowledgments

My special acknowledgment and thanks to *Ms. Patricia A. Russo* for her insightful editorial and style suggestions.

THANKS to *Dr. Irma H. Russo* for her critiques and delightful moments discussing the manuscript and ideas, to *Ms. Rosemary Sonlin* for verifying the accuracy of the references, and to the *Pathology Consultation Services* from Rydal, PA, that have financed the writing and editing of this book.

Philadelphia, PA, USA Jose Russo, MD

Contents

Contributors

Mary Helen Barcellos-Hoff Department of Radiation Oncology, New York University, Langone School of Medicine, New York, NY, USA
mhbarcellos-hoff@nyumc.org

Angela M. Betancourt Department of Pharmacology and Toxicology, University of Alabama at Birmingham, Birmingham, AL, USA

Frank M. Biro Division of Adolescent Medicine, Cincinnati Children's Hospital Medical Center, University of Cincinnati College of Medicine, Cincinnati, OH, USA
frank.biro@cchme.org

Irineu Illa Bochaca Department of Radiation Oncology, New York University, Langone School of Medicine, New York, NY, USA

Deborah J. Clegg Department of Internal Medicine, University of Texas Southwestern Medical Center, Touchstone Diabetes Center, Dallas, TX, USA
deborah.clegg@utsouthwestern.edu

Ricardo López de Cicco Breast Cancer and the Environment Research Center, Breast Cancer Research Laboratory, Fox Chase Cancer Center, Philadelphia, PA, USA

Suzanne E. Fenton National Toxicology Program, National Institute of Environmental Health Sciences, Research Triangle Park, NC, USA
suzanne.fenton@nih.gov

Sandra Z. Haslam Department of Biomedical and Integrative Physiology, Michigan State University, East Lansing, MI, USA

Breast Cancer and the Environment Research Center, Michigan State University, East Lansing, MI, USA
shaslam@msu.edu

Robert A. Hiatt University of California San Francisco,
San Francisco, CA, USA

Professor and Chair of Epidemiology and Biostatistics,
Director of Population Sciences and Deputy Director, Helen Diller Family Comprehensive Cancer Center, San Francisco, CA, USA
rhiatt@epi.ucsf.edu

Sarah Jenkins Department of Pharmacology and Toxicology,
University of Alabama at Birmingham, Birmingham, AL, USA

Coral A. Lamartiniere Department of Pharmacology and Toxicology,
University of Alabama at Birmingham, Birmingham, AL, USA

Division of Urology, Department of Surgery, University of Alabama at Birmingham, Birmingham, AL, USA
coral@uab.edu

Maricel V. Maffini Department of Anatomy and Cellular Biology,
Tufts University School of Medicine, Boston, MA, USA
maricel.maffini@tufts.edu

James A. Mobley Department of Pharmacology and Toxicology,
University of Alabama at Birmingham, Birmingham, AL, USA

UAB Comprehensive Cancer Center, University of Alabama at Birmingham, Birmingham, AL, USA

Division of Urology, Department of Surgery, University of Alabama at Birmingham, Birmingham, AL, USA

Raquel Moral Breast Cancer and the Environment Research Center,
Breast Cancer Research Laboratory, Fox Chase Cancer Center,
Philadelphia, PA, USA

Department of Cell Biology, Physiology and Immunology, Medicine School,
Universitat Autònoma de Barcelona, Barcelona, Spain

David H. Nguyen Molecular Endocrinology Program, University of California, Berkeley, CA, USA

Suraj Peri Department of Biostatistics, Fox Chase Cancer Center,
Philadelphia, PA, USA

Jennifer L. Rayner Toxicology and Hazard Assessment Group,
Oak Ridge National Laboratory, Oak Ridge, TN, USA

Irma H. Russo Breast Cancer and the Environment Research Center,
Breast Cancer Research Laboratory, Fox Chase Cancer Center,
Philadelphia, PA, USA
Irma.russo@fccc.edu

Jose Russo Breast Cancer Research Laboratory, Breast Cancer and the Environment Research Center, Fox Chase Cancer Center, Philadelphia, PA, USA
jose.russo@fccc.edu

Patrícia A. Russo Breast Cancer and the Environment Research Center, Breast Cancer Research Laboratory, Fox Chase Cancer Center, Philadelphia, PA, USA

Stephen Safe Department of Veterinary Physiology and Pharmacology, Texas A&M University, College Station, TX, USA

Institute of Biosciences and Technology, Texas A&M Health Sciences Center, Houston, TX, USA
ssafe@cvm.tamu.edu

Julia Santucci-Pereira Breast Cancer and the Environment Research Center, Breast Cancer Research Laboratory, Fox Chase Cancer Center, Philadelphia, PA, USA

Michael Slifker Department of Biostatistics, Fox Chase Cancer Center, Philadelphia, PA, USA

Carlos Sonnenschein Department of Anatomy and Cellular Biology, Tufts University School of Medicine, Boston, MA, USA

Ana M. Soto Department of Anatomy and Cellular Biology, Tufts University School of Medicine, Boston, MA, USA

Kelcey Walker Department of Veterinary Physiology and Pharmacology, Texas A&M University, College Station, TX, USA

Jun Wang Department of Pharmacology and Toxicology, University of Alabama at Birmingham, Birmingham, AL, USA

Richard Wang Breast Cancer and the Environment Research Center, Breast Cancer Research Laboratory, Fox Chase Cancer Center, Philadelphia, PA, USA

Sally S. White NIEHS, National Toxicology Program, Research Triangle Park, NC, USA

Mary S. Wolff Department of Community and Preventive Medicine, Mount Sinai School of Medicine, New York, NY, USA

Yong Xu Children's Nutrition Research Center, Department of Pediatrics, Baylor College of Medicine, Houston, TX, USA

Chengfeng Yang Department of Biomedical and Integrative Physiology, Michigan State University, East Lansing, MI, USA

Breast Cancer and the Environment Research Center, Michigan State University, East Lansing, MI, USA

Center for Integrative Toxicology, Michigan State University, East Lansing, MI, USA

Shu Zhang Institute of Biosciences and Technology, Texas A&M Health Sciences Center, Houston, TX, USA

Chapter 1
Epidemiologic Basis of the Role of Environmental Endocrine Disruptors in Breast Cancer

Robert A. Hiatt

Abstract What can be said about the role of environmental endocrine disruptors in breast cancer from epidemiologic studies of humans? To address this question, we define endocrine disruptors, consider their sources in the environment, document the breast cancer trends in incidence and mortality over time, place exposures in the context of "windows of susceptibility," discuss the strengths and limitations of the epidemiologic approach in environmental studies, and review studies in humans relevant to this question across a range of endocrine disruptors. We take a life-course perspective on breast cancer etiology that encompasses the known and potential impact of environmental factors early in development and during "windows of susceptibility" across the life span. Such an approach presents certain challenges for human epidemiologic studies, which are discussed. However, observational epidemiologic studies, natural experiments, and novel study designs, along with toxicological and mechanistic studies using animal models, are creating a fuller picture of the role of the environment in breast cancer. Recommendations for filling gaps in our current knowledge of this topic complete the chapter.

Keywords Epidemiology • Endocrine disrupting chemicals • Breast cancer • Environment

R.A. Hiatt (✉)
University of California San Francisco, 185 Berry Street, Lobby 5, Suite 5700, San Francisco, CA 94107-0560, USA

Professor and Chair of Epidemiology and Biostatistics,
Director of Population Sciences and Deputy Director,
Helen Diller Family Comprehensive Cancer Center,
Box 0560, San Francisco, CA 94143-0560, USA
e-mail: rhiatt@epi.ucsf.edu

J. Russo (ed.), *Environment and Breast Cancer*, DOI 10.1007/978-1-4419-9896-5_1,

1.1 Introduction

Breast cancer remains the most common cancer among women in industrialized countries and is the second leading cause of death from cancer (Kohler et al. 2011). While much is known about the etiology of breast cancer in women, estimates have suggested that only 40% of cases in the United States can be explained by established risk factors, such as earlier age at menarche and older age at first full-term pregnancy (Madigan et al. 1995), As a result there remain concerns about the role of the environment in the causal chain. This volume explores what we know now about the relationship between the environment and breast cancer from the perspective of the multiple disciplines engaged in solving this challenge. These disciplines include genetics, molecular biology, toxicology, endocrinology, and epidemiology, all of which are needed to adequately address the complex nature of this problem (Mabry et al. 2008).

We start with a view of what is known from epidemiologic studies in humans across a range of factors focusing on the chemical environment and substances known as endocrine disruptors. We take a life-course perspective on breast cancer etiology that encompasses the known and potential impact of environmental factors early in development and during "windows of susceptibility" (Diamanti-Kandarakis et al. 2009; Fenton 2006). Such an approach presents certain challenges for human epidemiologic studies, which will be discussed. However, observational epidemiologic studies, natural experiments, and novel study designs, along with toxicological and mechanistic studies using animal models, are creating a fuller picture of the role of the environment in breast cancer.

1.1.1 Statement of the Problem

What then can be concluded about the role of environmental factors, especially about endocrine disruptors and breast cancer, from epidemiologic studies of humans? To address this question we must first define endocrine disruptors, consider their sources in the environment, document the breast cancer trends in incidence and mortality over time, place exposures in the context of "windows of susceptibility," discuss the strengths and limitations of the epidemiologic approach in environmental studies, and review studies in humans relevant to this question. Although the "environment" is frequently defined broadly to include social factors, aspects of the human built environment, and exposures resulting from the so-called lifestyle behaviors (diet and physical activity), in this volume we focus more narrowly on the physical environment and exposures such as chemicals, toxicants, and radiation.

1.1.2 Definition of an Endocrine Disruptor

The National Institute of Environmental Health Sciences (NIEHS) defines endocrine disruptors as "chemicals that may interfere with the body's endocrine system and produce adverse developmental, reproductive, neurological, and immune effects in both humans and wildlife" (http://www.niehs.nih.gov/health/topics/agents/endocrine/ – accessed 11/13/10). Endocrine disrupting chemicals (EDCs) have effects on male and female reproduction, neuroendocrine targets, thyroid disruption, metabolism, and obesity as well as other effects (Rudel and Perovich 2009); (Diamanti-Kandarakis et al. 2009). Some endocrine disruptors that are xenoestrogens (foreign estrogens) may contribute to the development of hormone-dependent cancers such as breast cancer (Sonnenschein and Soto 1998). In many cases positive findings in animal models have stimulated new epidemiologic studies that examine the risks of cancer in humans associated with pharmaceutical and chemical exposures (Friedman et al. 2009; Rudel et al. 2007).

EDCs comprise a number of different chemical classes including exogenous hormones, pesticides, compounds used in plastics and consumer products, heavy metals, and plant constituents. Sources for EDCs are multiple but are primarily found in food, polluted water, and air, which includes indoor air pollution and house dust. Some of these substances are fat soluble and persist in the food chain and in human fat tissue for years. Other chemicals may have a lasting effect on physiologic systems, but be measurable only transiently after exposure, usually many years before cancer or other long-term outcomes are observed.

1.1.3 Rationale for Concern in Humans

Concern about the effects of EDCs in humans comes from a number of sources. First, there are numerous studies in animal systems where EDC exposure has produced reproductive system abnormalities both in terms of pathophysiologic and anatomical outcomes. For example, bisphenol A (BPA) exposure to rats during fetal development and perinatally results in precancerous mammary lesions, increased susceptibility to carcinogens, and increased number of terminal end buds and ducts or density of the breast (Crain et al. 2008; Fenton 2006). Second, in humans higher dose exposures in occupational settings and to pharmaceuticals have been associated with biologic/reproductive effects and some cancer outcomes. The best example here is in utero exposure to diethylstilbestrol (DES) which is an estrogen compound given to women between about 1940 and 1970 to prevent miscarriages and which resulted in rare cervicovaginal cancers (Herbst et al. 1971) and other reproductive system abnormalities, including breast cancer (Palmer et al. 2006). The toxicology of EDCs and other environmental carcinogens are discussed in detail in subsequent chapters, but examples from epidemiologic studies will be discussed below.

1.1.4 Breast Cancer

This volume focuses on the human burden of breast cancer, its etiology, and prevention. The most recent data from the United States estimate that given current trends, 207,090 women are expected to be diagnosed with breast cancer in 2010 and 39,840 women will die with this disease (Jemal et al. 2010a). No other cancer, except basal and squamous cell skin cancers, which tend not to invade and become fatal, is more common. Only lung cancer is more likely to take a woman's life (estimated 71,080 deaths in 2010) (Jemal et al. 2010a). On the basis of its prevalence alone, breast cancer is the most studied and among the best understood cancers in humans. The economic impact in terms of value of life lost from breast cancer was $121 billion in 2000 (Yabroff et al. 2008). Because it strikes women while they are in their most productive years, and because of myriad influences on the quality of life and impact on families, it has a huge impact on women's overall health and deserves the scientific attention it gets.

Since the early part of the last century there have been clear upward trends in both incidence and mortality, although in decades prior to the 1990s these trends were modest and in the range of 1%/year. The best data for trends earlier in the last century come from the Connecticut Cancer Registry, which has been reporting data from 1935 onward. Trends from this registry indicate a steady and marked increase in breast cancer incidence from age-standardized (to 1970 US population) rates of 56.6/100,00 from the years 1935 through 1939, to 114.5/100,000 in 1990–1991 (Polednak 1994). However, since the early 1990s there has been a downward trend in mortality from breast cancer, while incidence continued to increase in white women until about 2001 (age standardized to 2000 US population rate of 144.3/100,000 in white women). Cancer incidence rates decreased somewhat earlier in black women (around 1993) and somewhat later in Asian/Pacific Islanders, American Indians, and Hispanics (2002–2005) (http://seer.cancer.gov/csr/1975_2007/browse_csr.php?section=4&page=sect_04_zfig.04.html#graph – accessed 11/13/10) (Jemal et al. 2010). These trends have been echoed in other industrialized countries but not worldwide. In less-developed countries, breast cancer incidence and mortality rate trends seem to be increasing (Jemal et al. 2010b). International differences in breast cancer mortality are almost fivefold between the countries with the highest and lowest rates (Mettlin 1999). This difference, plus changes in incidence within one or two generations among immigrant populations, strongly points to environmental factors in the etiology of breast cancer. Even within countries like the United States rates vary substantially (Sturgeon et al. 2004) and certain communities and areas of the country with the highest rates have generated public concern and spurred advocacy to better understand the problem and do something to reduce excess risk in these areas (Gammon et al. 2002a; Hiatt et al. 2009). These surveillance data are all compatible with environmental causes of breast cancer, but the downward trend in breast cancer mortality in the US in the last few decades does not point to some inexorable increase in the environmental determinants of this cancer. Environmental toxicants may well still play a role, but the overall trends suggest progress in prevention, early detection, and treatment of this disease.

Although a few environmental factors are now reasonably well established as risk factors for breast cancer, most accepted risk factors fall into categories of reproductive history and genetic susceptibility (Hunter et al. 1997). A variety of attempts have been made to determine how much of breast cancer incidence can be explained from known or highly suspected risk factors like ages of menarche, menopause, and first full-term pregnancy (Madigan et al. 1995). Such estimates of population attributable risk suggest that only approximately 40% of breast cancer can be explained by what is already known. In this context concern remains that environmental factors may play a substantial role and that they would not be discovered by conventional epidemiologic studies in adult women. Studies in adult women rely on the recall of self-reported exposures earlier in life or on levels of putative chemicals in biospecimens (e.g., blood, urine) after the time of diagnosis. Both methods of assessment of exposure have their weaknesses. Women may not be able to accurately report known exposures in terms of duration or dose when they occurred many years before and they may not even know they were exposed to particular chemicals in question. When assays of chemicals are performed after the diagnosis of breast cancer, it is difficult to establish causality.

1.1.5 Mechanism of Exposure

Critical times for exposure to EDCs can occur at various points along the life-course, not just in adult life. This perspective is relatively new in our thinking about breast cancer etiology. Whereas the appreciation that cancer can take decades to develop after initiation has been a basic understanding about cancer etiology for many years, the focus on certain "windows of susceptibility," derived from an understanding of breast development and susceptibility to environmental insults, is more recent (Diamanti-Kandarakis et al. 2009). These windows, or periods, of susceptibility or vulnerability generally refer to the impact of exposures in utero (Soto et al. 2008), in childhood before puberty (Okasha et al. 2003), during adolescence and breast development, the period leading up to a first pregnancy, and during pregnancy itself (Fenton 2006). In all these phases of the female life-course, the breast, which is the only organ to develop after birth, is undergoing some stage of development during which EDCs and other environmental agents may have their effects. It behooves science, therefore, to study effects of exposures during these particular "windows" and not some more generalized concept of exposure at unspecified times prior to cancer diagnosis.

1.1.6 Occupational and Therapeutic Exposures vs. Population Exposures

Much of the evidence for the relationship between the chemical environment and cancer comes from exposures in occupational or therapeutic settings. Thus, lessons have been learned from exposure to pharmacologic doses of exogenous estrogens (i.e., DES) exposure in utero (Troisi et al. 2007) or from the accidental exposures of workers to dioxins (Bueno de Mesquita et al. 1993). Small selected populations exposed to very high doses of chemicals generally characterize such studies.

However, our primary interest is in evidence that can be derived from population studies where doses are much smaller across larger populations.

1.1.7 The Timing of Exposure: A Life-Course Approach

1.1.7.1 In Utero

It is not known when in the life span the initiation of breast cancer takes place, but it may be at the very beginning of life. Although past epidemiologic studies of the association between birth weight and breast cancer risk have yielded inconsistent results, a recent meta-analysis has demonstrated an increased risk with larger birth weights. Relative to birth weights between 2,500 and 2,999 g, those between 3,500 and 3,999 g and 4,000 g or more yielded statistically significant odds ratios of 1.15 and 1.24, respectively, for developing breast cancer as adults (Park et al. 2008). This suggests that the in utero hormonal milieu may influence breast cancer risk. A meta-analysis of epidemiologic evidence that included 57 studies confirmed this relationship (Xue and Michels 2007). A mechanism suggested by Trichopoulos et al. (2005) is that higher levels of hormones during pregnancy favor the generation of a higher number of susceptible stem cells with compromised genomic stability.

Backing up the epidemiologic observations, studies in animal models have found that stem cells in the fetal breast in utero are capable of cancer initiation (Russo and Russo 1996). The presence of a population of stem cells in the fetal breast and their continued presence in adult reproductive years have been demonstrated in rodent models (Chepko and Smith 1999). In human tissue, analysis of random X-chromosome inactivation supports the hypothesis that the mammary gland is organized into distinct stem cell-derived monoclonal patches (Diallo et al. 2001).

In utero exposures to estrogens, androgens, IGF-1, and possibly alpha-fetoprotein have all been postulated to be associated with increased breast cancer risk in later life (Ekbom et al. 1997; Forman et al. 2005). DES use by mothers during their pregnancies has led to elevated rates of breast cancer in their adult children (Troisi et al. 2007). Exposure of mice to BPA in utero has been associated with preneoplastic lesions and carcinoma in situ in the developing mammary gland (Soto et al. 2008). Thus, there is substantial evidence from both epidemiologic and animal studies that exposures and events in utero can influence adult breast cancer incidence, and this is one "window" during which EDCs may have an effect.

1.1.7.2 Puberty

Soon after birth and until the onset of puberty, the breast remains in a dormant state. Although the exact mechanisms responsible for breast development at puberty have not been defined, the initiation of puberty in girls is coincident with the activation of the hypothalamic-pituitary-gonadal (HPG) axis, or thelarche, and the activation of the hypothalamic pituitary adrenal (HPA) axis, or adrenarche, which are independent events. The relative timing of thelarche and adrenarche may differentially determine the onset of menarche (Biro et al. 2006).

Human puberty is the period of transition from childhood to adolescence and is characterized by a complex sequence of biologic events leading to the maturation of secondary sex characteristics, accelerated linear growth, and ultimately to the attainment of reproductive capacity (Buck Louis et al. 2008).

A focus on the "window of susceptibility" around puberty stems from the well-established observation that an earlier onset of menarche is associated with an increased risk of breast cancer (Hunter et al. 1997). In a pooled analysis of 7,764 premenopausal women from 19 studies, and 16,467 postmenopausal women from 18 studies, the percent decrease in breast cancer risk for each additional year of menarche delay was estimated to be 9 and 4%, for pre- and postmenopausal women, respectively (Clavel-Chapelon 2002).

That both the age when girls begin puberty and their age of menarche have declined over the last century is well established (Euling et al. 2008) and has been confirmed by recent observations from the Breast Cancer and the Environment Research Centers (BCERCs) (Biro et al. 2010). This strongly suggests that changes in lifestyle and/or environmental factors have influenced these trends. When menarche is accelerated without a concomitant acceleration in the timing of menopause, it is widely thought that increased duration of hormone exposure would promote the development of breast cancer (de Waard and Thijssen 2005). However, it may be that the pubertal transition itself is critical because of rapid breast development and the susceptibility of rapidly duplicating cells to environmental insults (Berkey et al. 1999). Compared to other times in life, the pubertal breast in the rodent contains the highest number and the greatest proliferative activity of the terminal duct lobular units (TDLUs), the functional units of the breast (Rudland 1993). This may be related to the apparent susceptibility of the breast to carcinogens during puberty (Knight and Sorensen 2001). In rats, administration of a carcinogen when the mammary tissue is dividing and differentiating during puberty and up to first pregnancy onset induces the greatest number of carcinomas (Colditz and Frazier 1995).

However, among environmental factors, the clearest evidence of an impact on breast cancer etiology at the time of puberty comes from the study of ionizing radiation exposure. This subject will be discussed in a later chapter, but an increased risk of breast cancer has been consistently reported for radiation exposure from various sources, including the atomic weapon explosions in Nagasaki-Hiroshima (Tokunaga et al. 1991), medical treatments such as radiotherapy for postpartum mastitis (Shore et al. 1986) and tuberculosis (Boice et al. 1991), Hodgkin's disease and childhood cancer, ankylosing spondylitis, tinea capitis, enlarged thymus (Shore et al. 1993), skin hemangioma (John and Kelsey 1993), and among radiologic technologists (Boice et al. 1995). Among atomic bomb survivors, increased risk clearly has been related to younger age at exposure around the time of puberty (Land et al. 2003). Finally, elevated breast cancer risk in areas that were most contaminated from the Chernobyl accident has been noted in Belarus (average cumulative dose ≥40 mSv) about 10 years after the incident, and risk was greater among women who were younger at the time of exposure (Pukkala et al. 2006).

Thus, endocrine disruptors found in the environment may influence both the timing and pace of the pubertal transition as well as female reproductive outcomes (Crain et al. 2008). More of a focus on environmental impact of exposures to EDCs is justified during puberty given the evidence that they interfere with normal hormonal synthesis and metabolic pathways during this "window of susceptibility."

1.1.7.3 Adult Life Prior to First Pregnancy

It is well known that a lower age of first full-term pregnancy confers substantial protection against postmenopausal breast cancer compared to first full-term pregnancy at a latter age (the cutoff is usually around 35 years), or nulliparous women (Hunter et al. 1997). This is thought to be because during pregnancy the breast cells and breast architecture will have fully matured, and there is less proliferative activity, and thus decreased sensitivity to environmental carcinogens (Russo et al. 2001). Parity is also directly associated with a protective effect as each successive live birth confers addition protection, presumably by the same mechanism (Kauppila et al. 2009). However, pregnancy also transiently increased the risk of breast cancer in the first 5 years or so after delivery (Williams et al. 1990). Thus the event of pregnancy and its frequency represent another window of susceptibility during which the human breast is at risk of environmental carcinogenesis including potentially risks associated with exposure to EDCs.

1.2 Epidemiologic Approaches

Given the challenges of exposure assessment, timing, and intermediate outcomes referred to above, what are the options for approaching these important questions in human populations using the discipline of epidemiology?

An ideal design would be prospective/longitudinal in nature and follow girls from interuterine life to maturity and until after menopause, when breast cancer incidence becomes most common. Assessments of exposure of various sorts, including self-reports from parents, the girls and later on the women themselves, as well as from biospecimen assays and other assessments of impact on biologic mechanisms, would be taken at frequent intervals over the life course and especially during critical windows of susceptibility. Likewise, assessments of intermediate outcomes that suggest increased risk of breast cancer such as early menarche, anovulatory menstrual cycles, maximum attained height, age at first pregnancy, number of pregnancies, and periods of breast-feeding would also be recorded. The obvious problem with this approach is the length of time and the expense needed to capture the data and then wait for breast cancer outcomes to occur. Other challenges include that the type of exposures assessed along the way may no longer be of interest or relevant a half century after its measurement. What then are the less than ideal, but realistic study design alternatives?

1.2.1 Cohort Studies

Cohort studies that assess exposures during particular windows of susceptibility with shorter lengths of follow-up to valid intermediate endpoints represent the next best design to a lifelong cohort. Thus studies that examine exposures in the prepubertal period with the outcomes of pubertal onset and menarche or studies during adolescence with the outcome of growth rates and maximum adult height are possible examples. With advances in science it may be possible to examine in utero exposures and outcomes measured in stem cell biology or breast development as a viable design. In some situations it may be possible to construct retrospective cohorts from populations with existing data from many years before. For example, exposure very early in life (0–2 years of life) to radiation for angiomata has yielded information on increased breast cancer risk in a Swedish retrospective cohort (Eidemuller et al. 2009). Also, assays for DDE and polychlorinated biphenyls (PCBs) in stored serum of young mothers have yielded data on increased breast cancer rates four decades later (Cohn et al. 2007).

1.2.2 Case-Control Studies

Case-control studies have the advantage of not requiring long periods of follow-up and expense. In such studies, women with the outcome of interest (e.g., cases with breast cancer) and women from the same population and similar to the cases but without breast cancer are evaluated for exposures of interest at some time in the past. The problem with such studies is a recall bias for self-reported exposures wherein women with breast cancer may be more likely to report exposures than controls (Zota et al. 2010). There is also the challenge of simply being able to remember exposures so long in the past or even not being aware of exposures earlier in life. Assays of biospecimens after a diagnosis of breast cancer may be influenced by preclinical malignant pathophysiology or treatment and even if taken immediately after diagnosis, may not reflect the relevant exposure level several decades earlier when a cancer was likely to have been initiated. This, of course, is especially true for putative carcinogens that may remain measurable in the body for only short periods after exposure.

1.2.3 Ecologic Correlation Studies

Some investigators attempt to find support for more definitive causal relationships by using ecologic correlation studies. In these types of designs group level characteristics instead of individual data are used. For example, characteristics of counties or other geographically or politically defined regions are chosen and correlated again breast cancer rates. In one such study, based on characteristics of counties in Kentucky, estimates of the herbicide triazine and breast cancer rates determined from the state cancer registry revealed an elevated risk of cancer associated with exposure to the herbicide (Kettles et al. 1997). Other studies in humans use available clinical populations with diagnoses of interest, but little information on important confounding or mediating factors (Takeuchi et al. 2004). However, such association or correlation studies cannot be considered as strong evidence for causality because of the potential for effects from unmeasured confounding factors, lack of information at the individual level and misclassification biases. Results from such studies are best used to generate hypotheses.

1.2.4 Cross-Sectional Studies

Cross-sectional studies are when the exposure and outcome are assessed at the same point in time and no "directionality" of the relationship or causality can be ascertained. Such studies produce information on the prevalence or frequency of the exposure of interest in a particular population at a given point in time. Although such studies can be done over a short term, and multiple associations can be assessed at one time, the problem lies not being able to say which came first, the exposure or the outcomes, making such studies of limited value in assessing causality.

1.2.5 Case Studies

Probably the simplest approach to data gathering in epidemiology is the case study wherein the investigator describes observations of an individual or group along with qualitative information on these observations. Such reports may generate interest and ideas for further investigation, but cannot themselves be used to determine causality.

1.3 Review of Studies

What then is the evidence from epidemiologic studies that have attempted to assess exposures to EDCs and either breast cancer or some intermediate outcome relevant to breast cancer (e.g., age at menarche, obesity)? This chapter is not meant to be a comprehensive systematic review, but rather a survey of the most important types and classes of EDCs currently identified. A very thorough systematic review of environmental pollutants and breast cancer has been recently published by Brody et al. (2007).

1.3.1 DES

DES exposure is a good place to start. First introduced in 1938 to prevent miscarriages, it was in use until 1971. This estrogenic compound was taken off the market when daughters of women who took it during pregnancy developed adenocarcinomas of the vagina (Herbst et al. 1971). Subsequently, as the women who took DES have aged multiple reproductive abnormalities have emerged including increased breast cancer rates (Palmer et al. 2006; Troisi et al. 2007). Women who were exposed to DES in utero have formed a highly informative group of adult women with a well-defined exposure and multiple outcomes identified over a 40-year follow-up period. Breast cancer rates among DES daughters have been elevated, especially for cancers occurring over age 50 years (RR 3.0, 95% CI, 1.01–8.98) (Palmer et al. 2006) The studies are nearly ideal epidemiologically in that they have been prospective with good follow-up, clear and precise levels of exposure, and careful ascertainment of several important outcomes, including breast cancer. We have learned that in utero exposures can have important and devastating effects on adult health many years later and, as mentioned above, that the period of organogenesis during fetal life is one of several periods of life ("windows of susceptibility") when humans are sensitive to the effects of carcinogens, in this case synthetic estrogens. The parallel effects of EDCs on estrogen signaling and other mechanisms have drawn on the lessons of DES studies, but from an epidemiologic standpoint the DES studies are difficult to duplicate in terms of the clarity of the exposure dose and time and the extremely long and costly period of follow-up. Also DES exposures were to high-dose pharmacological levels of a potent estrogen, whereas most of the EDCs with which we are now concerned represent much lower environmental doses, albeit to a much larger population at risk.

1.3.2 Organochlorines

Organochlorines are a group of synthetic chemicals, some of which have properties of EDCs. They include PCBs, dioxins and organochlorine pesticides such as DDT, lindane, heptachlor, dieldrin, aldrin and hexachlorobenzene, and triazine herbicides such as atrazine. Also referred to as persistent organic pollutants (POPs), they are lipophilic and resistant to degradation. POPs are persistent in individual fat stores, the food chain, and the environment and have become highly prevalent in industrialized countries since World War II. Since being banned from use in the late 1970s and 1980s because of toxicities, body burdens in the United States and other industrialized countries have diminished substantially (Wolff 2006). Nevertheless, POPs are still ubiquitous in the environment and can be measured in biospecimens from virtually all US adults and children. Compared to the other EDCs that follow, there have been a substantial number of epidemiologic studies of the effects of exposures to organochlorines on breast cancer. However, using traditional epidemiologic observational studies in adulthood (usually case-control or cohort studies), the association of organochlorines with breast cancer has been inconsistent (Salehi et al. 2008; Xu et al. 2010). Some cohort studies have found associations with one organochlorine, for example dieldrin, but not others (Hoyer et al. 1998). Even in studies of large populations logically at very high risk of exposure, such as farmer's wives in the Agricultural Health Study, no clear relationships between overall pesticide exposure and breast cancer have been established. Due to the small number of cases available for analysis, only a suggestive relationship with specific pesticides has been found (Engel et al. 2005). Associations with earlier menarche have been positive in several (Gladen et al. 2000; Ouyang et al. 2005; Vasiliu et al. 2004) but not all studies (Denham et al. 2005).

1.3.2.1 DDT

Most epidemiologic studies of organochlorines and breast cancer have included both DDT and PCBs, but most have focused on exposure to the pesticide *p,p′* DDT and its metabolite *p,p′* DDE. Despite the large number of studies in this area following the initial positive results in case-control studies (Falck et al. 1992; Wolff et al. 1993), the results are mostly negative and reviews have considered them unsupportive of the hypothesis that organochlorines are associated with increased breast cancer risk (Calle et al. 2002; Lopez-Cervantes et al. 2004).

Since 1993 there have been over 30 published studies and all but a few have been negative despite being well-conducted investigations using a variety of study designs, including case-control and historical follow-up approaches. These studies have also been conducted in a number of high income countries around the world and among a number of subgroups defined by race/ethnicity, reproductive and menopausal status, body mass index, and genetic predisposition, without yielding consistent results (Calle et al. 2002). Cohn et al. summarized 17 epidemiologic studies, 8 of which were prospective with as much as 14 years of follow-up (Krieger et al. 1994) among adult women (Cohn et al. 2003). Some of these studies were able to use prediagnostic stored serum, but were still unable to show any relationship between organochlorine exposure and breast cancer.

Then in 2007 Cohn et al. reported a study using stored sera from the Childhood Development Study on women at the time of childbirth (average age 26 years), 129 of whom went on to develop breast cancer before 50 years of age (i.e., premenopausal) (Cohn et al. 2007). Compared to 129 women from the same cohort who did not develop breast cancer those who were in the highest tertile of *p,p′* DDT exposure were 2.8 times (95% CI 1.2–6.7) as likely to develop breast cancer as those in the lowest tertile. The strongest relationship was seen in women who were <14 years in 1945 (OR=5.4, 95% CI 1.7–17.1), which was the earliest year when girls could have been exposed given the patterns of DDT use in the 1940s and 1950s. This study, which will be difficult to replicate because of the unusual nature of the data set, supports the concept that the timing of exposure (i.e., early development window) may be critical to the contribution of EDCs to carcinogenesis.

1.3.2.2 Polychlorinated Biphenyls

PCBs are a family of 209 possible organochlorine congers that were used as industrial coolants, insulators, and lubricants, as well as many other applications until the United States banned their use in 1979. Since then, decreasing human body burden concentrations have been documented over the last 20 years. As with DDT, PCBs have been inconsistently related to breast cancer in many studies of adult women using a variety of epidemiologic observational study designs, including occupational cohort studies (Engel et al. 2005). Reviews have concluded that the epidemiologic data do not support any association with breast cancer (Calle et al. 2002; Laden et al. 2001). However, there is evidence from at least four studies of a gene–environment interaction with CYP1A1 that suggest high levels of PCB exposure and expression of CYP1A1 confers a higher risk of breast cancer (Brody et al. 2007; Laden et al. 2002; Moysich et al. 1999).

Regulatory agencies have reviewed the evidence for organochlorines and breast cancer in depth based on human, animal, and mechanistic studies. The US National Toxicology Program still classifies both DDT and PCBs as "reasonably anticipated to be human carcinogens" despite weak human epidemiologic data. The International Agency for Research on Cancer (IARC) classifies DDT as "possibly carcinogenic to humans" and PCBs as "probably carcinogenic to humans," and the US Environmental Protection Agency considers both DDT and PCBs as "probable human carcinogens." Thus, faced with weak human data and relatively strong evidence in animal systems, it may be that future epidemiologic studies need to be designed to examine exposures in earlier periods of development such as was done by Cohn et al. (2007) and is being currently carried out in prospective studies with intermediate endpoints such as early puberty (Hiatt et al. 2009).

1.3.2.3 Dioxin

2,3,7,8-Tetrachlorodibenzo-*p*-dioxin (TCDD) is also an organochlorine, but one which is a product of combustion, metal processing, and chemical manufacturing. It is probably one of the most toxic substances known and, like DDT and PCBs, is persistent in nature. Effects on human health have included concerns for cancer and more general reproductive and endocrine effects (Kogevinas 2001). Exposures to this compound have largely taken place in occupational settings and accidents, so large scale epidemiologic studies have not been feasible to organize. Rather most human data on the impact of TCDD come from occupational health cohorts where doses are higher than in the general environment and the number of women is small (Manz et al. 1991). A major exception has been the widespread exposure of personnel in Vietnam to Agent Orange, which contained small amounts of TCDD as a contaminant. The EPA considers TCDD "carcinogenic to humans." The assessment is for all cancers together and lung cancer with little data specific to breast cancer.

A recent report from the National Academies' of Sciences discussed four occupational cohorts that had enrolled workers employed in industrial settings in which dioxin was a by-product. Two of these involved pesticide production and were fairly small in size. One study followed 243 men accidentally exposed in 1953 in which 13 cancer deaths occurred (Ott and Zober 1996); a second tracked 1,189 men involved in pesticide production in which 124 cancer deaths occurred (Becher et al. 1998); and a third followed a larger cohort of 5,132 employees in manufacturing companies in whom 377 cancer deaths occurred (Steenland et al. 1999). A fourth cohort study has also been reported from the Netherlands with 2,310 workers who prepared phenoxy herbicides in which 31 cancer deaths occurred (Bueno de Mesquita et al. 1993). In all cases results have generally not been statistically significant although they are slightly in the positive direction. Also with the small number of cancer deaths stable site-specific rates were not possible. Finally, these cohorts were for male workers and no useful data for breast cancer in women can be derived.

Evidence of another sort comes from the "Seveso Accident" in Italy in 1976 where a large population surrounding a chemical plant was exposed to TCDD. Twenty year follow-up of cancer incidence in 111,874 women with graded exposures to dioxin has resulted in no elevations overall, but in one zone after 15 years of follow-up five cases of breast cancer have occurred, which is significantly more than expected (RR 2.57: 95% CI 1.07–6.20) (Pesatori et al. 2009). Longer follow-up may reveal more cases and clearer relationships to the exposure.

Overall the weight of the epidemiologic evidence that TCDD is a human carcinogen is only suggestive and the designation of regulatory agencies (i.e., EPA, NTP, and IARC) that it is a carcinogen rests largely on positive animal and mechanistic studies. Further epidemiologic evidence will await long-term follow-up of existing cohort of exposed individuals.

1.3.3 Polycyclic Aromatic Hydrocarbons

Polycyclic aromatic hydrocarbons (PAHs) are a large class of chemicals formed by the incomplete combustion of coal, oil, and gas, as well as grilled meats, tobacco smoke, and other substances to which humans are exposed in ambient air. These substances are genotoxic and known to be potential breast carcinogens (Morris and Seifter 1992), perhaps by damaging DNA through oxidative stress. Some PAHs are also weakly estrogenic, thus presenting another mechanism by which they may influence breast cancer etiology (Santodonato 1997). Animal experiments indicate that puberty and early development may be the period when the breast is most sensitive to these effects (Fenton 2006). Also, since air pollution can vary by neighborhood environments, there may be an interaction between PAH exposure and the social environment (Morello-Frosch and Jesdale 2006).

Epidemiologic studies have used a number of design approaches to determine if PAHs are related to breast cancer risk but have been inconclusive. In western New York, occupational exposure to both benzene and PAHs was assessed from occupational histories that aimed to determine the probability and intensity of exposures in different job classifications. Data from the histories revealed a 2.3-fold elevated risk of estrogen receptor-positive (but not negative) breast cancer cases compared to women frequency matched by age and county of residence (Petralia et al. 1999). In the Long Island Breast Cancer Study using a similar case-control approach with frequency matching by age in a nonoccupational setting, PAH-DNA adducts were slightly, but not significantly, elevated among women with breast cancer with no dose–response relationship (Gammon et al. 2002b). Slightly elevated risks of around 30% in association with PAH-DNA adducts were also confirmed in a later analysis in the same study (Sagiv et al. 2009). In another study from western New York, measurements of total suspended particulates (TSP) in the air were used as a proxy for PAH exposure and linked to women with breast cancer and their controls at the time of their births based on residential histories. In women with postmenopausal breast cancer, exposure to high concentrations of TSPs was associated with a 2.4-fold elevated risk that was on the borderline of significance, although the relationship could have been related to unmeasured confounding factors (Bonner et al. 2005). A more recent study from the same group studied exposure to traffic emissions among women with breast cancer with residence serving as an indirect measure of exposure. The study determined exposures at various points in the life-course including the age of menarche. In this study, elevated risk, again slightly over twofold, was observed for exposures at the time of menarche and age at first birth for women with postmenopausal breast cancer (Nie et al. 2007). All of these studies have used case-control designs and depended on respondent recall of information from the past, proxy measures of exposure, or assays of PAH-DNA adducts after the diagnosis of breast cancer. PAH-DNA adducts may be more a measure of exposure rather than the host biologic response to PAH (Gammon and Santella 2008). Although the studies from western New York have been rather consistent in their levels of risk estimates and the studies from the Long Island Breast Cancer Study have suggested a link between PAH-DNA adducts and breast cancer, the role of PAHs in breast cancer etiology in humans remains unclear.

1.3.4 Bisphenol A

The widely used industrial monomer BPA is a weakly estrogenic chemical that is polymerized in the manufacture of polycarbonate plastic and epoxy resins. Human exposure occurs by the leaching of BPA from plastic-lined food and beverage cans and from some dental sealants, among many other common sources in modern life

(Brotons et al. 1995; Olea et al. 1996). BPA is used as an additive in many other products but may be less durable than commonly believed because the ester bond linking polymerized BPA molecules can be hydrolyzed, and hydrolysis increases dramatically at high or low pH and as temperature increases. BPA may, thus, leach into food and beverages under normal conditions of use from tin cans and polycarbonate plastic containers (Brotons et al. 1995; Howdeshell et al. 2003), and the rate of leaching may greatly increase when the polycarbonate polymer is scratched and discolored (Howdeshell et al. 2003).

Evidence for estrogenic effects of BPA has been reported in studies in rodent models showing that it activates estrogen receptors alpha (ERα) and beta (ERβ) (Matthews et al. 2001; Routledge et al. 2000) and stimulates MCF-7 breast cancer cell growth (Krishnan et al. 1993). Effects on weight gain, puberty, male and female reproductive tract abnormalities, and the mammary gland in animal models have been documented (Maffini et al. 2006; Ramos et al. 2001; Suzuki et al. 2002).

In human urine BPA levels in parts per billion (ng/mL) have been documented in many studies; one large study revealed that 95% of urinary samples tested contained BPA levels in parts per billion (ng/mL) (Calafat et al. 2005) as did and 94% of samples tested in a study of prepubertal 6–7-year-old girls in the BCERCs across the US (Wolff et al. 2007). However, there is uncertainty as to the level and risk of exposure to BPA in humans. There are currently no epidemiologic studies of BPA and breast cancer in humans, but in Japanese studies associations have been found between BPA, circulating androgens and polycystic ovarian syndrome, repeated miscarriage, and endometrial hyperplasia (Hiroi et al. 2004; Sugiura-Ogasawara et al. 2005; Takeuchi et al. 2004). These studies used available samples from clinical populations for comparisons without any effort to control for possible confounding factors between them. In one of the few epidemiologic prospective studies of the health effects of BPA in 1,151 girls between 6 and 8 years old, after 2 years of follow-up there was no statistically significant effect on pubertal onset as measured by the earliest Tanner Stage for both breast development and the appearance of pubic hair (Wolff et al. 2010).

1.3.5 Parabens

Parabens are antimicrobial preservatives found in personal care products, including underarm cosmetics, that can act like weak estrogens to bind to the estrogen receptor. Although there is human data documenting parabens in urine in almost all (>96%) of a demographically diverse sample of adults (Ye et al. 2006), and parabens have been documented in breast cancer specimens, the levels were substantially less than what is required to produce estrogenic effects (Witorsch and Thomas 2010). There are no epidemiologic studies to date that link their use to biologic outcomes or breast cancer in humans (Witorsch and Thomas 2010). A recent study has measured urine parabens levels in a diverse sample of 1,151 6–8-year-old girls as a possible determinant of pubertal onset 2 years later and found no relationship.

Parabens levels, which often occur together with benzophenome-3 (BP-3), a phenol found in sunscreens, were, however, significantly higher in the summer and among white girls (Wolff et al. 2010).

1.3.6 Phthalates

Personal care products and cosmetics may include EDCs in the categories of phthalates and organic solvents as well as parabens (Wolff et al. 1996). Butyl benzyl phthalate (BBP) is an estrogenic compound and a partial agonist for the ER (Andersen et al. 1999), which is widely used in plastic food wraps and other plastics as well as in cosmetic formulations. Adult intake has been estimated at 2 μg/kg body weight/day and exposure to infants and children could be as much as threefold higher. Animal studies in rats have shown that prenatal exposure to 500, or 1,000 mg/kg of BBP, or 250 or 375 mg/kg of its major metabolite, monobenzyl phthalate, induced significant alterations in the reproductive system of male offspring, including undescended testes and a decrease in the anogenital distance (Ema et al. 2003; Swan et al. 2005). Several in vitro tests, such as MCF-7 cell proliferation, ER binding in the rat uterus, and transfection of yeast with the human ER gene, have demonstrated the estrogenic activity of BBP (Andersen et al. 1999; Hong et al. 2005). However, there is poor evidence on the mechanism mediating BBP's effect on cell proliferation. It is likely that the estrogenic response is not only elicited via the ER, but also through the activation of other still unknown pathways (Baker et al. 1999). In humans, a recent case-control study in northern Mexico compared 233 breast cancer cases to 221 age-matched controls on urinary levels of phthalates obtained (in the cases) prior to treatment. Cases had significantly higher levels of monoethyl phthalate (MEP), but controls had higher levels of other phthalates. Adjustments for other phthalates and breast cancer risk factors resulted in statistically significant elevated odds of breast cancer with higher MEP levels (OR 2.20; 95% CI 1.33–3.63) and was stronger for premenopausal women (OR 4.13; 95% CI 1.60–10.70) (Lopez-Carrillo et al. 2010) This is a provocative finding because there are no other known epidemiologic studies attempting to relate phthalate exposure to breast cancer, but it is not clear whether the levels of phthalates measured after diagnosis (even though it was before treatment) reflect the relevant time of exposure. Studies, not of breast cancer, but of pubertal timing in girls have been done in Taiwan and the US In a small Taiwanese case-control study 30 girls with premature thelarche (breast development) were compared to 26 girls with central precocious puberty and 33 normal controls and found to have higher levels of monomethyl phthalate (MMP) than the control group ($p=0.005$) (Chou et al. 2009). Another much larger study, again from the BCERCs, has assessed a panel of nine phthalate metabolites by grouping similar metabolites into either high or low molecular weight with similar biologic activity. In 1,149 girls analyzed, there was a weak nonstatistically significant relationship to pubertal onset as measured by the appearance of either breast or pubic hair development with 2 years of follow-up associated with low molecular weight phthalates and a weakly inverse association relationship for high molecular weight phthalates and pubic hair development ($p = 0.04$ for trend in quintiles) (Wolff et al. 2010). Additional follow-up in this on-going longitudinal study may clarify these relationships. Overall, however, there seems to be some suggestive evidence that phthalate exposure may be associated with breast cancer and breast cancer risk factors early in development, although the direction of the relationship for different phthalates is not consistent.

1.3.7 Polybrominated Diphenyl Ethers

A study of brominated flame retardants (polybrominated biphenyls, PBBs) among accidentally exposed farm workers in Michigan revealed an association with earlier pubic hair, but not breast development, in the daughters of exposed mothers (Blanck et al. 2000). Polybrominated diphenyl ethers (PBDEs) are a subgroup of flame retardants, which are now being phased out because of proven toxicity, but a number are still in common use and are under study in relationship to pubertal development. Although no epidemiologic studies have been done in adults, serum levels in girls in the BCERC study of six congeners of PBDEs were detected in 70% of the sample of girls from California and Ohio. Levels were higher for girls from California and for black when compared to white girls (Windham et al. 2010). This was probably due to California's fire regulations and safety codes. Further analysis will examine the relationship of these PBDE levels to pubertal onset and maturation.

1.3.8 Perfluoroalkyl Acids

Perfluoroalkyl acids (PFAAs) are a family of perfluorinated chemicals that have also found their way into the environment and have EDC properties. Two of the most widely studied are perfluorocatanoic acid (PFOA) and perfluorooctane sulfate (PFOS) (Lau et al. 2007). PFOA is a synthetic compound introduced halfway through the last century for use in many industrial and consumer products including Teflon and Gore-Tex (Steenland et al. 2010). Detectable levels can be found in the serum of most persons tested in the US with a median level of 4 ng/mL (Calafat et al. 2007). Drinking water seems to be the main source of exposure. In animal systems PFOA has been associated with tumor development, probably via effects on the immune and endocrine systems rather than genotoxicity (Steenland et al. 2010). Epidemiologic studies are very limited to date for cancer relevant outcomes in general and especially for breast cancer (Olsen et al. 2009; Steenland et al. 2010). One occupational study used questionnaires to ask workers in perfluorooctane-sulfonyl fluoride production (past and present) about breast cancer and several other conditions and estimated PFOS exposure from a job exposure matrix up to the year of diagnosis. No association was found among 1,400 persons returning questions of any of the conditions of interest (Grice et al. 2007). Olsen et al. (2009) comprehensively reviewed eight epidemiologic studies that related PFOA and PFOS to human fetal development (i.e., gestational age, birth weight, birth length, head circumference, chest circumference, ponderal index, and placental weight) and found no consistent relationships.

1.3.9 Phytoestrogens

Epidemiologic studies on the effects of phytoestrogens and breast cancer have been mixed, but tend toward being protective if consumed in sufficiently high doses (Patisaul and Jefferson 2010). Phytoestrogens in food have weak estrogenic or antiestrogenic effects and fall into three major classes: isoflavones, lignans and coumestans. Isoflavones are found mainly in soy products and are largely in two forms, genistein and daidzein, with glycetin a third less common variety. Lignans are found primarily in grain products. Soy intake is substantially higher among Asian populations and since dose is a critical factor, discussion of epidemiologic results for isoflavones needs to take the population studied into account. Several well-conducted epidemiologic studies, mostly using case-control designs, have addressed this issue. Those conducted in Asia, where intake of soy products is high, have tended to show a protective effect (Wu et al. 2008). A meta-analysis of eight studies in Asian countries showed a significant trend of decreasing risk with increasing soy intake. In Western countries, in contrast, 11 studies showed no protective effect.

For breast cancer survival, Guha et al. have examined recurrence of breast cancer among survivors of early stage postmenopausal disease in a cohort of 1,954 women in California and Utah and found substantially reduced risks of around 60% among women taking tamoxifen, even though the highest quintile of risk (>1,453 μg/day) was still very low compared to Asian countries (Guha et al. 2009). In a prospective population-based study in Shanghai, China, among 5,042 breast cancer survivors soy protein was also protective for both mortality (hazard ration 0.71, 95% 0.54–0.92) and breast cancer recurrence (hazard ratio 0.68, 95% 0.54–0.87), irrespective of estrogen receptor status or tamoxifen use. In this study the highest quartile of consumption was >15.31 g/day, 100 times higher than in the US study (Shu et al. 2009).

Well-conducted epidemiologic studies of adolescent soy intake are fairly consistent in showing a graded protective effect with dose (Korde et al. 2009; Lee et al. 2009; Shu et al. 2001; Wu et al. 2002). Finally, in young girls, in a cross-sectional study of 192 healthy 9 year olds in New York urinary phytoestrogen levels were associated with later breast development; these effects were strongest for the isoflavones daidzein (prevalence ratio 0.89 [0.83–0.96]) and genistien (PR 0.94 [0.88–1.01]) (Wolff et al. 2008).

1.3.10 Other Suspected EDCs

Heavy metals such as cadmium and lead are both known or probable carcinogens and also have estrogenic properties (Choe et al. 2003). Lead exposure has been associated with later pubertal onset or menarche in several studies (Denham et al. 2005; Selevan et al. 2003; Wu et al. 2003). Both lead and cadmium have been associated with breast cancer incidence in case-control (Cantor et al. 1995; McElroy et al. 2006).

Environmental tobacco smoke (ETS) has been assessed in girls and associated with early menarche (Reynolds et al. 2004; Windham et al. 2004). However, mechanisms by which ETS might contribute to earlier menarche remain to be elucidated especially by examining possible gene–environment interactions such as those with NAT2 slow acetylator and GSTMI null genotypes that may be associated with breast cancer in adults (Ambrosone et al. 2008; Terry and Goodman 2006).

1.4 Gaps in Knowledge

This review of the human epidemiologic data illustrates that there is enough substantial evidence for a role of EDCs in the etiology of breast cancer that additional research is needed. Given the limitations of such studies, however, multiple approaches to filling current gaps in knowledge need to be pursued:

- Traditional epidemiologic approaches to examining single chemicals, especially with novel study designs (Cohn et al. 2007), need to be supported. There are numerous understudied EDCs with common exposures including PFAA, phenols, phthalates, diesel exhaust, and chlorinated solvents (Rudel et al. 2007).
- Exposures, however, are inadequately assessed by looking at one chemical at a time. More research is needed to inform epidemiologic inquiry using measures of relevant mixtures of chemicals. Although this necessarily increases the number of exposures to be studied, common mixtures could be identified for toxicologic studies for use in human investigations.
- New methods of assessing cumulative exposure are needed and there have been recent suggestions to examine “internal environmental dose” in terms of the impact of environmental chemicals on molecules, pathways, and systems inside the body. This includes processes of inflammation, oxidative stress, lipid peroxidation, infections, gut flora, and other pathophysiologic processes. This so-called “exposome” approach could be a transformative in terms of assessing environmental exposure and should be vigorously pursued (Rappaport and Smith 2010).
- Support for long-term longitudinal studies that assess exposures early in life and follow participants over a lifetime is expensive and require long periods of time but can provide invaluable data. Examples are the Fels Longitudinal Study (Demerath et al. 2007) and the recently initiated National Children’s Study (Kuehn 2010). Such long-term longitudinal studies with multiple measurements over the life-course should be fully funded.

- Finally, it is clear that many of the limitations to the study of breast cancer and the environment stem from the difficulties of assessing past exposures and doses in adults. These include problems of faulty memories, lack of knowledge of exposures, recall bias, short half-life of exposure biomarkers, and the rapid turnover of chemicals in the environment. All of which argue for a life-course approach that recognizes that environmental chemicals and EDCs in particular have effects on stages of development or "windows of susceptibility" that begin in intrauterine life and include the prepubertal and pubertal phases of life, as well as pregnancy. Studies directed at endpoints during these periods that are known to influence breast cancer risk in adult life (e.g., the age of pubertal onset or menarche) can be conducted in a prospective fashion with much higher quality data on exposures and outcomes (Hiatt et al. 2009).

1.5 Conclusion

This chapter has introduced the topic of this book with a focus on epidemiologic studies of endocrine disrupting chemicals (EDCs) and breast cancer in women. There is no substitute for evidence in human populations for establishing causation and establishing the basis for public health action and policy. The nature and limitations of epidemiology as discussed in this introduction set up the need for linking studies in human populations to evidence from mechanistic and toxicologic studies in animals that will be discussed in subsequent chapters. Epidemiologic studies of particular EDCs have been briefly reviewed. The compounds for which some evidence exists include DDT in early life, PAHs, phytoestrogens in sufficiently high doses, and PCBs in subgroups with particular genetic characteristics. Studies are currently in progress to assess the effects of exposures to these and other EDCs early in the life-course. Much remains to be elucidated, not only in terms of the risks for breast cancer and intermediate outcomes as assessed by human epidemiology, but also the biologic effects of these compounds in animal models. Main effects from assessing the role of one chemical at a time may be insufficient. It is likely that chemicals interact with each other and that their effect is modified by the presence of genetic polymorphisms and by the social context in which the exposure plays out. It should be clear that only with a transdisciplinary approach we can find solutions to the complex problem of understanding and mitigating the effect of the environment on the etiology of breast cancer.

References

Ambrosone CB et al (2008) Cigarette smoking, N-acetyltransferase 2 genotypes, and breast cancer risk: pooled analysis and meta-analysis. Cancer Epidemiol Biomarkers Prev 17:15–26

Andersen HR et al (1999) Comparison of short-term estrogenicity tests for identification of hormone-disrupting chemicals. Environ Health Perspect 107(suppl 1):89–108

Baker VA et al (1999) Safety evaluation of phytosterol esters. Part 1. Assessment of oestrogenicity using a combination of in vivo and in vitro assays. Food Chem Toxicol 37:13–22

Becher H et al (1998) Quantitative cancer risk assessment for dioxins using an occupational cohort. Environ Health Perspect 106(suppl 2):663–670
Berkey CS et al (1999) Adolescence and breast carcinoma risk. Cancer 85:2400–2409
Biro FM et al (2006) Pubertal correlates in black and white girls. J Pediatr 148:234–240
Biro FM et al (2010) Pubertal assessment method and baseline characteristics in a mixed longitudinal study of girls. Pediatrics 126:e583–e590
Blanck HM et al (2000) Age at menarche and tanner stage in girls exposed in utero and postnatally to polybrominated biphenyl. Epidemiology 11:641–647
Boice JD et al (1991) Diagnostic x-ray procedures and risk of leukemia, lymphoma, and multiple myeloma. J Am Med Assoc 265:1290–1294
Boice JD Jr et al (1995) Breast cancer among radiologic technologists. JAMA 274:394–401
Bonner MR et al (2005) Breast cancer risk and exposure in early life to polycyclic aromatic hydrocarbons using total suspended particulates as a proxy measure. Cancer Epidemiol Biomarkers Prev 14:53–60
Brody JG et al (2007) Environmental pollutants and breast cancer: epidemiologic studies. Cancer 109:2667–2711
Brotons JA et al (1995) Xenoestrogens released from lacquer coatings in food cans. Environ Health Perspect 103:608–612
Buck Louis GM et al (2008) Environmental factors and puberty timing: expert panel research needs. Pediatrics 121(suppl 3):S192–S207
Bueno de Mesquita HB et al (1993) Occupational exposure to phenoxy herbicides and chlorophenols and cancer mortality in The Netherlands. Am J Ind Med 23:289–300
Calafat AM et al (2005) Urinary concentrations of bisphenol A and 4-nonylphenol in a human reference population. Environ Health Perspect 113:391–395
Calafat AM et al (2007) Polyfluoroalkyl chemicals in the U.S. population: data from the National Health and Nutrition Examination Survey (NHANES) 2003–2004 and comparisons with NHANES 1999-2000. Environ Health Perspect 115:1596–1602
Calle EE et al (2002) Organochlorines and breast cancer risk. CA Cancer J Clin 52:301–309
Cantor KP et al (1995) Occupational exposures and female breast cancer mortality in the United States. J Occup Environ Med 37:336–348
Chepko G, Smith GH (1999) Mammary epithelial stem cells: our current understanding. J Mammary Gland Biol Neoplasia 4:35–52
Choe SY et al (2003) Evaluation of estrogenicity of major heavy metals. Sci Total Environ 312:15–21
Chou YY et al (2009) Phthalate exposure in girls during early puberty. J Pediatr Endocrinol Metab 22:69–77
Clavel-Chapelon F (2002) Differential effects of reproductive factors on the risk of pre- and postmenopausal breast cancer. Results from a large cohort of French women. Br J Cancer 86:723–727
Cohn BA et al (2003) DDT and DDE exposure in mothers and time to pregnancy in daughters. Lancet 361:2205–2206
Cohn BA et al (2007) DDT and breast cancer in young women: new data on the significance of age at exposure. Environ Health Perspect 115:1406–1414
Colditz GA, Frazier AL (1995) Models of breast cancer show that risk is set by events of early life: prevention efforts must shift focus. Cancer Epidemiol Biomarkers Prev 4:567–571
Crain DA et al (2008) Female reproductive disorders: the roles of endocrine-disrupting compounds and developmental timing. Fertil Steril 90:911–940
de Waard F, Thijssen JH (2005) Hormonal aspects in the causation of human breast cancer: epidemiological hypotheses reviewed, with special reference to nutritional status and first pregnancy. J Steroid Biochem Mol Biol 97:451–458
Demerath EW et al (2007) Genetic and environmental influences on infant weight and weight change: the Fels Longitudinal Study. Am J Hum Biol 19:692–702
Denham M et al (2005) Relationship of lead, mercury, mirex, dichlorodiphenyldichloroethylene, hexachlorobenzene, and polychlorinated biphenyls to timing of menarche among Akwesasne Mohawk girls. Pediatrics 115:e127–e134

Diallo R et al (2001) Monoclonality in normal epithelium and in hyperplastic and neoplastic lesions of the breast. J Pathol 193:27–32
Diamanti-Kandarakis E et al (2009) Endocrine-disrupting chemicals: an Endocrine Society scientific statement. Endocr Rev 30:293–342
Eidemuller M et al (2009) Breast cancer risk among Swedish hemangioma patients and possible consequences of radiation-induced genomic instability. Mutat Res 669:48–55
Ekbom A et al (1997) Intrauterine environment and breast cancer risk in women: a population-based study. J Natl Cancer Inst 89:71–76
Ema M et al (2003) Decreased anogenital distance and increased incidence of undescended testes in fetuses of rats given monobenzyl phthalate, a major metabolite of butyl benzyl phthalate. Reprod Toxicol 17:407–412
Engel LS et al (2005) Pesticide use and breast cancer risk among farmers' wives in the agricultural health study. Am J Epidemiol 161:121–135
Euling SY et al (2008) Examination of US puberty-timing data from 1940 to 1994 for secular trends: panel findings. Pediatrics 121:S172–S191
Falck F Jr et al (1992) Pesticides and polychlorinated biphenyl residues in human breast lipids and their relation to breast cancer. Arch Environ Health 47:143–146
Fenton SE (2006) Endocrine-disrupting compounds and mammary gland development: early exposure and later life consequences. Endocrinology 147:S18–S24
Forman MR et al (2005) Through the looking glass at early-life exposures and breast cancer risk. Cancer Invest 23:609–624
Friedman GD et al (2009) Pharmaceuticals that cause mammary gland tumors in animals: findings in women. Breast Cancer Res Treat 116:187–194
Gammon MD, Santella RM (2008) PAH, genetic susceptibility and breast cancer risk: an update from the Long Island Breast Cancer Study Project. Eur J Cancer 44:636–640
Gammon MD et al (2002a) The Long Island Breast Cancer Study Project: description of a multi-institutional collaboration to identify environmental risk factors for breast cancer. Breast Cancer Res Treat 74:235–254
Gammon MD et al (2002b) Environmental toxins and breast cancer on Long Island. I. Polycyclic aromatic hydrocarbon DNA adducts. Cancer Epidemiol Biomarkers Prev 11:677–685
Gladen BC et al (2000) Pubertal growth and development and prenatal and lactational exposure to polychlorinated biphenyls and dichlorodiphenyl dichloroethene. J Pediatr 136:490–496
Grice MM et al (2007) Self-reported medical conditions in perfluorooctanesulfonyl fluoride manufacturing workers. J Occup Environ Med 49:722–729
Guha N et al (2009) Soy isoflavones and risk of cancer recurrence in a cohort of breast cancer survivors: the Life After Cancer Epidemiology study. Breast Cancer Res Treat 118:395–405
Herbst AL et al (1971) Adenocarcinoma of the vagina. Association of maternal stilbestrol therapy with tumor appearance in young women. N Engl J Med 284:878–881
Hiatt RA et al (2009) The breast cancer and the environment research centers: transdisciplinary research on the role of the environment in breast cancer etiology. Environ Health Perspect 117:1814–1822
Hiroi H et al (2004) Differences in serum bisphenol a concentrations in premenopausal normal women and women with endometrial hyperplasia. Endocr J 51:595–600
Hong EJ et al (2005) Conflict of estrogenic activity by various phthalates between in vitro and in vivo models related to the expression of Calbindin-D9k. J Reprod Dev 51:253–263
Howdeshell KL et al (2003) Bisphenol A is released from used polycarbonate animal cages into water at room temperature. Environ Health Perspect 111:1180–1187
Hoyer AP et al (1998) Organochlorine exposure and risk of breast cancer. Lancet 352:1816–1820
Hunter DJ et al (1997) Non-dietary factors as risk factors for breast cancer, and as effect modifiers of the association of fat intake and risk of breast cancer. Cancer Causes Control 8:49–56
Jemal A et al (2010a) Cancer statistics, 2010. CA Cancer J Clin 60:277–300
Jemal A et al (2010b) Global patterns of cancer incidence and mortality rates and trends. Cancer Epidemiol Biomarkers Prev 19:1893–1907

John EM, Kelsey JL (1993) Radiation and other environmental exposures and breast cancer. Epidemiol Rev 15:157–162
Kauppila A et al (2009) Birth intervals and breast cancer risk. Br J Cancer 101:1213–1217
Kettles MK et al (1997) Triazine herbicide exposure and breast cancer incidence: an ecologic study of Kentucky counties. Environ Health Perspect 105:1222–1227
Knight CH, Sorensen A (2001) Windows in early mammary development: critical or not? Reproduction 122:337–345
Kogevinas M (2001) Human health effects of dioxins: cancer, reproductive and endocrine system effects. Hum Reprod Update 7:331–339
Kohler BA et al (2011) Annual report to the nation on the status of cancer, 1975–2007, featuring tumors of the brain and other nervous system. J Natl Cancer Inst 103:714–736
Korde LA et al (2009) Childhood soy intake and breast cancer risk in Asian American women. Cancer Epidemiol Biomarkers Prev 18:1050–1059
Krieger N et al (1994) Breast cancer and serum organochlorines: a prospective study among white, black, and Asian women. J Natl Cancer Inst 86:589–599
Krishnan AV et al (1993) Bisphenol-A: an estrogenic substance is released from polycarbonate flasks during autoclaving. Endocrinology 132:2279–2286
Kuehn BM (2010) National Children's Study expands. JAMA 304:1776
Laden F et al (2001) 1,1-Dichloro-2,2-bis(p-chlorophenyl)ethylene and polychlorinated biphenyls and breast cancer: combined analysis of five U.S. studies. J Natl Cancer Inst 93:768–776
Laden F et al (2002) Polychlorinated biphenyls, cytochrome P450 1A1, and breast cancer risk in the Nurses' Health Study. Cancer Epidemiol Biomarkers Prev 11:1560–1565
Land CE et al (2003) Incidence of female breast cancer among atomic bomb survivors, Hiroshima and Nagasaki, 1950-1990. Radiat Res 160:707–717
Lau C et al (2007) Perfluoroalkyl acids: a review of monitoring and toxicological findings. Toxicol Sci 99:366–394
Lee SA et al (2009) Adolescent and adult soy food intake and breast cancer risk: results from the Shanghai Women's Health Study. Am J Clin Nutr 89:1920–1926
Lopez-Carrillo L et al (2010) Exposure to phthalates and breast cancer risk in northern Mexico. Environ Health Perspect 118:539–544
Lopez-Cervantes M et al (2004) Dichlorodiphenyldichloroethane burden and breast cancer risk: a meta-analysis of the epidemiologic evidence. Environ Health Perspect 112:207–214
Mabry PL et al (2008) Interdisciplinarity and systems science to improve population health: a view from the NIH Office of Behavioral and Social Sciences Research. Am J Prev Med 35:S211–S224
Madigan MP et al (1995) Proportion of breast cancer cases in the United States explained by well-established risk factors. J Natl Cancer Inst 87:1681–1685
Maffini MV et al (2006) Endocrine disruptors and reproductive health: the case of bisphenol-A. Mol Cell Endocrinol 254–255:179–186
Manz A et al (1991) Cancer mortality among workers in chemical plant contaminated with dioxin. Lancet 338:959–964
Matthews JB et al (2001) In vitro and in vivo interactions of bisphenol A and its metabolite, bisphenol A glucuronide, with estrogen receptors alpha and beta. Chem Res Toxicol 14:149–157
McElroy JA et al (2006) Cadmium exposure and breast cancer risk. J Natl Cancer Inst 98:869–873
Mettlin C (1999) Global breast cancer mortality statistics. CA Cancer J Clin 49:138–144
Morello-Frosch R, Jesdale BM (2006) Separate and unequal: residential segregation and estimated cancer risks associated with ambient air toxics in U.S. metropolitan areas. Environ Health Perspect 114:386–393
Morris JJ, Seifter E (1992) The role of aromatic hydrocarbons in the genesis of breast cancer. Med Hypotheses 38:177–184
Moysich KB et al (1999) Polychlorinated biphenyls, cytochrome P4501A1 polymorphism, and postmenopausal breast cancer risk. Cancer Epidemiol Biomarkers Prev 8:41–44
Nie J et al (2007) Exposure to traffic emissions throughout life and risk of breast cancer: the Western New York Exposures and Breast Cancer (WEB) study. Cancer Causes Control 18:947–955

Okasha M et al (2003) Exposures in childhood, adolescence and early adulthood and breast cancer risk: a systematic review of the literature. Breast Cancer Res Treat 78:223–276
Olea N et al (1996) Estrogenicity of resin-based composites and sealants used in dentistry. Environ Health Perspect 104:298–305
Olsen GW et al (2009) Perfluoroalkyl chemicals and human fetal development: an epidemiologic review with clinical and toxicological perspectives. Reprod Toxicol 27:212–230
Ott MG, Zober A (1996) Cause specific mortality and cancer incidence among employees exposed to 2,3,7,8-TCDD after a 1953 reactor accident. Occup Environ Med 53:606–612
Ouyang F et al (2005) Serum DDT, age at menarche, and abnormal menstrual cycle length. Occup Environ Med 62:878–884
Palmer JR et al (2006) Prenatal diethylstilbestrol exposure and risk of breast cancer. Cancer Epidemiol Biomarkers Prev 15:1509–1514
Park SK et al (2008) Intrauterine environments and breast cancer risk: meta-analysis and systematic review. Breast Cancer Res 10:R8
Patisaul HB, Jefferson W (2010) The pros and cons of phytoestrogens. Front Neuroendocrinol 31(4):400–419
Pesatori AC et al (2009) Cancer incidence in the population exposed to dioxin after the "Seveso accident": twenty years of follow-up. Environ Health 8:39
Petralia SA et al (1999) Risk of premenopausal breast cancer and patterns of established breast cancer risk factors among teachers and nurses. Am J Ind Med 35:137–141
Polednak AP (1994) Trends in cancer incidence in Connecticut, 1935-1991. Cancer 74:2863–2872
Pukkala E et al (2006) Breast cancer in Belarus and Ukraine after the Chernobyl accident. Int J Cancer 119:651–658
Ramos JG et al (2001) Prenatal exposure to low doses of bisphenol A alters the periductal stroma and glandular cell function in the rat ventral prostate. Biol Reprod 65:1271–1277
Rappaport SM, Smith MT (2010) Epidemiology. Environment and disease risks. Science 330:460–461
Reynolds P et al (2004) Active smoking, household passive smoking, and breast cancer: evidence from the California Teachers Study. J Natl Cancer Inst 96:29–37
Routledge EJ et al (2000) Differential effects of xenoestrogens on coactivator recruitment by estrogen receptor (ER) alpha and ERbeta. J Biol Chem 275:35986–35993
Rudel RA, Perovich LJ (2009) Endocrine disrupting chemicals in indoor and outdoor air. Atmos Environ 43:170–181
Rudel RA et al (2007) Chemicals causing mammary gland tumors in animals signal new directions for epidemiology, chemicals testing, and risk assessment for breast cancer prevention. Cancer 109:2635–2666
Rudland PS (1993) Epithelial stem cells and their possible role in the development of the normal and diseased human breast. Histol Histopathol 8:385–404
Russo IH, Russo J (1996) Mammary gland neoplasia in long-term rodent studies. Environ Health Perspect 104:938–967
Russo J et al (2001) Cancer risk related to mammary gland structure and development. Microsc Res Tech 52:204–223
Sagiv SK et al (2009) Polycyclic aromatic hydrocarbon-DNA adducts and survival among women with breast cancer. Environ Res 109:287–291
Salehi F et al (2008) Review of the etiology of breast cancer with special attention to organochlorines as potential endocrine disruptors. J Toxicol Environ Health B Crit Rev 11:276–300
Santodonato J (1997) Review of the estrogenic and antiestrogenic activity of polycyclic aromatic hydrocarbons: relationship to carcinogenicity. Chemosphere 34:835–848
Selevan SG et al (2003) Blood lead concentration and delayed puberty in girls. N Engl J Med 348:1527–1536
Shore RE et al (1986) Breast cancer among women given X-ray therapy for acute postpartum mastitis. J Natl Cancer Inst 77:689–696
Shore RE et al (1993) Thyroid cancer among persons given x-ray treatment in infancy for an enlarged thymus gland. Am J Epidemiol 137:1068–1080

Shu XO et al (2001) Association of body size and fat distribution with risk of breast cancer among Chinese women. Int J Cancer 94:449–455
Shu XO et al (2009) Soy food intake and breast cancer survival. JAMA 302:2437–2443
Sonnenschein C, Soto AM (1998) An updated review of environmental estrogen and androgen mimics and antagonists. J Steroid Biochem Mol Biol 65:143–150
Soto AM et al (2008) Does breast cancer start in the womb? Basic Clin Pharmacol Toxicol 102:125–133
Steenland K et al (1999) Cancer, heart disease, and diabetes in workers exposed to 2,3,7,8-tetrachlorodibenzo-p-dioxin. J Natl Cancer Inst 91:779–786
Steenland K et al (2010) Epidemiologic evidence on the health effects of perfluorooctanoic acid (PFOA). Environ Health Perspect 118:1100–1108
Sturgeon SR et al (2004) Trends in breast cancer mortality rates by region of the United States, 1950-1999. Cancer Causes Control 15:987–995
Sugiura-Ogasawara M et al (2005) Exposure to bisphenol A is associated with recurrent miscarriage. Hum Reprod 20:2325–2329
Suzuki A et al (2002) Developmental effects of perinatal exposure to bisphenol-A and diethylstilbestrol on reproductive organs in female mice. Reprod Toxicol 16:107–116
Swan SH et al (2005) Decrease in anogenital distance among male infants with prenatal phthalate exposure. Environ Health Perspect 113:1056–1061
Takeuchi T et al (2004) Positive relationship between androgen and the endocrine disruptor, bisphenol A, in normal women and women with ovarian dysfunction. Endocr J 51:165–169
Terry PD, Goodman M (2006) Is the association between cigarette smoking and breast cancer modified by genotype? A review of epidemiologic studies and meta-analysis. Cancer Epidemiol Biomarkers Prev 15:602–611
Tokunaga M et al (1991) Follow-up studies of breast cancer incidence among atomic bomb survivors. J Radiat Res (Tokyo) 32 suppl:201–211
Trichopoulos D et al (2005) Towards an integrated model for breast cancer etiology: the crucial role of the number of mammary tissue-specific stem cells. Breast Cancer Res 7:13–17
Troisi R et al (2007) Cancer risk in women prenatally exposed to diethylstilbestrol. Int J Cancer 121:356–360
Vasiliu O et al (2004) In utero exposure to organochlorines and age at menarche. Hum Reprod 19:1506–1512
Williams EM et al (1990) Short term increase in risk of breast cancer associated with full term pregnancy. BMJ 300:578–579
Windham GC et al (2004) Age at menarche in relation to maternal use of tobacco, alcohol, coffee, and tea during pregnancy. Am J Epidemiol 159:862–871
Windham GC et al (2010) Body burdens of brominated flame retardants and other persistent organo-halogenated compounds and their descriptors in US girls. Environ Res 110:251–257
Witorsch RJ, Thomas JA (2010) Personal care products and endocrine disruption: a critical review of the literature. Crit Rev Toxicol 40(suppl 3):1–30
Wolff MS (2006) Endocrine disruptors: challenges for environmental research in the 21st century. Ann N Y Acad Sci 1076:228–238
Wolff MS et al (1993) Blood levels of organochlorine residues and risk of breast cancer. J Natl Cancer Inst 85:648–652
Wolff MS et al (1996) Breast cancer and environmental risk factors: epidemiological and experimental findings. Annu Rev Pharmacol Toxicol 36:573–596
Wolff MS et al (2007) Pilot study of urinary biomarkers of phytoestrogens, phthalates, and phenols in girls. Environ Health Perspect 115:116–121
Wolff MS et al (2008) Environmental exposures and puberty in inner-city girls. Environ Res 107:393–400
Wolff MS et al (2010) Investigation of relationships between urinary biomarkers of phytoestrogens, phthalates, and phenols and pubertal stages in girls. Environ Health Perspect 118:1039–1046
Wu T et al (2002) Ethnic differences in the presence of secondary sex characteristics and menarche among US girls: the Third National Health and Nutrition Examination Survey, 1988-1994. Pediatrics 110:752–757

Wu T et al (2003) Blood lead levels and sexual maturation in U.S. girls: the Third National Health and Nutrition Examination Survey, 1988-1994. Environ Health Perspect 111:737–741
Wu AH et al (2008) Epidemiology of soy exposures and breast cancer risk. Br J Cancer 98:9–14
Xu X et al (2010) Associations of serum concentrations of organochlorine pesticides with breast cancer and prostate cancer in U.S. adults. Environ Health Perspect 118:60–66
Xue F, Michels KB (2007) Intrauterine factors and risk of breast cancer: a systematic review and meta-analysis of current evidence. Lancet Oncol 8:1088–1100
Yabroff KR et al (2008) Estimates and projections of value of life lost from cancer deaths in the United States. J Natl Cancer Inst 100:1755–1762
Ye X et al (2006) Parabens as urinary biomarkers of exposure in humans. Environ Health Perspect 114:1843–1846
Zota AR et al (2010) Self-reported chemicals exposure, beliefs about disease causation, and risk of breast cancer in the Cape Cod Breast Cancer and Environment Study: a case-control study. Environ Health 9:40

Chapter 2
Puberty as a Window of Susceptibility

Frank M. Biro and Mary S. Wolff

Abstract Recent studies have begun to address the relationship between environmental exposures to pubertal development and to later risk of breast cancer. This chapter will review how physiologic changes could define puberty as a window of susceptibility. For example, although many studies have reported the relationship between age of menarche and breast cancer, the underlying physiologic mechanism may be related to pubertal growth characteristics, such as timing of or degree of peak height velocity. The maturing breast also contains cells that might be especially susceptible to toxic exogenous agents. The chapter will also discuss how environmental exposures, including dietary factors, could impact timing of puberty or subsequent risk of breast cancer.

Keywords Endocrine disrupting chemicals • Puberty • Pubertal growth • Breast cancer risk factors

2.1 Puberty as a Window of Susceptibility

Environmental exposures have long been invoked to explain incidence of breast cancer. Both lifestyle and xenobiotic exposures might be implicated in the wide variation of breast cancer incidence worldwide. Additional interest in environmental factors was raised during the late twentieth century with the recognition that genetics and lifestyle did not explain all the variability in breast cancer risk and with concern about the increasing rates of the disease (Madigan et al. 1995; Wolff and Weston 1997). Recently, research has also begun to examine environmental exposures in

F.M. Biro (✉)
Division of Adolescent Medicine, Cincinnati Children's Hospital Medical Center, University of Cincinnati College of Medicine, 3333 Burnet Avenue, Cincinnati, OH 45229-3039, USA
e-mail: frank.biro@cchmc.org

J. Russo (ed.), *Environment and Breast Cancer*, DOI 10.1007/978-1-4419-9896-5_2,

relation to female pubertal development, given the epidemiologic associations noted between breast cancer and age of menarche.

This chapter will examine the concept of puberty as a window of susceptibility. It will examine the hormonal events and anthropometric changes associated with puberty, potential mechanisms to explain how pubertal and reproductive events are associated with risk of breast cancer, and how environmental exposures – through chemicals, diet, and activity – may impact pubertal events as well as risk of breast cancer.

2.2 Physiologic Principles Underlying Puberty as a Window of Susceptibility

The development of the mammary gland is regulated at three critical periods of development: during fetal life, at the time of puberty, and with pregnancy. Similarly, critical windows for breast cancer exist throughout a woman's lifespan. Recognized risk factors of breast cancer include age at menarche, age at first full term pregnancy, and age at menopause, which suggests that timing of hormonally related events are relevant to the pathogenesis of breast cancer. The breast undergoes progressive changes from birth through menopause. In the peri-pubertal period, the mammary gland undergoes elongation and branching of the ductal tree, regulated by growth hormone and insulin-like growth factor (IGF-1), as well as estrogen, progesterone, and prolactin (Asselin-Labat et al. 2010). The primary ducts grow and divide with the formation of terminal end buds; terminal end buds divide into smaller ductules, or alveolar buds, which cluster around the terminal duct and form lobule type 1. Further growth and differentiation into lobules 2 and 3 is a gradual process throughout later puberty and into adulthood. Full differentiation into lobule type 4 occurs as a result of pregnancy, through permanent alterations in gene expression pattern (Russo et al. 2005). Thus, parity is protective for breast cancer (Kelsey et al. 1993). In addition, regardless of the number of pregnancies, breastfeeding reduces breast cancer risk by about 4% (Collaborative Group on Hormonal Factors in Breast Cancer 2002), possibly by further altering the architecture of mammary tissue. Breastfeeding is also the most efficient means of elimination of many environmental toxins (LaKind et al. 2001).

Breast epithelium exhibits maximal proliferative activity during the luteal phase of the menstrual cycle, and the highest level of cell proliferation is observed in undifferentiated lobule type 1 (Russo et al. 2000). Expansion of mammary epithelium suggests a stem-like cell with regenerative capacity (Visvader 2009). Rapidly developing breast tissue is felt to have the greatest susceptibility to environmental exposures (Berkey et al. 1999). Mammary stem cells or early progenitors are thought to be the critical cellular target in carcinogenesis (Reya et al. 2001). An empiric observation endorses this perspective; girls and young women exposed to radiation before age 20 years are at higher risk of breast cancer than women exposed to radiation later in life (Ronckers et al. 2005). Of note, mammary tumorigenesis is a multifactorial process, with cumulative damage occurring over a long period of time (Armitage and Doll 1954). Mathematical models suggest six or more successive critical events involved in premenopausal breast cancer. In a similar fashion, the shortest recognized latency period has been found with ionizing radiation. The greatest risk was found between atomic bomb exposure early in life and premenopausal breast cancer, with a latency period of at least 10 years. Because tumorigenesis is a cumulative process, latency is likely longer than 10 years for multiple weak carcinogenic events, including risks for breast cancer such as age at menarche and alcohol use (relative risks < 1.5). Of interest, earlier puberty in girls has been observed after radiation treatment (Table 2.1). Because latency for puberty is shorter than that for breast cancer, it may be easier to detect the impact of environmental exposures with onset of puberty than with associations with breast cancer.

Critical windows of breast cancer risk span the lifetime. Known factors include anthropometric changes and hormonal events associated with puberty, such as age at menarche, age at peak height velocity, and age at first term pregnancy. Strong epidemiologic studies support a 30% increased risk by younger age at menarche (Kelsey et al. 1993; Peeters et al. 1995; Petridou et al. 1996; Garland et al. 1998; Clavel-Chapelon 2002; Okasha et al. 2003). A pooled analysis noted that the risk of premenopausal breast cancer was reduced by 9% for each year that menarche was delayed, and the risk of postmenopausal breast cancer was reduced by 4% for each year that menarche was delayed (Clavel-Chapelon 2002). Menarche is the most well-established early-life risk factor, in part because it is an accurately recalled developmental milestone. Associations between menarche and breast cancer are especially strong with premenopausal breast cancer, which recently has been better characterized as basal-like breast cancer subtype (Yang et al. 2007; Millikan et al. 2008). Similarly, early menarche has been proposed to explain higher rates of premenopausal and basal-like breast cancer among blacks, whose pubertal development occurs earlier than whites. Blacks experienced menarche about 6 months earlier than whites throughout the twentieth century, and the difference in first breast development was about a year earlier (Wolff et al. 2008). Earlier puberty and premenopausal breast cancer in blacks further suggest a possible link with environment, as some minority groups may have higher exposures to many chemicals than other racial/ethnic groups. Previous studies noted a high correlation between age of menarche and breast cancer among American women over the past century, which has decreased in more recent studies (from 0.9 to 0.39) (Biro et al. 2006).

Earlier pubertal maturation, associated with an earlier ability to reproduce, would have provided a selective reproductive advantage, especially 5,000 or more years ago. This trait would have been selected and preserved and did not become a disadvantage until women began to live beyond their fifth decade (Biro et al. 2009). In addition, caloric restriction and physical activity of hunter-gatherers would be protective for breast cancer. Such a "thrifty phenotype" may explain why selected polymorphisms involved with sex steroid metabolism have been associated with onset of puberty (Kadlubar et al. 2003). A number of studies have examined the effect of sex hormones, particularly estrogens, relative to breast cancer risk. Endogenous estrogen levels were higher in women who subsequently developed

Table 2.1 Selected chemical and radiation exposures in relation to puberty and breast cancer

Exposure	Strength of evidence	Puberty/menarche	Strength of evidence	Breast cancer	References
Radiation (atomic bomb)			++	Pre-Japan bomb survivors (younger age, greater risk) (premenopausal after exposure <10 year)	Shore (2009), Tokunaga et al. (1979)
Secondary to RT	+	Earlier after childhood cancer treatment	++	After chest radiation (younger age, greater risk)	Armstrong et al. (2009), Chow (2008), Henderson et al. (2010), John et al. (2007), Noorda et al. (2001), Ron (2003)
Light at night, blindness	+	Earlier	+	Increased risk	Flynn-Evans et al. (2009), Stevens (2002)
Cigarette smoke	+	Earlier	±	May increase	Flynn-Evans et al. (2009), Reynolds et al. (2004), Rubin et al. (2009), Terry and Goodman (2006), Terry and Rohan (2002), Windham et al. (2004)
Zearalenone	+	Clinically early	–	No association, small study	Massart et al. (2008), Pillay et al. (2002)
Lavendar and tea tree oil	+	Gynecomastia in boys			Henley et al. (2007)
Soy/isoflavones	+	Delay menarche and breast development	+	Reduced risk	Cheng et al. (2010), Lee et al. (2009), Shu et al. (2001, 2009), Wolff et al. (2008, 2010)
Enterolactone/ lignans	+	Later menarche and breast development	+	Reduced risk	Buck et al. (2010), Wolff et al. (2008, 2010)

Pb (lead)	+	Delay of menarche and breast development			Wu et al. (2003)
PCBs	±	Delay*	+	May increase in susceptible subgroups	Brody et al. (2007), Rogan and Ragan (2007), Wolff et al. (2008)
Dioxin	±	Advance/delay	±	May increase	Brody et al. (2007), Leijs et al. (2008), Rogan and Ragan (2007)
DDT/E	±	Advance/delay	±	May increase recurrence	Brody et al. (2007), Cohn et al. (2007), Rogan and Ragan (2007)
PBB	+		–	Increased	Blanck et al. (2000), Henderson et al. (2010), Rogan and Ragan (2007)
PAH/AP including PAH-DNA adducts			±	Increased	Brody et al. (2007)
Phthalates	±	Advance/delay	±	Increased	Aschengrau et al. (1998), Chou et al. (2009), Lopez-Carrillo et al. (2010), Wolff et al. (2010)

Chemicals were chosen if we found (1) parallel data for puberty (usually menarche age) and breast cancer and/or (2) compelling evidence for one of the outcomes

– or *Grayed area* signifies poor/no/weak evidence, ± equivocal or conflicting evidence, + good evidence, ++ strong evidence

Breast cancer – environment references are mainly from Brody et al. (2007) and puberty – environment from Rogan and Ragan (2007), except where indicated,

* published data are not consistent regarding impact on timing of maturation; most data suggest delay

postmenopausal breast cancer (Thomas et al. 1997). Both pubertal onset and risk for breast cancer are associated with increased estradiol, estrone, estrone sulfate, and DHEAS (Toniolo et al. 1995; Hankinson et al. 1998; Cauley et al. 1999). In addition to genetics, obesity, alcohol intake, and some dietary patterns have been linked to variation in hormone levels.

Other maturation time points, such as age at peak height velocity, have been introduced as risk factors for breast cancer. Early age of menarche, as noted, is associated with age of onset of puberty, which, in turn, is associated with earlier age of the pubertal growth spurt. Earlier age of the pubertal growth spurt is associated with greater growth velocity (Biro et al. 2001), and obese and tall children have greater levels of IGF-1 in response to growth hormone (Bouhours-Nouet et al. 2007). This evidence may explain the apparent disparity in the epidemiologic observations that women with greater height have a greater risk of breast cancer (Friedenreich 2001), whereas those with earlier menarche also have a greater risk of breast cancer, but are shorter as adults. Previous studies have noted that the age of menarche is associated with risk of breast cancer, but not when age at peak growth is included in the analysis; menarche may serve as a proxy for age at peak growth, or both factors may reflect age at onset of puberty (Ahlgren et al. 2006). Similarly, women who reached maximum height at a young age (under 12 years) had a much greater risk of breast cancer (Li et al. 2007). Of note, the association of growth velocity with breast cancer is stronger for women with early menarche (De Stavola et al. 2004).

A last factor associated with earlier age of menarche is a longer interval from menarche to first pregnancy, as well as a greater number of lifetime menstrual cycles; both factors are thought to indicate increased cumulative endogenous hormone levels. As noted earlier, pregnancy induces permanent alterations in gene expression patterns (Russo et al. 2005) and full differentiation into lobule type 4. A longer interval from menarche to pregnancy would increase the duration of exposure of breast tissue to endogenous hormones and endocrine disrupting chemicals during the greatest susceptibility to potential carcinogens. Additionally, as noted above, earlier age of menarche would increase the number of menstrual cycles that occur prior to pregnancy, as well as number of cycles across the life span. A greater number of ovulatory cycles over the lifetime is correlated with increased risk of breast cancer.

2.3 Environmental Exposures

Another potential explanation for increased breast cancer risk is that exogenous (or xenobiotic) environmental exposures may lead to earlier menarche and thus could also increase subsequent risk of breast cancer. Strong experimental data support the idea that environmental chemicals can influence both sexual maturation and breast carcinogenesis, including breast development (Rudel et al. 2007; Schoeters et al. 2008). The mechanistic pathways linking environment to puberty and breast cancer include hormone receptors, P450 enzyme modification, GNRH action, immunomodification, and imprinting (Moral et al. 2007, 2008; Schoeters et al. 2008).

More recently, there has been emphasis on hormonally active environmental exposures which might enhance the production and/or activity of endogenous hormones, resulting in advanced puberty and increased breast cancer risk.

Laboratory findings suggest that the combination of exposure window, dose, and type of chemical impacts the age of sexual maturation in animals. As a result, later or earlier development can occur with the same chemical, or with mixtures, if the dose and timing of exposure are appropriate. An example of this relationship is found in the genistein literature; genistein exposure during pubertal maturation, not fetal or midadult exposure, decreases later breast cancer risk (Warri et al. 2008). During the past 20 years, limited epidemiologic data have emerged to support these environmental hypotheses, as summarized in Table 2.1. For breast cancer, there is ample evidence that radiation induces the disease, probably through a genotoxic mechanism. In general, studies of the environment and breast cancer have placed more emphasis on hormonally active exposures because of the dependence of breast cancer on steroid hormones and because many new-age chemicals have "endocrine-disrupting" properties. Such exposures are equally relevant to pubertal development which also requires estrogen. For puberty, two clinical studies indicate a strong association of chemical exposures and breast development. A case study of prepubertal boys with gynecomastia was explained by the use of highly estrogenic body oils (Henley et al. 2007). Another study attributed precocious puberty to exposure to the phytoestrogen zearalenone, a mycotoxin (Massart et al. 2008). These two examples include three elements relevant to research on hormonally active environmental exposures: a sufficiently high estrogen-equivalent or genotoxic dose of xenobiotic is required for premature breast development; associations with such exposures may be more easily detectable in an estrogen-deprived hormonal state (prepubertal boys or girls); and removal of exposure can lead to remission. The possibility of exposure remediation suggests that prevention may be possible, if environment contributes substantially to risk. On the other hand, if exposures are intermittent, they may be difficult to measure accurately and may limit the ability to detect associations in relation to intermediate outcomes or disease.

Other evidence in the Table 2.1 provides some support for a role of the environment in both breast cancer and female puberty. Some of the weaker associations are due to study limitations, including cross-sectional design, low exposures, and small numbers. Still, available evidence demonstrates consistency for the direction of findings with both puberty and breast cancer. Thus, advance/delay of puberty is seen in parallel with increased/reduced breast cancer risk for radiation, light-at-night, and phytoestrogens (Table 2.1). The best examples of these studies include relatively high exposures that may also be fairly consistent over time, so that issues about the windows of susceptibility are less influential for study design. For example, in breast cancer research, high soy intake in adulthood has been found to reflect dietary intake around adolescence (Shu et al. 2001). There are a number of cross-sectional studies that have used environmental biomarkers or dietary intake to study onset of female development or breast cancer and in general reflect the experimental literature. Examples include lead, TCDD ("dioxin"), and halogenated biphenyls (which show advanced and delayed puberty (Table 2.1)). However, almost all of these studies of are crosssectional, and not all reports are consistent.

Both animal and human studies indicate the importance of multiple exposures and prenatal exposures in relation to puberty (Blanck et al. 2000; Denham et al. 2005; Christiansen et al. 2008), but little work has been done in this area. Of additional importance are exposure and disease modifiers, such as genetics, geography, socioeconomic factors, physical activity, and diet. These factors may alter the metabolism of environmental chemicals, DNA repair, hormone receptor activation, or innate hormone profiles.

2.4 Dietary Factors

In a review of prospective studies, the only dietary factors strongly associated with breast cancer were alcohol consumption, obesity, and weight gain (Michels et al. 2007). All are thought to be surrogates for higher circulating hormones. As noted by the authors, the failure to observe a relationship among most dietary agents and breast cancer may be a true lack of association between diet and breast cancer, inadequate follow-up, or evaluation during an inappropriate window of susceptibility (Michels et al. 2007). While not all the evidence on soy intake and breast cancer is consistent (Trock et al. 2006), research that undertook a more complete assessment of dietary soy reported a strong protective effect with greater soy intake (Wu et al. 2008). Timing of soy intake may be important; in the Shanghai Women's Health Study, high intake of soy foods was associated with a reduced risk of premenopausal breast cancer (relative risk 0.57), and the risk appeared to be further reduced when considering soy/isoflavone consumption as an adult (RR 0.41–0.44) (Lee et al. 2009). In another study among Asian-American women, soy intake during childhood was associated with a greater reduction in risk of breast cancer, contrasted to intake during adolescence or adulthood (Korde et al. 2009). These findings of greater reduction with childhood exposure are consistent with animal data that have demonstrated reduced risk of breast cancer with early soy exposure (Lamartiniere et al. 2000). Several mechanisms have been proposed to account for the relationship between phytoestrogens and breast cancer, including binding to estrogen receptor (ER) β and inhibition of the enzyme that converts androgens to estrogens, aromatase. More recently, researchers have proposed other novel mechanisms, such as reduction of DNA hypermethylation in key genes through DNA methyltransferase inhibition (Li and Tollefsbol 2010).

There have been several publications that have addressed issues regarding fiber intake and timing of puberty, as well as fiber intake and breast cancer. Dietary fiber has been demonstrated to delay onset of maturation, presumably through reducing bioavailable estrogen (Hughes and Jones 1985; Soriguer et al. 1995; Berkey et al. 2000; Koo et al. 2002). The majority of prospective studies have not demonstrated an association between dietary fiber and breast cancer risk. In the European Prospective Investigation into Cancer and Nutrition (EPIC), there was a decreased incidence of cancers overall among vegetarians, but there was no impact on breast cancer (Key et al. 2009). In the NIH-AARP Diet and Health Study, dietary fiber was associated with reduced risk of breast cancer, and the association was strongest for ER-/PR-tumors (Park et al. 2009). The inconsistent results regarding fiber and breast cancer may be due to several factors – as noted above in the potential relationship between phytoestrogen intake and breast cancer – weak or lack of association, inadequate follow-up, low cancer incidence at the time of assessment, or inappropriate timing of dietary factors.

2.5 Physical Activity

Lifetime physical activity is associated with lower risk of breast cancer, especially physical activity during late adolescence and early adulthood (ages 14–20) (Kruk 2007). In another study, household and occupational activity was associated with reduction of breast cancer risk, but recreational activity was less helpful (Friedenreich 2001), although two other groups noted that recreational activity was helpful (Verloop et al. 2000; Bernstein et al. 2005). In a prospective cohort, women who engaged in regular strenuous activity at age 35 had a reduced risk of breast cancer (RR 0.86), and there were similar findings, although of lower impact, for strenuous activity at ages 18 and 50 years, respectively (McTiernan et al. 2003).

2.6 Conclusions

As summarized in this chapter, puberty may serve as a critical window of susceptibility for the development of breast cancer. A number of mechanisms may contribute to this relationship. Overall, the lifetime burden of steroid hormones is considered most critical, although variations within the pubertal window may also influence specific cellular structures that render the mammary gland more susceptible to tumorigenesis later in life. Therefore cumulative hormone and hormonally active chemical exposures may increase risk for breast cancer, but they may also alter the onset and duration of early windows of susceptibility, including breast development, age at menarche, rate of growth and achieved height, and timing of pregnancy.

References

Ahlgren M, Melbye M, Wohlfahrt J, Sorensen TIA (2006) Growth patterns and the risk of breast cancer in women. Int J Gynecol Cancer 16 (suppl 2):569–575

Armitage P, Doll R (1954) The age distribution of cancer and a multi-stage theory of carcinogenesis. Br J Cancer 8(1):1–12

Armstrong GT, Whitton JA, Gajjar A et al (2009) Abnormal timing of menarche in survivors of central nervous system tumors: a report from the Childhood Cancer Survivor Study. Cancer 115:2562–2570

Aschengrau A, Coogan PF, Quinn M et al (1998) Occupational exposure to estrogenic chemicals and the occurrence of breast cancer: an exploratory analysis. Am J Ind Med 34(1):6–14
Asselin-Labat ML, Vaillant F, Sheridan JM et al (2010) Control of mammary stem cell function by steroid hormone signalling. Nature 465:798–802
Berkey CS, Frazier AL, Gardner JD et al (1999) Adolescence and breast carcinoma risk. Cancer 85:2400–2409
Berkey CS, Gardner JD, Lindsay Frazier A et al (2000) Relation of childhood diet and body size to menarche and adolescent growth in girls. Am J Epidemiol 152:446–452
Bernstein L, Patel AV, Ursin G et al (2005) Lifetime recreational exercise activity and breast cancer risk among black women and white women. J Natl Cancer Inst 97:1671–1679
Biro FM, McMahon RP, Striegel-Moore R et al (2001) Impact of timing of pubertal maturation on growth in black and white female adolescents: the NHLBI Growth and Health Study. J Pediatr 138:636–643
Biro FM, Khoury P, Morrison JA (2006) Influence of obesity on timing of puberty. Int J Androl 29(1):272–277
Biro FM, Wolff MS, Kushi LH (2009) Impact of yesterday's genes and today's diet and chemicals on tomorrow's women. J Pediatr Adolesc Gynecol 22(1):3–6
Blanck HM, Marcus M, Tolbert PE et al (2000) Age at menarche and tanner stage in girls exposed in utero and postnatally to polybrominated biphenyl. Epidemiology 11:641–647
Bouhours-Nouet N, Gatelais F, Boux de Casson F et al (2007) The insulin-like growth factor-I response to growth hormone is increased in prepubertal children with obesity and tall stature. J Clin Endocrinol Metab 92:629–635
Brody JG, Rudel RA, Michels KB et al (2007) Environmental pollutants, diet, physical activity, body size, and breast cancer: where do we stand in research to identify opportunities for prevention? Cancer 15(12 suppl):2627–2634
Buck K, Zaineddin AK, Vrieling A et al (2010) Meta-analyses of lignans and enterolignans in relation to breast cancer risk. Am J Clin Nutr 92(1):141–153
Cauley JA, Lucas FL, Kuller LH et al (1999) Elevated serum estradiol and testosterone concentrations are associated with a high risk for breast cancer. Study of Osteoporotic Fractures Research Group. Ann Intern Med 130(4 pt 1):270–277
Cheng G, Remer T, Prinz-Langenohl R et al (2010) Relation of isoflavones and fiber intake in childhood to the timing of puberty. Am J Clin Nutr 92(3):556–564
Chou YY, Huang PC, Lee CC et al (2009) Phthalate exposure in girls during early puberty. J Pediatr Endocrinol Metab 22(1):69–77
Chow EJ, Friedman DL, Yasui Y, et al. (2008) Timing of menarche among survivors of childhood acute lymphoblastic leukemia: a report from the Childhood Cancer Survivor Study 50(4):854–8
Christiansen S, Scholze M, Axelstad M et al (2008) Combined exposure to anti-androgens causes markedly increased frequencies of hypospadias in the rat. Int J Androl 31:241–248
Clavel-Chapelon F (2002) Differential effects of reproductive factors on the risk of pre-and postmenopausal breast cancer. Results from a large cohort of French women. Br J Cancer 86:723–727
Cohn BA, Wolff MS, Cirillo PM et al (2007) DDT and breast cancer in young women: new data on the significance of age at exposure. Environ Health Perspect 115:1406–1414
Collaborative Group on Hormonal Factors in Breast Cancer (2002) Breast cancer and breastfeeding: collaborative reanalysis of individual data from 47 epidemiological studies in 30 countries, including 50302 women with breast cancer and 96973 women without the disease. Lancet 360:187–195
De Stavola BL, dos Santos SI, McCormack V et al (2004) Childhood growth and breast cancer. Am J Epidemiol 159:671–682
Denham M, Schell LM, Deane G et al (2005) Relationship of lead, mercury, mirex, dichlorodiphenyldichloroethylene, hexachlorobenzene, and polychlorinated biphenyls to timing of menarche among Akwesasne Mohawk girls. Pediatrics 115:e127–e134
Flynn-Evans EE, Stevens RG, Tabandeh H et al (2009) Effect of light perception on menarche in blind women. Ophthalmic Epidemiol 16(4):243–248

Friedenreich CM (2001) Review of anthropometric factors and breast cancer risk. Eur J Cancer Prev 10:15–32
Garland M, Hunter DJ, Colditz GA et al (1998) Menstrual cycle characteristics and history of ovulatory infertility in relation to breast cancer risk in a large cohort of US women. Am J Epidemiol 147:636–643
Hankinson SE, Willett WC, Manson JE et al (1998) Plasma sex steroid hormone levels and risk of breast cancer in postmenopausal women. J Natl Cancer Inst 90:1292–1299
Henderson TO, Amsterdam A, Bhatia S et al (2010) Systematic review: surveillance for breast cancer in women treated with chest radiation for childhood, adolescent, or young adult cancer. Ann Intern Med 152:444–455
Henley DV, Lipson N, Korach KS et al (2007) Prepubertal gynecomastia linked to lavender and tea tree oils. N Engl J Med 356:479–485
Hughes RE, Jones E (1985) Intake of dietary fibre and the age of menarche. Ann Hum Biol 12:325–332
John EM, Phipps AI, Knight JA et al (2007) Medical radiation exposure and breast cancer risk: findings from the Breast Cancer Family Registry. Int J Cancer 121:386–394
Kadlubar FF, Berkowitz GS, Delongchamp RR et al (2003) The CYP3A4* 1B variant is related to the onset of puberty, a known risk factor for the development of breast cancer. Cancer Epidemiol Biomarkers Prev 12:327–331
Kelsey JL, Gammon MD, John EM (1993) Reproductive factors and breast cancer. Epidemiol Rev 15(1):36–47
Key TJ, Appleby PN, Spencer EA et al (2009) Cancer incidence in vegetarians: results from the European Prospective Investigation into Cancer and Nutrition (EPIC-Oxford). Am J Clin Nutr 89(5):1620S–1626S
Koo MM, Rohan TE, Jain M et al (2002) A cohort study of dietary fibre intake and menarche. Public Health Nutr 5:353–360
Korde LA, Wu AH, Fears T et al (2009) Childhood soy intake and breast cancer risk in Asian American women. Cancer Epidemiol Biomarkers Prev 18:1050–1059
Kruk J (2007) Lifetime physical activity and the risk of breast cancer: a case-control study. Cancer Detect Prev 31(1):18–28
LaKind JS, Berlin CM, Naiman DQ (2001) Infant exposure to chemicals in breast milk in the United States: what we need to learn from a breast milk monitoring program. Environ Health Perspect 109(1):75–88
Lamartiniere CA, Zhao YX, Fritz WA (2000) Genistein: mammary cancer chemoprevention, in vivo mechanisms of action, potential for toxicity and bioavailability in rats. J Womens Cancer 2:11–19
Lee SA, Shu XO, Li H et al (2009) Adolescent and adult soy food intake and breast cancer risk: results from the Shanghai Women's Health Study. Am J Clin Nutr 89:1920–1926
Leijs MM, Koppe JG, Olie K et al (2008) Delayed initiation of breast development in girls with higher prenatal dioxin exposure: a longitudinal cohort study. Chemosphere 73:999–1004
Li Y, Tollefsbol TO (2010) Impact on DNA methylation in cancer prevention and therapy by bioactive dietary components. Curr Med Chem 17:2141–2151
Li CI, Littman AJ, White E (2007) Relationship between age maximum height is attained, age at menarche, and age at first full-term birth and breast cancer risk. Cancer Epidemiol Biomarkers Prev 16:2144–2149
Lopez-Carrillo L, Hernandez-Ramirez RU, Calafat AM et al (2010) Exposure to phthalates and breast cancer risk in northern Mexico. Environ Health Perspect 118:539–544
Madigan MP, Ziegler RG, Benichou J et al (1995) Proportion of breast cancer cases in the United States explained by well-established risk factors. J Natl Cancer Inst 87:1681–1685
Massart F, Meucci V, Saggese G et al (2008) High growth rate of girls with precocious puberty exposed to estrogenic mycotoxins. J Pediatr 152:690–695
McTiernan A, Kooperberg C, White E et al (2003) Recreational physical activity and the risk of breast cancer in postmenopausal women: the Women's Health Initiative Cohort Study. JAMA 290:1331–1336

Michels KB, Mohllajee AP, Roset-Bahmanyar E et al (2007) Diet and breast cancer: a review of the prospective observational studies. Cancer 109:2712–2749
Millikan RC, Newman B, Tse CK et al (2008) Epidemiology of basal-like breast cancer. Breast Cancer Res Treat 109(1):123–139
Moral R, Wang R, Russo IH et al (2007) The plasticizer butyl benzyl phthalate induces genomic changes in rat mammary gland after neonatal/prepubertal exposure. BMC Genomics 8:453
Moral R, Wang R, Russo IH et al (2008) Effect of prenatal exposure to the endocrine disruptor bisphenol A on mammary gland morphology and gene expression signature. J Endocrinol 196(1):101–112
Noorda EM, Somers R, van Leeuwen FE et al (2001) Adult height and age at menarche in childhood cancer survivors. Eur J Cancer 37:605–612
Okasha M, McCarron P, Gunnell D et al (2003) Exposures in childhood, adolescence and early adulthood and breast cancer risk: a systematic review of the literature. Breast Cancer Res Treat 78:223–276
Park Y, Brinton LA, Subar AF et al (2009) Dietary fiber intake and risk of breast cancer in postmenopausal women: the National Institutes of Health-AARP Diet and Health Study. Am J Clin Nutr 90(3):664–671
Peeters PHM, Verbeek ALM, Krol A et al (1995) Age at menarche and breast cancer risk in nulliparous women. Breast Cancer Res Treat 33(1):55–61
Petridou E, Syrigou E, Toupadaki N et al (1996) Determinants of age at menarche as early life predictors of breast cancer risk. Int J Cancer 68:193–198
Pillay D, Chuturgoon AA, Nevines E et al (2002) The quantitative analysis of zearalenone and its derivatives in plasma of patients with breast and cervical cancer. Clin Chem Lab Med 40:946–951
Reya T, Morrison SJ, Clarke MF et al (2001) Stem cells, cancer, and cancer stem cells. Nature 414:105–111
Reynolds P, Hurley SE, Hoggatt K et al (2004) Correlates of active and passive smoking in the California Teachers Study cohort. J Womens Health (Larchmt) 13(7):778–790
Rogan WJ, Ragan NB (2007) Some evidence of effects of environmental chemicals on the endocrine system in children. Int J Hyg Environ Health 210(5):659–667
Ron E (2003) Cancer risks from medical radiation. Health Phys 85(1):47–59
Ronckers CM, Erdmann CA, Land CE (2005) Radiation and breast cancer: a review of current evidence. Breast Cancer Res 7(1):21–32
Rubin C, Maisonet M, Kieszak S et al (2009) Timing of maturation and predictors of menarche in girls enrolled in a contemporary British cohort. Paediatr Perinat Epidemiol 23(5):492–504
Rudel RA, Attfield KR, Schifano JN et al (2007) Chemicals causing mammary gland tumors in animals signal new directions for epidemiology, chemicals testing, and risk assessment for breast cancer prevention. Cancer 109(12 suppl):2635–2666
Russo J, Hu YF, Yang X et al (2000) Developmental, cellular, and molecular basis of human breast cancer. J Natl Cancer Inst Monogr 27:17–37
Russo J, Mailo D, Hu YF et al (2005) Breast differentiation and its implication in cancer prevention. Clin Cancer Res 11:931s–936s
Schoeters G, Den Hond E, Dhooge W et al (2008) Endocrine disruptors and abnormalities of pubertal development. Basic Clin Pharmacol Toxicol 102:168–175
Shore RE (2009) Low-dose radiation epidemiology studies: status and issues. Health Phys 97(5):481–486
Shu XO, Jin F, Dai Q et al (2001) Soyfood intake during adolescence and subsequent risk of breast cancer among Chinese women. Cancer Epidemiol Biomarkers Prev 10:483–488
Shu XO, Zheng Y, Cai H et al (2009) Soy food intake and breast cancer survival. JAMA 302:2437–2443
Soriguer FJ, Gonzalez-Romero S, Esteva I et al (1995) Does the intake of nuts and seeds alter the appearance of menarche? Acta Obstet Gynecol Scand 74:455–461
Stevens RG (2002) Lighting during the day and night: possible impact on risk of breast cancer. Neuro Endocrinol Lett 23(suppl 2):57–60

Terry PD, Goodman M (2006) Is the association between cigarette smoking and breast cancer modified by genotype? A review of epidemiologic studies and meta-analysis. Cancer Epidemiol Biomarkers Prev 15(4):602–611

Terry PD, Rohan TE (2002) Cigarette smoking and the risk of breast cancer in women: a review of the literature. Cancer Epidemiol Biomarkers Prev 11(10 pt 1):953–971

Thomas HV, Reeves GK, Key TJ (1997) Endogenous estrogen and postmenopausal breast cancer: a quantitative review. Cancer Causes Control 8:922–928

Tokunaga M, Norman JE Jr, Asano M et al (1979) Malignant breast tumors among atomic bomb survivors, Hiroshima and Nagasaki, 1950-74. J Natl Cancer Inst 62(6):1347–1359

Toniolo PG, Levitz M, Zeleniuch-Jacquotte A et al (1995) A prospective study of endogenous estrogens and breast cancer in postmenopausal women. J Natl Cancer Inst 87:190–197

Trock BJ, Hilakivi-Clarke L, Clarke R (2006) Meta-analysis of soy intake and breast cancer risk. J Natl Cancer Inst 98:459–471

Verloop J, Rookus MA, van der Kooy K et al (2000) Physical activity and breast cancer risk in women aged 20-54 years. J Natl Cancer Inst 92:128–135

Visvader JE (2009) Keeping abreast of the mammary epithelial hierarchy and breast tumorigenesis. Genes Dev 23:2563–2577

Warri A, Saarinen NM, Makela S et al (2008) The role of early life genistein exposures in modifying breast cancer risk. Br J Cancer 98:1485–1493

Windham GC, Bottomley C, Birner C et al (2004) Age at menarche in relation to maternal use of tobacco, alcohol, coffee, and tea during pregnancy. Am J Epidemiol 159(9):862–871

Wolff MS, Weston A (1997) Breast cancer risk and environmental exposures. Environ Health Perspect 105(suppl 4):891–896

Wolff MS, Britton JA, Boguski L et al (2008) Environmental exposures and puberty in inner-city girls. Environ Res 107:393–400

Wolff MS, Teitelbaum SL, Pinney SM et al (2010) Investigation of relationships between urinary biomarkers of phytoestrogens, phthalates, and phenols and pubertal stages in girls. Environ Health Perspect 118(7):1039–1046

Wu T, Buck GM, Mendola P (2003) Blood lead levels and sexual maturation in US girls: the Third National Health and Nutrition Examination Survey, 1988-1994. Environ Health Perspect 111:737–741

Wu AH, Koh WP, Wang R et al (2008) Soy intake and breast cancer risk in Singapore Chinese Health Study. Br J Cancer 99(1):196–200

Yang XR, Sherman ME, Rimm DL et al (2007) Differences in risk factors for breast cancer molecular subtypes in a population-based study. Cancer Epidemiol Biomarkers Prev 16:439–443

Chapter 3
In Search of the Optimal Experimental Model

Irma H. Russo and Jose Russo

Abstract The increasing concern that environmental exposures may affect mammary gland differentiation and their potential for cancer risk has placed greater emphasis on the standardization of morphometric methods for the evaluation of mammary gland development in experimental animal models. Traditional morphological studies of whole mount preparations and histological sections have provided an enormous amount of information on the degree of mammary gland development and its response to diet, endogenous and exogenous hormones, and exposures to environmental chemicals, xenoestrogens, or physical agents. Their usefulness for assessing the effect of environmental exposures on mammary gland development and differentiation at specific stages of growth will depend upon optimal specimen selection and standardization of data for comparisons among laboratories. Past and present work has clearly indicated that the study of the rat mammary gland whole mount preparations under the stereomicroscope, combined with microscopic analysis, represents an important tool for evaluating risk assessment. The identification of the terminal end bud in the mammary glands of rodents and the intermediate cell (IC) as specific targets for carcinogens indicate that the adequate identification and quantification of these structures during specific windows of development would provide sufficient information for evaluating carcinogenic response. This classical model serves as a useful tool for incorporating state-of-the-art technologies that permit the microdissection of stem cells from their specific location sites for their genomic and proteomic analysis. Knowledge gained through these studies will serve for predicting the probabilities of developing cancer by detecting early genomic or epigenetic damage occurring in stem and progenitor cells.

I.H. Russo (✉)
Breast Cancer Research Laboratory, Fox Chase Cancer Center, 333 Cottman Avenue, Philadelphia, PA 19111-2497, USA
e-mail: Irma.russo@fccc.edu

J. Russo (ed.), *Environment and Breast Cancer*, DOI 10.1007/978-1-4419-9896-5_3,

Keywords Cancer stem cell • Mammary cancer • Environmental pollutants • Site of origin of cancer • Terminal end buds • Lobule type 1 • Whole mount preparations • Mammary gland morphometric analysis

Abbreviations

AB	Alveolar bud
BCSC	Breast cancer stem cell
CIS	Carcinoma in situ
CSC	Cancer stem cell
DMBA	7,12-Dimethylbenz(a)anthracene
HBEC	Human breast epithelial cell
IC	Intermediate cell
IDP	Intraductal proliferation
NMU	*N*-Methyl-*N*-nitrosourea
PAH	Polycyclic aromatic hydrocarbon
TDLU	Terminal ductal lobular unit
TEB	Terminal end bud

3.1 Introduction

Advances in biology are rapidly elucidating the molecular mechanisms that modulate cellular-response networks. The need to uncover the manner in which environmental agents perturb pathways to cause toxicity has been previously addressed (Committee on Toxicity Testing 2007). In this report it was acknowledged that for the foreseeable future, any in vitro strategy will need to include a provision to assess likely metabolites with whole-animal testing. Basic and translational researchers seeking to elucidate the cause(s) of breast cancer, and the role played by environmental agents on breast cancer causation and progression, have reached similar conclusions in the Mammary Gland Whole Mount Round Robin meeting held in Oakland, CA, on November 16, 2009. The objective of this meeting – the improvement of the reliability and standardization of mammary gland whole mount assessments – seemed to radically differ from the vision of the report issued by the Committee on Toxicity Testing (2007) which sought to find new conceptual and technological approaches for identifying at molecular level better predictors of potential human health effects in sensitive populations. However, both disciplines benefit by collaborating to address the global increase in incidence of breast cancer in women from all ethnic backgrounds in most industrialized countries (Althuis et al. 2005; Gibson 2010; Moorman et al. 2010). Although environmental pollutants such as chimney soot have been known to cause cancer since the middle 1700s (Waldron 1983), no such an agent has been found to be linked to the occurrence of breast cancer. Up to now only frequent exposure to radiation, either accidental (McGregor et al. 1977) or for diagnostic or therapeutic purposes (Boice et al. 1991; Boice 2001; Clemons et al. 2000; Cutuli et al. 2001), has been causally associated with breast cancer development. A positive association has been found with unopposed exposure to endogenous or exogenous estrogens (MacMahon 2006; Russo et al. 2010), either as the result of early menarche (Leung et al. 2008), late menopause (Moron et al. 2009), and use of hormone replacement therapy (HRT) (Menes et al. 2009). A definitive association has been found with alcohol consumption (Hamajima et al. 2002); however, the relevance of these findings in the overall population and the mechanisms through which they could de novo initiate cancer or promote preexisting lesions remain to be clarified. In spite of these uncertainties, worldwide epidemiological data have reached consensus on the fact that early pregnancy, before age 24, and multiple pregnancies protect women from developing breast cancer at postmenopause (de Waard and Thijssen 2005; Hinkula et al. 2001; MacMahon et al. 1970). Breastfeeding has been found to confer additional protection to women from most ethnic groups (Collaborative Group on Hormonal Factors in Breast Cancer 2002), including carriers of inherited *BRCA1* or *BRCA2* deleterious mutations (Anderson et al. 2008; Andrieu et al. 2006).

Breast cancer is considered to be an age-related disease, since the highest number of invasive new cases are diagnosed in postmenopausal Caucasian women over 60 years of age. The incidence of breast cancer is lower in premenopausal women and even lower in women under 40. This latter group is composed of carriers of inherited *BRCA1* or *BRCA2* deleterious mutations, predominantly women of Ashkenazi Jewish or African-American ancestry (Anderson et al. 2008; Lund et al. 2009). Tumor characteristics differ between pre- and postmenopausal women. Tumors that develop in postmenopausal women tend to be more differentiated and estrogen receptor (ER) positive, being therefore amenable to respond to antiestrogen therapy with selective estrogen receptor modulators (SERMs) or aromatase inhibitors. Tumors developed in younger women are diagnosed at later stages, are more aggressive, and are of basal-like triple negative type, characterized by lack of ER, progesterone receptor (PR), and histochemical expression of HER-2 growth factor (Schneider et al. 2008), characteristics that make them ineligible for antiestrogen therapy and that require chemotherapy for treatment (Freres et al. 2010). The observations that in these populations early age at menarche significantly increases breast cancer risk and early parity does not confer protection (Kotsopoulos et al. 2005) indicate that age at diagnosis is an important criterion for categorizing the disease into two different types that respond differently to early life risk factors (Clavel-Chapelon and Gerber 2002) and might differ in their pathogenesis. The demonstration of this postulate requires the identification of the time and site of origin of breast cancer. The search for the time and site of origin of breast cancer in women has been pursued through numerous studies involving hundreds of normal and pathological breast tissues from surgical and autopsy specimens (Alpers and Wellings 1985; Russo and Russo 1987, 2004; Steeg 2008); however, normal breast tissues representative of the critical stages of development, or windows of high susceptibility during which breast cancer could be initiated, are largely unavailable, thus the need for identifying an ideal animal tumor model that mimics the human disease still continues. In addition to the widely used rodent models, several species, including dogs (Selman et al. 1994), cats (Stolwijk et al. 1989), and monkeys (Broerse et al. 1991, 2000; Wood et al. 2006, 2007), are being evaluated for their ability to answer specific questions on the mechanisms of initiation and progression of mammary cancer. The usefulness of these models depends upon similarities between human and the chosen model's characteristics, such as normal anatomy of the mammary gland and its development during infantile and pubertal growth and reproduction; the influence of reproductive, aging, and nongenotoxic factors on the susceptibility of the gland to neoplasia; and the impact of hormones and growth factors on mammary carcinogenesis (Russo and Russo 1996). This knowledge will contribute to an increased understanding of how these parameters are influenced by the genetic makeup of the model utilized, as well as by environmental and dietetic interactions and reproductive factors (Russo and Russo 1996, 2004; Russo et al. 1990).

The understanding of the mechanisms of cancer initiation has in great part being accomplished through the study of the basic architecture of the rat mammary glands in whole mount preparations (Russo et al. 1989b). The use of this classical procedure has provided essential information on the location of specific structures that are characterized by their morphology, rate of cell proliferation, and hormone responsiveness, features that determine their susceptibility to be transformed by a given carcinogen (Russo and Russo 1980). The study of this model should allow researchers to test the influence of host factors such as age at the time of exposure, effect of hypothalamic (DiVall and Radovick 2008) and pituitary hormones on the initiation of ovarian function, i.e., age at the time of vaginal opening, a mimic of menarche (Sisk et al. 2001), and reproductive history on the initiation of tumorigenesis, and to assess the response of induced tumors to chemotherapy or other therapeutic modalities. This knowledge will contribute to clarifying the increasingly complex picture of breast cancer that is emerging from current epidemiological, clinical, pathological, and molecular data.

3.2 Correlative Study of Human and Rodent Breast Development and Differentiation

An important concept in human breast development is that in women, like in all mammalian species, this organ is not completely developed at birth. Furthermore, its development is influenced by the same dietetic and environmental influences that affect whole body growth from intrauterine life to adulthood. Because breast tissues from infants and prepubertal girls are not available for the study of their morphology and development, a gap exists in the knowledge of changes occurring during those critical phases of development (Russo and Russo 1987). By the time girls reach puberty the ductal and lobular structures of the breast reflect different stages of development. Extrapolations from rodent studies have allowed us to predict that the stages of breast development are similar to those observed in rodents. The most immature structure identified in whole mount preparations of breast tissues from peripubertal girls is the lobule type 1 (Lob 1) (Russo et al. 1990), which is considered to be similar to the rodent terminal end bud (TEB) and also similar to or the precursor of the terminal ductal lobular unit (TDLU) (Wellings et al. 1975). The TDLU/Lob 1 has been identified as the site of origin of the most common breast malignancy, the ductal carcinoma, as demonstrated in comparative studies of normal and cancer-bearing breasts obtained at autopsy and from cancer-bearing lumpectomy or mastectomy specimens (Russo et al. 1990). The hormonal stimulus of ovarian hormones and the establishment of regular menstrual cycles induce significant changes in breast morphology. The previously described Lob 1 progresses to the more developed lobule type 2 (Lob 2) and type 3 (Lob 3), but full development will be attained only through pregnancy. During pregnancy a rapid increase in the number of newly formed ductules accelerates the progression of Lob 2 to Lob 3; this growth phase is followed by the functional or secretory phase with the formation of secretory acini that characterize the milk-producing fully differentiated Lob 4. After postlactational involution, Lob 4 regresses to Lob 3, which remain present as the predominant structure in the breast until a woman reaches the fourth decade of life, decreasing thereafter due to their involution to Lob 2 and Lob 1 (Russo and Russo 1987, 2004). The breasts of women who have never been pregnant, on the other hand, are predominantly composed of Lob 1, whose percentage remains almost constant throughout their lifespan. A moderate number of Lob 2 and occasional Lob 3 develop during the early reproductive years, but they regress to Lob 1 after menopause. At the end of the fifth decade of life, the breast of both nulliparous and parous women contains predominantly Lob 1. Despite the similarity in the lobular composition of the breast, the fact that nulliparous women are at higher risk of developing breast cancer than parous women indicates that Lob 1 differs biologically and therefore exhibits different susceptibility to carcinogenesis in these two groups of women. This postulate has been supported by the differences in gene expression observed between the breast of parous and nulliparous women even after menopause (Russo et al. 2008). Additional support is provided by the findings that normal-appearing breast tissues from cancer patients contain significantly higher number of hyperplastic terminal ducts, atypical Lob 1 and ductal carcinomas in situ (DCIS) that originate in Lob 1 than breast tissues of women free of cancer. More differentiated structures, such as the lobule types 2, 3 and 4, on the other hand, originate either hormone-dependent lobular carcinomas in the former, or benign hyperplastic lobules, cysts, fibroadenomas, adenomas, and lactating adenomas in Lob 3 and Lob 4, respectively (Russo and Russo 1987, 2004).

3.2.1 The Stem Cell of Mammary Cancer

The realization that a definitive identification of the breast cancer stem cell (BCSC) has not been accomplished as yet is discouraging. Eighty years ago Sabin et al. (1932) reported that radioactive material damaged the chromatin of stem cells in lymphoid tissues. It took almost another 50 years to discover that environmental polycyclic aromatic hydrocarbons (PAH) caused mammary cancer by damaging the highly proliferating undifferentiated cells of TEBs (Russo et al. 1983).

Nevertheless, the debate on the site and cell of origin of breast cancer still continues today. The difficulties that hinder advances in the identification of the BCSC are rooted in the basic biology of breast development. Currently, two broad types of mammalian stem cells are recognized: *embryonic stem cells* that are isolated from the inner cell mass of blastocysts and *adult stem cells* that are found in adult tissues. However, the epithelium lining the ducts of the mammary parenchyma does not belong to any of these categories. Whereas in a developing embryo stem cells can differentiate into all of the specialized embryonic tissues, in adult organisms stem cells and progenitor cells replenish specialized cells and maintain the normal turnover of regenerative organs. In the mammary gland, which is an immature organ until the second or third decade of life, stem cells with the properties of embryonic stem cells present in TEBs coexist with progenitor/label-retaining cells that extend along the ductal tree from the nipple to the distal branches of the mammary parenchyma (Fernandez-Gonzalez et al. 2010). Electron microscopic analysis of TEBs provides information on the cellular composition of these structures based upon cell and nuclear size, nuclear-cytoplasmic ratio, amount of chromatin condensation, electron density of the cytoplasm, number and distribution of organelles, and presence or absence of Mg^{2+}- and $Na^{+}K^{+}$-dependent ATPases (Russo et al. 1977). These criteria permitted the identification of myoepithelial cells and three types of epithelial cells: light, intermediate, and dark cells. The analysis of the DNA labeling index revealed that all the cell types proliferated, although at different rates, depending upon the type of cells and of their location within the mammary gland tree. Cell proliferation was maximal in intermediate cells (IC) located in TEBs, being significantly lower in dark and myoepithelial cells found in the same location. High cell proliferation was associated with greater incorporation of H^3-DMBA and a progressive dominance of IC in 7,12-Dimethylbenz(a)anthracene (DMBA)-induced intraductal proliferations (IDPs) and in ductal carcinomas. Intermediate cells have been isolated from cultured DMBA-induced mammary tumors that also originated dark cells, which represented a terminally differentiated cell or a class in transition to differentiation (Bennett et al. 1978). A pluripotent stem cell population that lacks differentiated features such as cytoplasmic polarity, cell junctions, and organized cytoskeletal elements but that is capable of differentiating into both mammary ductal and mammary myoepithelial cell types has been described in the cap cells of the end bud in the mouse mammary gland (Hinck and Silberstein 2005; Daniel et al. 1987). Extensive work performed for characterizing progenitor and stem cells utilizing immunohistochemical (IHC) and genomic markers has been reviewed in other publications (Russo et al 2006); therefore, this topic will not be further discussed here.

3.2.2 *Stem Cells as Moving Targets of Carcinogens*

Experimentally induced mammary cancer in rodent models is the result of the interaction of a carcinogen with a structure that has to fulfill specific biological conditions in order to become a "target" that responds to the carcinogenic stimulus through transformation and tumor development. Thus, in susceptible rat strains, such as Sprague–Dawley or Wistar–Furth, administration of the PAH 7,12-dimethyl-benz(a)anthracene (DMBA) or the alkylating agent *N*-methyl-*N*-nitrosourea (NMU) stimulate the initiation of mammary cancer by binding to the TEB's epithelial cells that have been primed by the stimulus of ovarian steroid hormones (Russo and Russo 1996). The susceptibility of the mammary gland to these chemical carcinogens is strongly sex and age dependent; it is maximal when the carcinogens are administered to virgin females between the ages of 40 and 46 days, coincident with the period in which the mammary gland exhibits active organogenesis and the TEBs high proliferative activity (Russo et al. 1983), features that characterize a "high risk window." Mammary tumors induced by DMBA or NMU are in general hormone-dependent adenocarcinomas whose incidence, number of tumors per animal, tumor latency, and tumor type are influenced by the age, reproductive history, and endocrinological milieu of the host at the time of carcinogen exposure, as well as by prenatal and postnatal environmental exposures. The natural course of development of TEBs is cleavage and further branching into alveolar buds (ABs) and these develop into lobules, progressively developing a fully functional organ by the end of pregnancy (Russo et al. 1989a). The binding of the carcinogenic agent to the highly proliferating IC interferes with the TEBs' normal process of differentiation (Russo et al. 1983); as a consequence, the proportion of IC progressively increases and they become the dominant cell type in IDPs, the earliest multilayered and papillary preneoplastic lesions that are identified morphologically by 14 days after DMBA administration. IDPs are precursors of DCIS and invasive ductal carcinomas. These observations confirmed that under normal conditions the IC acts as a progenitor stem cell, which by dividing asymmetrically would generate daughter cells that differ in their specific characteristics and potential, becoming either an identical stem cell and another that will be committed to differentiation (Russo et al. 2010). These observations support the postulate that exposure to a carcinogen during a "high risk window" disrupts this process, as it has been demonstrated in human breast epithelial cells (HBEC) transformed in vitro by 17β-estradiol treatment (Russo et al. 2010). The TEB in the rat mammary gland is the target of carcinogens and originates ductal carcinomas prior to the formation of lobules, whereas in the woman's breast the TDLU is surrounded by lobular structures (Wellings et al. 1975). The most undifferentiated structure that has been already characterized in the breast of young nulliparous women is the Lob 1. Correlative studies have shown an equivalence between the TEB of the young virgin rat mammary gland and the Lob 1 of the woman's breast in their carcinogenic potential. However, human data are still insufficient to draw a complete picture of the pathogenesis of breast cancer. The knowledge of the architecture and cell kinetic characteristics of the breast at the time of carcinogen administration constitutes a necessary initial step for understanding the pathogenesis of the disease. It is also required for distinguishing those changes induced by the carcinogen from changes reflecting normal gland development, especially when evaluating early tumorigenic response in short-term studies. The fact that each specific compartment of the breast gives origin to a specific type of lesion lends support to the biological concept that the differentiation of the breast determines its susceptibility to neoplastic transformation and the type of lesions developed in response to the same carcinogenic insult. Further work needs to be done to clarify in both women and rodent models the ultimate mechanism(s) through which the basal-like cell in Lob 1 and the IC in TEB become the BCSC in response to a carcinogenic stimulus (Russo et al. 1983, 2006).

3.3 Conclusions and Future Directions

In the absence of human data rodent mammary carcinoma models have been particularly useful for dissecting the initiation, promotion, and progression steps of carcinogenesis. The susceptibility of the rodent mammary gland to develop neoplasms through exposure to chemicals, radiation, viruses, hormones, or through genetic modifications makes this a useful model for testing a variety of agents that could possibly be etiologic agents of cancer in women. These models have provided valuable information on the dose and route of administration to be used and optimal host conditions for eliciting maximal tumorigenic response. Studies of the influence of normal gland development on the pathogenesis of chemically induced mammary carcinomas have clarified the role of differentiation in cancer initiation. An additional advantage of these models is the particular morphological characteristics of their mammary glands, since the growth of the ductal tree along flat sheets of the fat pad facilitates the visual inspection and morphometric analysis of the parenchyma and the identification of target sites of carcinogen action.

Current knowledge on breast cancer incidence and on the pathogenesis of the disease is based on data collected from mammographically detectable or palpable breast masses whose time of initiation and rate of growth are not known. There is an obvious need for experimental animal models that closely reproduce human disease in order to establish valid extrapolations when testing the carcinogenic potential of chemicals, drugs, environmental agents, or dietetic compounds, as well as the response of mammary tumors to chemotherapeutic or chemopreventive compounds. Studies of the pathogenesis of chemically induced mammary cancer in rodents have served for identifying the TEB as the site of origin of ductal carcinomas, providing the tools for determining that the stem cells that originate mammary cancer are the same that originate the normal mammary parenchyma. Furthermore, rodent studies have confirmed that the fate of developing a normal ductal and lobular system or a tumor is set early in life by the influence of endogenous or environmental genotoxic or nongenotoxic influences that negatively affect the normal pattern of development imprinted in the mammary epithelium. A second important contribution of the study of this model is the verification that mammary cancer starts "de novo" as a malignant lesion initiated in the highly proliferating IC or stem cells 1, the cancer stem cell (CSC) present in the TEB. These neoplastic lesions are established and already progressing before lobular structures such as those identified surrounding TDLUs are formed. Besides, more differentiated lobular structures affected by a carcinogen originate more benign lesions whose characteristics are determined by the type of structure affected and its degree of differentiation (Russo and Russo 1996). This concept has been revisited in a recent publication indicating that various genes that regulate self-renewal in normal stem cells are also found in CSC. This implies that cancers may occur because of damage in normal stem cells and early progenitor cells. Further refinement of experimental models is required to mimic more closely the lifetime cumulative exposures that modulate the susceptibility of the breast to undergo malignant transformation. Drawbacks in currently used rodent models for long-term carcinogenicity studies are the lack of inclusion of the analysis of the mammary gland when evaluating the carcinogenic potential of given drugs and the lack of consideration of specific windows of susceptibility during breast development that are crucial for the assessment of environmental effect on lifetime cancer risk. Altogether our present and past work has clearly indicated that the study of the rat mammary gland whole mount preparations under the stereomicroscope, either alone or in combination with its microscopic analysis, represents an important tool for evaluating risk assessment. The fact that the mammary gland in rodents has a specific target that is the TEB, and that in that structure the intermediate cell is the one affected by a carcinogen indicates that the study of these two parameters could suffice for evaluating carcinogenic response. The advantage of utilizing rodent models for risk assessment is the particular morphological characteristics of their mammary glands, since the growth of the ductal tree along flat sheets of the fat pad facilitates the visual inspection and morphometric analysis of the parenchyma and the identification of target sites of carcinogen action. The TEB being the specific target affected by carcinogenic agents, the adequate identification and quantification of these structures during specific windows of development and therefore susceptibility of the animal to exogenous agents must be emphasized. This postulate is supported by the high correlation coefficient between the presence of these structures and the incidence of malignant lesions, as has been demonstrated in numerous experimental studies (Brown et al. 1998; Hilakivi-Clarke et al. 2001; Messina and Hilakivi-Clarke 2009; Moral et al. 2008; Russo and Russo 1996). Thus, this classical model serves as a useful tool for incorporating state-of-the-art technologies that permit the microdissection of stem cells from their specific location sites for their genomic and proteomic analysis. Knowledge gained through these studies will serve to predict the probabilities of developing cancer by detecting early genomic or epigenetic damage occurring in stem and progenitor cells.

Conflict of Interest Statement

There are no competing interests to disclose.

Acknowledgments This work was supported by grants R21 ES015148 and ES012771 from the National Institute Environmental Health Sciences (NIEHS) and R21 CA124522 from the National Cancer Institute (NCI).

References

Alpers CE, Wellings SR (1985) The prevalence of carcinoma in situ in normal and cancer-associated breasts. Hum Pathol 16:796–807

Althuis MD, Dozier JM, Anderson WF, Devesa SS, Brinton LA (2005) Global trends in breast cancer incidence and mortality 1973-1997. Int J Epidemiol 34:405–412

Anderson WF, Rosenberg PS, Menashe I, Mitani A, Pfeiffer RM (2008) Age-related crossover in breast cancer incidence rates between black and white ethnic groups. J Natl Cancer Inst 100:1804–1814

Andrieu N, Goldgar DE, Easton DF, Rookus M, Brohet R, Antoniou AC et al (2006) Pregnancies, breast-feeding, and breast cancer risk in the International BRCA1/2 Carrier Cohort Study (IBCCS). J Natl Cancer Inst 98:535–544

Bennett DC, Peachey LA, Durbin H, Rudland PS (1978) A possible mammary stem cell line. Cell 15:283–298

Boice JD Jr, Preston D, Davis FG, Monson RR (1991) Frequent chest X-ray fluoroscopy and breast cancer incidence among tuberculosis patients in Massachusetts. Radiat Res 125:214–222

Boice JD Jr (2001) Radiation and breast carcinogenesis. Med Pediatr Oncol 36:508–513

Broerse JJ, van Bekkum DW, Zoetelief J, Zurcher C (1991) Relative biological effectiveness for neutron carcinogenesis in monkeys and rats. Radiat Res 128:S128–S135

Broerse JJ, Bartstra RW, van Bekkum DW, van der Hage MH, Zurcher C, van Zwieten MJ et al (2000) The carcinogenic risk of high dose total body irradiation in non-human primates. Radiother Oncol 54:247–253

Brown NM, Wang J, Cotroneo MS, Zhao YX, Lamartiniere CA (1998) Prepubertal genistein treatment modulates TGF-alpha, EGF and EGF-receptor mRNAs and proteins in the rat mammary gland. Mol Cell Endocrinol 144:149–165

Clavel-Chapelon F, Gerber M (2002) Reproductive factors and breast cancer risk. Do they differ according to age at diagnosis? Breast Cancer Res Treat 72:107–115

Clemons M, Loijens L, Goss P (2000) Breast cancer risk following irradiation for Hodgkin's disease. Cancer Treat Rev 26:291–302

Collaborative Group on Hormonal Factors in Breast Cancer (2002) Breast cancer and breastfeeding: collaborative reanalysis of individual data from 47 epidemiological studies in 30 countries, including 50302 women with breast cancer and 96973 women without the disease. Lancet 360:187–195

Committee on Toxicity Testing and Assessment of Environmental Agents (2007) Toxicity testing in the 21st century: a vision and a strategy. The National Academy Press, Washington, DC

Cutuli B, Borel C, Dhermain F, Magrini SM, Wasserman TH, Bogart JA et al (2001) Breast cancer occurred after treatment for Hodgkin's disease: analysis of 133 cases. Radiother Oncol 59:247–255

Daniel CW, Silberstein GB, Strickland P (1987) Direct action of 17β-estradiol on mouse mammary ducts analyzed by sustained release implants and steroid autoradiography. Cancer Res 47:6052–6057

de Waard F, Thijssen JH (2005) Hormonal aspects in the causation of human breast cancer: epidemiological hypotheses reviewed, with special reference to nutritional status and first pregnancy. J Steroid Biochem Mol Biol 97:451–458

DiVall SA, Radovick S (2008) Pubertal development and menarche. Ann N Y Acad Sci 1135:19–28

Fernandez-Gonzalez R, Illa-Bochaca I, Shelton DN, Welm BE, Barcellos-Hoff MH, Ortiz-de-Solorzano C (2010) In situ analysis of cell populations: long-term label-retaining cells. Methods Mol Biol 621:1–28

Freres P, Collignon J, Gennigens C, Scagnol I, Rorive A, Barbeaux A et al (2010) "Triple negative" breast cancer. Rev Med Liege 65:120–126

Gibson JE (2010) An integrated summary of commentary on the National Academy of Sciences report on "Toxicity testing in the 21st century: a vision and a strategy". Hum Exp Toxicol 29:33–35

Hamajima N, Hirose K, Tajima K, Rohan T, Callee EE, Heath CW Jr et al (2002) Alcohol, tobacco and breast cancer – collaborative reanalysis of individual data from 53 epidemiological studies, including 58,515 women with breast cancer and 95,067 women without the disease. Br J Cancer 87:1234–1245

Hilakivi-Clarke L, Cho E, deAssis S, Olivo S, Ealley E, Bouker KB et al (2001) Maternal and prepubertal diet, mammary development and breast cancer risk. J Nutr 131:154S–157S

Hinck L, Silberstein GB (2005) Key stages in mammary gland development: the mammary end bud as a motile organ. Breast Cancer Res 7:245–251

Hinkula M, Pukkala E, Kyyrönen P, Kauppila A (2001) Grand multiparity and the risk of breast cancer: population-based study in Finland. Cancer Causes Control 12:491–500

Kotsopoulos J, Lubinski J, Lynch HT, Neuhausen SL, Ghadirian P, Isaacs C et al (2005) Age at menarche and the risk of breast cancer in BRCA1 and BRCA2 mutation carriers. Cancer Causes Control 16:667–674

Leung AW, Mak J, Cheung PS, Epstein RJ (2008) Evidence for a programming effect of early menarche on the rise of breast cancer incidence in Hong Kong. Cancer Detect Prev 32:156–161

Lund MJ, Trivers KF, Porter PL, Coates RJ, Leyland-Jones B, Brawley OW et al (2009) Race and triple negative threats to breast cancer survival: a population-based study in Atlanta, GA. Breast Cancer Res Treat 113:357–370

MacMahon B (2006) Epidemiology and the causes of breast cancer. Int J Cancer 118:2373–2378

MacMahon B, Cole P, Lin TM, Lowe CR, Mirra AP, Ravnihar B et al (1970) Age at first birth and breast cancer risk. Bull World Health Organ 43:209–221

McGregor DH, Land CE, Choi K, Tokuoka S, Liu PI, Wakabayashi I et al (1977) Breast cancer incidence among atomic bomb survivors, Hiroshima and Nagasaki, 1950–1969. J Natl Cancer Inst 59:799–811

Menes TS, Kerlikowske K, Jaffer S, Seger D, Miglioretti DL (2009) Rates of atypical ductal hyperplasia have declined with less use of postmenopausal hormone treatment: findings from the Breast Cancer Surveillance Consortium. Cancer Epidemiol Biomarkers Prev 18:2822–2828

Messina M, Hilakivi-Clarke L (2009) Early intake appears to be the key to the proposed protective effects of soy intake against breast cancer. Nutr Cancer 61:792–798

Moorman PG, Iversen ES, Marcom PK, Marks JR, Wang F; Kathleen Cuningham Consortium for Research into Familial Breast Cancer et al (2010) Evaluation of established breast cancer risk factors as modifiers of BRCA1 or BRCA2: a multi-center case-only analysis. Breast Cancer Res Treat 124:441–451

Moral R, Wang R, Russo IH, Lamartiniere CA, Pereira J, Russo J (2008) Effect of prenatal exposure to the endocrine disruptor bisphenol A on mammary gland morphology and gene expression signature. J Endocrinol 196:101–112

Moron FJ, Ruiz A, Galan JJ (2009) Genetic and genomic insights into age at natural menopause. Genome Med 1:76

Russo J, Balogh GA, Russo IH; FCCC Hospital Network Participants (2008) Full-term pregnancy induces a specific genomic signature in the human breast. Cancer Epidemiol Biomarkers Prev 17:51–66

Russo J, Russo IH (1980) Influence of differentiation and cell kinetics on the susceptibility of the mammary gland to carcinogenesis. Cancer Res 40:2677–2687

Russo J, Russo IH (1987) Development of human mammary gland. In: Neville MC, Daniel CW (eds) The mammary gland development, regulation and function. Plenum, New York, pp 67–93

Russo IH, Russo J (1996) Mammary gland neoplasia in long-term rodent studies. Environ Health Perspect 104:938–967

Russo J, Russo IH (2004) Molecular basis of breast cancer: prevention and treatment. Springer, Berlin

Russo J, Wells P, Russo IH (1977) Adenosine triphosphatases as histochemical markers for cell of origin in experimental mammary carcinoma. Cancer Res 37:1088–1098
Russo J, Tait L, Russo IH (1983) Susceptibility of the mammary gland to carcinogenesis III. The cell of origin of mammary carcinoma. Am J Pathol 113:50–66
Russo IH, Medado J, Russo J (1989a) Endocrine influences on mammary gland structure and development. In: Jones TC, Mohr U, Hunt RD (eds) Integument and mammary gland of laboratory animals. Springer, Berlin, pp 252–266
Russo IH, Tewari M, Russo J (1989b) Morphology and development of rat mammary gland. In: Jones TC, Mohr U, Hunt RD (eds) Integument and mammary gland of laboratory animals. Springer, Berlin, pp 233–252
Russo J, Gusterson BA, Rogers AE, Russo IH, Wellings SR, Van Zwieten MJ (1990) Comparative study of human and rat mammary tumorigenesis. Lab Invest 62:1–32
Russo J, Balogh GA, Chen J, Fernandez SV, Fernbaugh R, Heulings R et al (2006) The concept of stem cell in the mammary gland and its implication in morphogenesis, cancer and prevention. Front Biosci 11:151–172
Russo J, Snider K, Pereira JS, Russo IH (2010) Estrogen induced breast cancer is the result of disruption of asymmetric cell division of the stem cell. Horm Mol Biol Clin Investig 1:53–65
Sabin FR, Doan CA, Forkner CE (1932) The production of osteogenic sarcomata and the effects on lymph nodes and bone marrow of intravenous injections of radium chloride and mesothorium in rabbits. J Exp Med 56:267–289
Schneider BP, Winer EP, Foulkes WD, Garber J, Perou CM, Richardson A et al (2008) Triple-negative breast cancer: risk factors to potential targets. Clin Cancer Res 14:8010–8018
Selman PJ, Mol JA, Rutterman GR, Garderen EV, Rijnberk A (1994) Progestin-induced growth hormone excess in the dog originates in the mammary gland. Endocrinology 134:287–292
Sisk CL, Richardson HN, Chappell PE, Levine JE (2001) In vivo gonadotropin-releasing hormone secretion in female rats during peripubertal development and on proestrus. Endocrinology 142:2929–2936
Steeg PS (2008) Heterogeneity of drug target expression among metastatic lesions: lessons from a breast cancer autopsy program. Clin Cancer Res 14:3643–3645
Stolwijk JAM, Minke JMHM, Rutteman GR, Hoekstra J, Prop FJA, Misdorp W (1989) Feline mammary carcinomas as a model for human breast cancer. II. Comparison of in vivo and in vitro adriamycin sensitivity. Anticancer Res 9:1045–1048
Waldron HA (1983) A brief history of scrotal cancer. Br J Ind Med 40:390–401
Wellings SR, Jensen HM, Marcum RG (1975) An atlas of subgross pathology of the human breast with special reference to possible precancerous lesions. J Natl Cancer Inst 55:231–273
Wood CE, Usborne AL, Starost MF, Tarara RP, Hill LR, Wilkinson LM, Geisinger KR, Feiste EA, Cline JM (2006) Hyperplastic and neoplastic lesions of the mammary gland in macaques. Vet Pathol 43:471–483
Wood CE, Hester JM, Cline JM (2007) Mammary gland development in early pubertal female macaques. Toxicol Pathol 35:795–805

Chapter 4
Early Life Exposure to Bisphenol A and Breast Neoplasia

Maricel V. Maffini, Carlos Sonnenschein, and Ana M. Soto

Abstract Excess estrogen exposure in developing individuals increases the risk of developing breast cancer later in life. This excess estrogen can originate from high levels of maternal endogenous estrogens or from exposure to exogenous endocrine disrupting compounds that mimic estrogen actions. One of those compounds is the ubiquitous bisphenol A or BPA, a chemical that has been found in over 90% of the American population tested and that mimics the actions of estradiol both in vitro and in vivo. The breast is a target organ for both estradiol and BPA. In this chapter we will discuss the effects of BPA on the developing mammary gland and its long-lasting consequences on the organ's health, and we will argue that prenatal and early life exposure to endocrine disrupting chemicals contributes to the increased incidence of breast cancer observed during the last decades.

Keywords Endocrine disruptors • Bisphenol A • Estrogen mimic • Mammary gland • Prenatal exposures • Carcinoma in situ • Precancerous lesions • Breast cancer incidence

4.1 Mammary Gland Development

The mammary gland is a highly plastic organ that undergoes recurrent growth, differentiation, and regression. The prenatal and postnatal developments are the results of harmonious interactions among cells, between cells and extracellular

M.V. Maffini (✉)
Department of Anatomy and Cellular Biology, Tufts University School of Medicine, 136 Harrison Avenue, Boston, MA 02111, USA
e-mail: maricel.maffini@tufts.edu

J. Russo (ed.), *Environment and Breast Cancer*, DOI 10.1007/978-1-4419-9896-5_4,

matrix, and between cells and hormones. The exceedingly high capacity of the mammary gland to remodel the connective and epithelial tissues and re-shape itself, especially during puberty, pregnancy and postlactation involution, is remarkable and is shared by all mammals (Maffini et al. 2010).

4.1.1 Human Breast Development

The thickening of the epidermis (milk lines) on the ventral surface of the 5-week old human fetus is the first sign of breast development. By the 15th week of gestation, the breast buds grow in length, producing cords of epithelium which invade the underlying mesenchyme. The collagenous mesenchyme differentiates into fatty stroma between weeks 20 and 32. The epithelial cords become hollow during the last 2 months of gestation; at this time, ductal and lobulo-alveolar branching also occurs. Near birth, the nipple is formed by evagination of the mammary skin surface (Rosen 2008). Both male and female mammary glands develop in a similar manner and no morphological differences are observed during fetal development and the first 2 years of age (Anbazhagan et al. 1991). After birth, the mammary gland remains in a resting state until puberty. The earliest stages of fetal breast formation appear to be independent of steroid hormones. Estrogen receptor (ER)-α protein has been detected using immunohistochemical techniques in epithelial cell nuclei in the fetal breast starting at gestational week 30 (Keeling et al. 2000). From birth to puberty, this receptor was heterogeneously expressed in the breast epithelial cells (Bartow 1998; Keeling et al. 2000). The earliest that progesterone receptor (PR) has been detected in the human breast epithelial cells is between 3 and 7 years of age (Bartow 1998).

With the onset of puberty and its cyclical secretion of estrogen and progesterone, the ducts grow by invading the adjacent connective tissue; lobulo-alveolar differentiation and growth also occur at this time. Other hormones contributing to the growth and differentiation of the gland are growth hormone, insulin, and glucocorticoids (Rosen 2008). Stroma-epithelium interactions are responsible for these organizational changes (Cunha et al. 1985). The adult breast is composed of 15–25 defined lobes associated with each of the major lactiferous ducts that open in the nipple (Rosen 2008). The smallest functional unit of the resting nonpregnant breast is the terminal ductal lobular unit (TDLU) which consists of a group of alveoli connected by ductules that drain into a larger duct (Fig. 4.1). Changes in cell proliferation, cell size, and tissue appearance are observed throughout the menstrual cycle. ER-β is the most abundant ER in the non-pregnant adult breast being expressed in approximately 70% of the epithelial cells (Weihua et al. 2000) while ER-α is expressed in only 4–15% of the ductal and lobular epithelial cells in the adult breast. Unlike ER-β, ER-α is not expressed in the breast stroma (Shyamala et al. 2002). Once the menstrual cycle is established, ER expression in the adult breast is also cyclical.

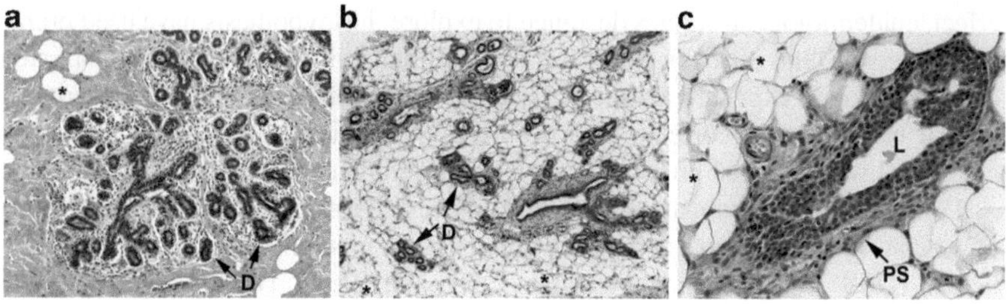

Fig. 4.1 Representative histological sections of mammary glands. (**a**) Terminal ductal lobular unit (TDLU) of human breast; (**b**) Rat mammary gland ductal network; (**c**) Terminal end bud (TEB) in rat mammary gland. *Fat cells; *PS* periductal stroma; *L* lumen; *D* ducts

4.1.1.1 Mammary Gland Development in Rodents

The development of the rodent mammary gland closely resembles that of the human breast, which makes these animals suitable surrogate models to study mammary gland biology. The mouse mammary gland development begins at embryonic day 10.5 (E10.5) with the appearance of presumptive mammary lines. Mammary placodes invaginate into the dermis at E13.5 as the mammary mesenchyme surrounding the epithelium becomes increasingly dense (Robinson et al. 1999). At E15.5 the precursor to the underlying fat pad is invaded by the mammary bud as it elongates into a cord called the mammary sprout. By E18, the mammary sprout begins to branch and lumen develops (Vandenberg et al. 2007). At this point, the growth of the mammary gland parallels the growth of the organism as a whole until puberty, at which time the gland undergoes substantial remodeling. In mice, ER-α and ER-β mRNAs are first expressed at E12.5 in the mesenchymal cells that surround the bud (Lemmen et al. 1999). By E16 these receptors were shown to be functional as they bind to radiolabeled estrogen (Narbaitz et al. 1980).

At puberty, rising levels of estrogens cause a rapid increase in ductal growth that is characterized by high levels of both cellular proliferation and apoptosis (cell death) at the terminal end buds (TEB); the bulbous TEBs lead the migration of the ducts into the stroma. The combination of proliferation and apoptosis is essential for the development of a lumen (Humphreys et al. 1996). The ductal tree develops into a network of ducts, terminal ducts, and alveolar buds as it completely fills the stroma, also referred to as the mammary fat pad. ER-α expression is mainly localized in the epithelium in adulthood (Saji et al. 2000).

4.1.2 Developmental Origins of Breast Cancer

Epidemiological studies suggest that fluctuating estrogen levels in the fetal environment have long-term consequences regarding the risk of developing breast cancer (Trichopoulos 1990). Given the long latency period between exposure and effect, epidemiological studies designed to explore this hypothesis have used prenatal markers of fetal estrogen exposure; for example, twin pregnancy as an indicator of high-estrogen exposure and preeclampsia for low-estrogen exposure. Increased risk of breast cancer correlated with twin dizygotic birth and preeclampsia was associated with lowered breast cancer risk (Potischman and Troisi 1999).

Direct evidence of prenatal estrogen exposure and associated breast cancer risk is now being collected from a cohort of women born to mothers treated with diethylstilbestrol (DES) during pregnancy in the 1950s and 1960s. These women, exposed during gestation to DES, are now reaching the age at which the incidence of breast cancer becomes prevalent. In the group of women aged 40 years and older exposed during gestation to this synthetic estrogen, there is a 2.5-fold increase in the incidence of breast cancer compared to unexposed women of similar age (Palmer et al. 2006). Likewise, experiments in rats showed that prenatal exposure to DES resulted in increased mammary gland cancer incidence during adulthood (Boylan and Calhoon 1983). These data are consistent with the hypothesis that excessive fetal estrogen exposure increases the risk of breast cancer. However, in the above-mentioned studies, DES was administered at pharmacological doses, while twinning and preeclampsia represent a physiological range of endogenous hormone levels to which fetuses are exposed. Additionally, there is a third type of exposure that ought to be addressed, which is the inadvertent and continuous exposure of fetuses to xenoestrogens.

4.1.2.1 Environmental Endocrine Disruptors Alter Mammary Gland Development

Although alterations in the mammary gland observed in animals exposed to endocrine disrupting compounds during adulthood are of great concern (Markey et al. 2003; White et al. 2007), exposures to those same compounds during the perinatal period have grave consequences long after the exposure has ended. Several endocrine disrupting chemicals alter mammary gland development subsequent to perinatal exposure. For instance, atrazine, dioxins, and perfluorooctanoic acid delay mammary gland development (Rayner et al. 2005; White et al. 2007; Fenton et al. 2002). In contrast, other endocrine disruptors such as bisphenol A (BPA) and DES resulted in the long-term increase of epithelial structures and the development of precancerous and cancerous lesions that manifested in adulthood (Tomooka and Bern 1982; Vandenberg et al. 2009). Because of its widespread presence in the environment and chronic human exposure, BPA was chosen as a model chemical to study developmental effects of xenoestrogens and to date is the best studied endocrine disrupting chemical regarding low-dose effects on the developing mammary gland.

4.1.2.2 BPA Alters Mammary Gland Development

BPA is used in the manufacture of polycarbonate plastics and epoxy resins; it leaches from food (Brotons et al. 1994) and beverage containers (Biles et al. 1997) and dental sealants and composites (Olea et al. 1996) under normal conditions of use (Markey et al. 2003). There are over 80 human biomonitoring studies in which BPA was measured in blood, urine, amniotic fluids and tissues such as placenta (Vandenberg et al. 2010). In 2005, BPA was found in over 90% of urine samples from a reference US population (Calafat et al. 2005). The higher levels were found in children and adolescents. BPA is regulated by the US Environmental Protection Agency and the reference daily intake, i.e., the dose that is considered safe for human exposure, was set at 50 μg/kg/day.

Prenatal exposure of mice to environmentally relevant levels of BPA resulted in alterations in both compartments of the mammary gland, namely the stroma and epithelium. At embryonic day 18 the mammary gland of BPA-exposed animals showed advanced maturation of the mammary fat pad, and ductal alterations including decreased cell size, delayed lumen formation, and increased ductal area (Vandenberg et al. 2007). At puberty, there was an increased number of TEBs relative to the ductal area, decreased apoptosis in the TEBs, and an increased number of epithelial cells expressing progesterone receptor (Munoz de Toro et al. 2005). At 4 months of age, there was a significant increase in lateral branching (Munoz de Toro et al. 2005). By 6 months, there was an overall increase in epithelial structures including terminal ends and a premature appearance of alveolar buds, normally associated with pregnancy in the mouse (Markey et al. 2001a). When the gestational exposure to low doses of BPA was extended through the lactation period, the offspring of the BPA-treated mothers had mammary glands with an increased volume fraction of alveolar buds at 3 and 9 months of age, and an increased volume fraction of ducts at 9 months of age; these changes occurred at 0.25 μg BPA/kg/day. Animals exposed to 2.5 μg/kg/day also showed an increase in alveolar buds at 9 months of age (Vandenberg et al. 2008).

The offspring of CD1 mice treated with four daily subcutaneous injections of either 0.5 or 10 mg BPA/kg/day starting at gestational day 15 showed altered development of the mammary gland at 4 weeks of age (Nikaido et al. 2004). Prenatal exposure (from gestational day 10 to birth) of Sprague–Dawley CD rats to 250 μg BPA/kg/day via gavage resulted in an increase in the number of TEBs at 21 days of age, an increased number of terminal ducts at 21 and 100 days of age, and an increased number of lobules type 1 at 35 days of age. Although morphological changes were only observed with the high-dose exposure, changes in gene expression were observed after exposure to both low (25 μg BPA/kg/day) and high BPA doses (Moral et al. 2008). BPA exposure also altered gene expression in a dose-dependent manner in these rats, and the number of genes varied with the animal's age. Using a similar exposure regimen, Betancourt et al. analyzed the proteomic profile of the mammary glands of female offspring before and during puberty. At postnatal day 21, 11 proteins identified by mass spectroscopy were differentially expressed in the BPA group compared to control (Betancourt et al. 2010); at PND50, ten proteins were differentially expressed in the BPA animals compared to control. Interestingly, among those proteins which showed significantly different expression from the treated animals were stromal proteins such as vimentin, adiponectin, and desmin, and the matricellular protein SPARC.

Scientific reports addressing the effects of BPA exposure conclude with a high degree of certainty that BPA induces alterations in the mammary gland that are manifested at different levels of biological organization regardless of route of exposure (oral vs. subcutaneous), the type of exposure (once a day vs. continuous), the timing of exposure (gestational vs. postnatal), and the species (mouse vs. rat). These outcomes can be obvious, such as altered tissue architecture, or more subtle, such as differential gene and/or protein expression. However, conventional toxicological studies have reported that BPA produces no effects on the mammary gland. The reported negative histopathological effects in the mammary gland of CD1 mouse offspring exposed to a broad range of BPA doses (from 0.003 to 600 mg/kg/day) did not include a description of which parameters were assessed or which time points were analyzed (Tyl et al. 2008). The main limitation of these conventional toxicological studies is the use of out-of-date, low sensitivity assays and lack of end points to detect low dose effects (Myers et al. 2009). For instance, routine toxicological studies do not provide details regarding how the mammary tissue was prepared (i.e., as whole mount or paraffin-embedded), or the type of analysis used to measure the quantity and quality of epithelial structures, and growth patterns. Whole-mounted mammary glands provide a unique view of the whole organ in three-dimensions, a feature that facilitates the identification of microscopic abnormalities swiftly. This omission may explain why the Tyl et al. study reported that BPA caused no effects on the mammary glands. Separately, the National Toxicology Program report on the potential effects of BPA on human health stated minimal concern for exposures in fetuses, children, and infants to low levels of BPA based on the effects observed in the mammary gland of laboratory animals (National Toxicology Program 2008). However, the report also asked for additional research in order to better understand the implications of human exposure to BPA.

A relatively small number of laboratories have reported effects of developmental exposure to BPA or other hormonally active pollutants on the mammary gland; this is a surprising fact considering that exposure to estrogen mimics and other endocrine disrupting compounds during critical windows of susceptibility has been associated with an increased risk of breast cancer in humans (Cohn et al. 2007; Palmer et al. 2006; Warner et al. 2002). One possible explanation for both the low number of reports and the disparities found in published data may be the lack of standardized analytical methods to assess the rodent's mammary glands. More specifically, the mammary gland tree undergoes normal physiological changes during puberty and adulthood; for instance, ductal extension and ductal and alveolar bud densities vary with age, species, and strains (Wadia et al. 2007). These normal features are easily identified only when the mammary gland can be observed in its entirety, which is achieved by the preparation of whole mounts (Fig. 4.2). The whole mount preparation consists of the entire organ spread onto a glass slide and processed in a way in which the three dimensional architecture is preserved. On the contrary, once the gland is embedded in a paraffin block and sectioned into thin slices, the spatial growth pattern and the size and distribution of epithelial structures are impossible to identify and subsequently to quantify. A first step toward improving the standardization of mammary gland evaluation was the organization of the interdisciplinary

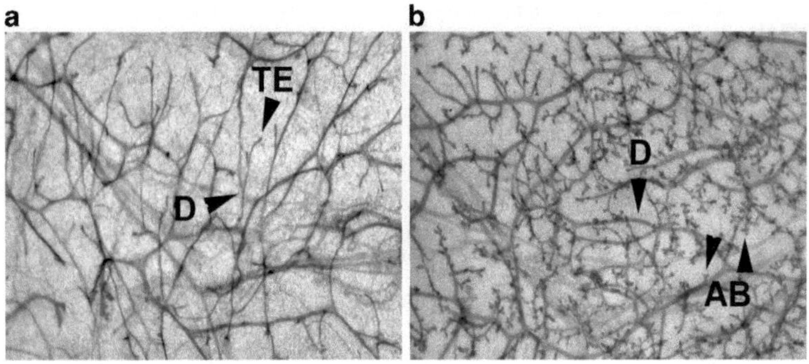

Fig. 4.2 The three-dimensional architecture of the mammary gland is easily observed in whole mount preparations. (**a**) Normal mouse mammary gland; (**b**) Mammary gland from a bisphenol A (BPA)-exposed mouse (from gestational day 8 to postnatal day 16). *TE* Terminal end; *D* duct; *AB* alveolar bud

workshop "Mammary gland evaluation and risk assessment" in November 2009 in Oakland (CA); the conclusions from that meeting were presented at the Society of Toxicology meeting in 2010 (Rudel et al. 2010; Fenton and Rudel 2010). Briefly, scientists from three countries participated in a round robin evaluation of mammary gland whole mounts from rodents (mice and rats) treated during gestation with chemicals or left untreated. The workshop participants unanimously agreed that "mammary gland whole mount preparations should be routinely incorporated into test protocols that include in utero or early life exposures in order to determine potential effects of chemicals on early life mammary gland development." They also noted that "histopathology alone was not suitable for detecting altered mammary gland morphology, but could be useful in conjunction with whole mounts" (Rudel et al. 2010; Fenton and Rudel 2010). Thus, standardized protocols should be developed and implemented by regulatory agencies for chemical toxicity testing and risk assessment of low dose effects of environmental endocrine disruptors.

4.1.2.3 Exposure to BPA During Organogenesis Induces Mammary Gland Neoplasias

The main risk factor for breast cancer is lifetime exposure to ovarian hormones. In addition to the altered morphology, the mammary glands of BPA-exposed mice showed an enhanced sensitivity to estradiol. Female mice exposed to BPA during gestation that subsequently were ovariectomized before puberty had a much stronger response to exogenous estradiol compared to animals not exposed to BPA in utero (Fig. 4.3). The BPA-exposed mice had an increased number of TEBs, TEB area, TEB density, and ductal extension (Wadia et al. 2007). TEBs are thought to be the site where cancer arises (Russo and Russo 1996). By extrapolating the effects observed in mice to humans, they would suggest that BPA exposure during early life may increase the risk of breast cancer.

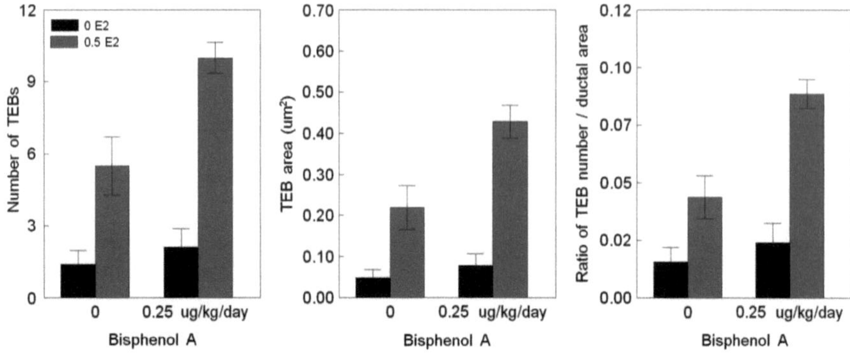

Fig. 4.3 Prenatal exposure to low dose BPA increases the sensitivity to estradiol. *TEBs* Terminal end buds

To explore the hypothesis that developmental exposure to low doses of BPA is able to induce mammary neoplasias long after the exposure ended, we used a rat model. The rat mammary gland responds to carcinogens by developing tumors that mimic the human breast disease regarding estrogen dependence and histopathology (Singh et al. 2000) more closely than the available mouse models (Nandi et al. 1995). BPA was administered at doses ranging from 2.5 to 1,000 μg/kg/day (the reference daily intake was set at 10 μg/kg/day by the European Commission and 50 μg/kg/day by the US EPA). Fetal exposure to BPA resulted in the development of carcinomas in situ in the mammary glands of 33% of the rats exposed to 250 and 1,000 μg BPA while none of the unexposed animals developed carcinomas in situ (Murray et al. 2007). Neoplasias were observed in young adult rats (50 and 95 days of age). Fetal exposure to BPA also increased the number of intraductal hyperplasias by 3- to 4-fold. Intraductal hyperplasia is a type of precancerous lesion that gives rise to mammary adenocarcinomas after transplantation into syngeneic mice (Medina 2000). The number of intraductal hyperplasias observed at 50 days of age was quantitatively similar in all the BPA doses tested, but they persisted longer in the animals exposed to the lowest dose. Moreover, prenatal exposure to 25 μg BPA/kg/day, followed by treatment of these animals at puberty with a "subcarcinogenic" dose of the chemical carcinogen *N*-nitrosomethylurea, resulted in the development of tumors only in the animals exposed to BPA in utero (Durando et al. 2007). The lesions observed in the BPA-exposed animals were highly proliferative and contained abundant ER-α positive cells (Murray et al. 2007), suggesting that the proliferative activity in these lesions may be estrogen-mediated. As mentioned previously, mammary carcinomas in rats as well as in humans are predominantly estrogen dependent, a feature that strengthens the relevance of these findings.

Similar to the results observed in the rat models, intraductal hyperplasias were observed in female mice exposed to all BPA doses (0.25, 2.5, and 25 μg BPA/kg/day) in a model of low dose exposure from gestational day 8 through lactation. The earliest precancerous lesions appeared at 3 months of age in animals exposed to the lowest dose (Vandenberg et al. 2008). These lesions were characterized by the presence of epithelial cells growing inside the ductal lumen, forming bridges between the duct's walls; the proliferation index of these cells was 5 times higher compared to normal ducts. Interestingly, epithelial cells from alveolar buds adjacent to the hyperplastic ducts also had a high proliferation index. The stroma associated with the intraductal hyperplasias showed macrophages and mast cells and it was high in fibrous collagen (Vandenberg et al. 2008).

These hyperproliferative and extensively disorganized mammary structures in both rats and mice buttress the link between perinatal exposure to BPA and the development of cancer and precancerous lesions in the adult mammary gland. Tissue architecture and homeostasis are established during development; the altered morphogenesis that occurs in the fetus during the period of BPA exposure is likely to lead to tissue disorganization and disease later in life (Vandenberg et al. 2007). Additionally, these data support the hypothesis that exposure to xenoestrogens during early development contributes to the increased incidence of breast cancer observed over the past several decades.

4.1.3 Is BPA a Carcinogen?

According to the US EPA, a carcinogen is a chemical or physical agent capable of causing cancer (http://www.epa.gov/airtoxics/nata/gloss1.html), a definition that does not specify the mechanism(s) by which the cancer is induced or the time lapse between the exposure and the diagnosis; it only identifies the consequence of an insult. Thus, by this definition BPA, like estradiol, is a carcinogen.

Due to the strong influence of the somatic mutation theory on explaining carcinogenesis during the last half a century, the term carcinogen has been used as a synonym for mutagen even though this is a very narrow definition that excludes proven carcinogens that are not mutagens (Sonnenschein and Soto 1999). BPA has failed to induce mutations in many different in vitro systems, including various *Salmonella typhimurium* strains (Andersen et al. 1975; Ashby and Tennant 1988; Schweikl et al. 1998; Masuda et al. 2005), Syrian hamster embryo cells (Tsutsui et al. 1998), and Chinese hamster V79 cells (Schweikl et al. 1998). In 2009, it was reported that exposure to very high doses of BPA (200 mg BPA/kg/day) induced DNA adducts in liver and mammary gland cells of CD1 mice dosed for 8 days (Izzotti et al. 2009). Because mutagenic effects or genotoxicity observed in vitro and/or in vivo using extraordinarily high doses does not necessarily correlate with cancer development, it is important to discuss the proposed modes of action of BPA in vivo.

There is evidence that BPA acts through ERs (Markey et al. 2001b; Vandenberg et al. 2009), that it causes modification of the DNA methylation patterns (Ho et al. 2006; Bromer et al. 2010), and that it directly perturbs tissue organization in the fetal mammary gland (Vandenberg et al. 2007). Direct effects of estrogens like BPA on the morphogenesis of their target organs are thought to be regulated through target gene expression involved in tissue patterning and in cell and tissue differentiation.

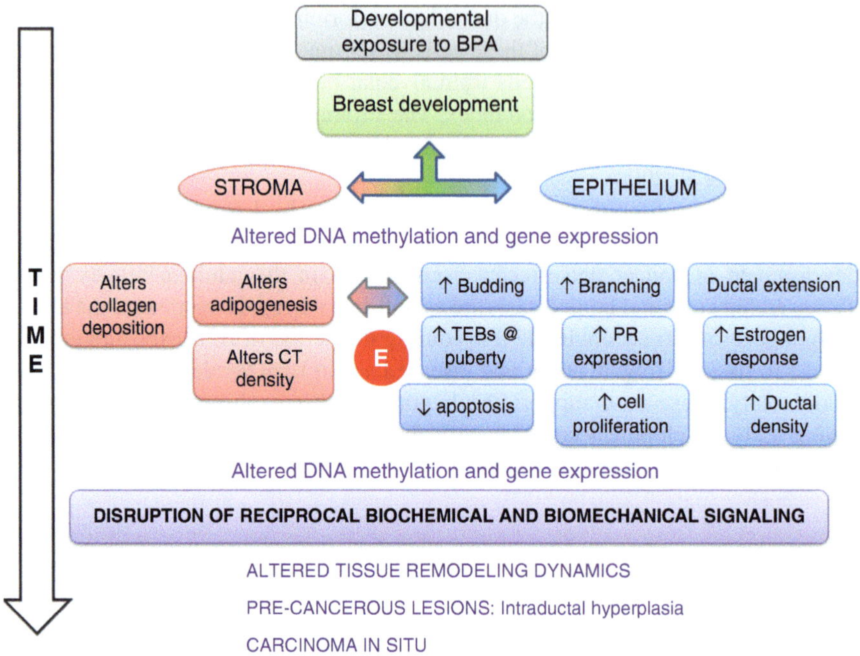

Fig. 4.4 Summary of the adverse effects observed in the mammary gland after developmental exposure to BPA. *E* Endogenous estrogens at puberty; *PR* progesterone receptor; *CT* connective tissue

For example, neonatal exposure to DES exerts an estrogenic effect in the female reproductive tract through altered expression of the Wnt7a signaling pathway (Ma and Sassoon 2006) and several Hox genes (Ma et al. 1998). Prenatal BPA exposure has also been shown to decrease DNA methylation in the promoter region and the intron of Hoxa10, a homeobox gene involved in uterine organogenesis (Bromer et al. 2010). Similarly, we have proposed that BPA alters the expression of estrogen-responsive genes normally expressed during mammary development, like msx2 and several Wnt family genes (Veltmaat et al. 2003), by acting through the ER present in the stroma of the fetal mammary gland (Murray et al. 2007; Soto and Sonnenschein 2010). Furthermore, the expression of some of these genes is regulated by estrogens in the adult mammary gland (Vandenberg et al. 2006). The untimely expression and/or repression of genes responsible for maintaining the reciprocal interactions between stroma and epithelium that mediate tissue morphogenesis and homeostasis may cause altered tissue development and ultimately neoplasia either by alteration in DNA methylation patterns or transcriptional regulation (Fig. 4.4). Additionally, remodeling of the mammary gland during each ovarian cycle may also contribute to neoplastic development; this remodeling activity is likely to be augmented due to the increased sensitivity to estradiol observed in perinatally exposed animals.

Finally BPA affects the hypothalamic-pituitary-ovarian axis by altering the estrous cyclicity of exposed individuals. This in turn may abnormally affect the development and remodeling of the mammary gland thus exacerbating the observed phenotypes of these individuals.

4.2 Conclusions

The link between fetal exposure to estrogens and the development of breast cancer that was first suggested by epidemiologists has now been confirmed as women exposed in fetal life to DES are shown to have an increased risk of developing breast cancer during adulthood. Fetal and neonatal exposures to endocrine disruptors have been shown to cause persistent alterations in the mammary glands of rodents, including pre- and neoplastic lesions, long after the exposure ended. In the case of BPA, mammary neoplasias may have their origin in the altered morphogenesis that occurs in the fetus and neonate during the period of exposure. The data obtained from laboratory animals support the hypothesis that exposure to BPA and other xenoestrogens during organogenesis may contribute to the rapid increase in the incidence of breast cancer observed over the past several decades.

References

Anbazhagan R, Bartek J, Monaghan P, Gusterson BA (1991) Growth and development of the human infant breast. Am J Anat 192:407–417

Andersen M, Kiel P, Larsen H, Maxild U (1975) Mutagenic action of arobatic epoxy resins. Nature 276:391–392

Ashby J, Tennant RW (1988) Chemical structure, *Salmonella* mutagenicity, and extent of carcinogenicity as indicators of genotoxic carcinogenesis among 222 chemicals tested in rodents by the US NCI/NTP. Mutat Res 204:17–115

Bartow SA (1998) Use of the autopsy to study ontogeny and expression of the estrogen receptor gene in human breast. J Mammary Gland Biol Neoplasia 3:37–48

Betancourt AM, Mobley JA, Russo J, Lamartiniere CA (2010) Proteomic analysis in mammary glands of rat offspring exposed in utero to bisphenol A. J Proteomics 73:1241–1253

Biles JE, McNeal TP, Begley TH, Hollifield HC (1997) Determination of bisphenol-A in reusable polycarbonate food-contact plastics and migration to food simulating liquids. J Agric Food Chem 45:3541–3544

Boylan ES, Calhoon RE (1983) Transplacental action of diethylstilbestrol on mammary carcinogenesis in female rats given one or two doses of 7,12-dimethylbenz(a)anthracene. Cancer Res 43:4879–4884

Bromer JG, Zhou Y, Taylor MB, Doherty L, Taylor HS (2010) Bisphenol-A exposure in utero leads to epigenetic alterations in the developmental programming of uterine estrogen response. FASEB J 24:2273–2280

Brotons JA, Olea-Serrano MF, Villalobos M, Olea N (1994) Xenoestrogens released from lacquer coating in food cans. Environ Health Perspect 103:608–612

Calafat AM, Kuklenyik Z, Reidy JA, Caudill SP, Ekong J, Needham JL (2005) Urinary concentrations of bisphenol A and 4-nonylphenol in a human reference population. Environ Health Perspect 113:391–395

Cohn BA, Wolff MS, Cirillo PM, Sholtz RI (2007) DDT and breast cancer in young women: new data on the significance of age at exposure. Environ Health Perspect 115:1406–1414
Cunha GR, Bigsby RM, Cooke PS, Sugimura Y (1985) Stromal-epithelial interactions in adult organs. Cell Differ 17:137–148
Durando M, Kass L, Piva J, Sonnenschein C, Soto AM, Luque EH, Munoz de Toro MM (2007) Prenatal bisphenol A exposure induces preneoplastic lesions in the mammary gland in Wistar rats. Environ Health Perspect 115:80–86
Fenton SE, Hamm JT, Birnbaum L, Youngblood GL (2002) Persistent abnormalities in the rat mammary gland following gestational and lactational exposure to 2,3,7,8-tetrachlorodibenzo-p-dioxin (TCDD). Toxicol Sci 67:63–74
Fenton SE, Rudel RA (2010) A multi-laboratory round robin comparison of mammary gland whole mounts contributes to protocol standardization. Society of Toxicology Annual Meeting Abstract #2372
Ho S-M, Tang WY, Belmonte de Frausto J, Prins GS (2006) Developmental exposure to estradiol and bisphenol a increases susceptibility to prostate carcinogenesis and epigenetically regulates phosphodiesterase type 4 variant 4. Cancer Res 66:5624–5632
Humphreys RC, Krajewska M, Krnacik S, Jæger R, Weiher H, Krajewski S, Reed JC, Rosen JM (1996) Apoptosis in the terminal end bud of the murine mammary gland: a mechanism of ductal morphogenesis. Development 122:4013–4022
Izzotti A, Kanitz S, D'Agostini F, Camoirano A, De Flora S (2009) Formation of adducts by bisphenol A, an endocrine disruptor, in DNA *in vitro* and in liver and mammary tissue of mice. Mutat Res 679:28–32
Keeling JW, Özer E, King G, Walker F (2000) Oestrogen receptor alpha in female fetal, infant, and child mammary tissue. J Pathol 191:449–451
Lemmen JG, Broekhof JLM, Kuiper GGJM, Gustafsson JA, Van Der Saag PT, van der Burg B (1999) Expression of estrogen receptor alpha and beta during mouse embryogenesis. Mech Dev 81:163–167
Ma L, Benson GV, Lim H, Dey SK, Maas RL (1998) Abdominal B (AbdB) Hoxa genes: regulation in adult uterus by estrogen and progesterone and repression in mullerian duct by the synthetic estrogen diethylstilbestrol (DES). Dev Biol 197:141–154
Ma R, Sassoon DA (2006) PCBs exert an estrogenic effect through repression of the Wnt7a signaling pathway in the female reproductive tract. Environ Health Perspect 114:898–904
Maffini MV, Sonnenschein C, Soto AM (2010) Breast. In: Woodruff TJ, Janssen SJ, Guillette LJ Jr, Giudice LC (eds) Environmental impacts on reproductive health and fertility. Cambridge University Press, Cambridge
Markey CM, Luque EH, Munoz de Toro MM, Sonnenschein C, Soto AM (2001a) *In utero* exposure to bisphenol A alters the development and tissue organization of the mouse mammary gland. Biol Reprod 65:1215–1223
Markey CM, Michaelson CL, Sonnenschein C, Soto AM (2001b) Alkylphenols and bisphenol A as environmental estrogens. In: Metzler M (ed) The handbook of environmental chemistry, vol 3, part L, Endocrine disruptors – part I. Springer, Berlin
Markey CM, Rubin BS, Soto AM, Sonnenschein C (2003) Endocrine disruptors from Wingspread to environmental developmental biology. J Steroid Biochem Mol Biol 83:235–244
Masuda S, Terashima Y, Sano A, Kuruto R, Sugiyama Y, Shimoi K, Tanji K, Yoshioka H, Terao Y, Kinae N (2005) Changes in the mutagenic and estrogenic activities of bisphenol A upon treatment with nitrite. Mutat Res 585:137–146
Medina D (2000) The preneoplastic phenotype in murine mammary tumorigenesis. J Mammary Gland Biol Neoplasia 5:393–407
Moral R, Wang R, Russo IH, Lamartiniere CA, Pereira J, Russo J (2008) Effect of prenatal exposure to the endocrine disruptor bisphenol A on mammary gland morphology and gene expression signature. J Endocrinol 196:101–112
Munoz de Toro MM, Markey CM, Wadia PR, Luque EH, Rubin BS, Sonnenschein C, Soto AM (2005) Perinatal exposure to bisphenol A alters peripubertal mammary gland development in mice. Endocrinology 146:4138–4147

Murray TJ, Maffini MV, Ucci AA, Sonnenschein C, Soto AM (2007) Induction of mammary gland ductal hyperplasias and carcinoma in situ following fetal bisphenol A exposure. Reprod Toxicol 23:383–390
Myers JP, vom Saal FS, Akingbemi BT et al (2009) Why public health agencies cannot depend on good laboratory practices as a criterion for selecting data: the case of bisphenol A. Environ Health Perspect 117:309–315
Nandi S, Guzman R, Yang J (1995) Hormones and mammary carcinogenesis in mice, rats, and humans: a unifying hypothesis. Proc Natl Acad Sci U S A 92:3650–3657
Narbaitz R, Stumpf WE, Sar M (1980) Estrogen receptors in the mammary gland primordia of fetal mouse. Anat Embryol 158:161–166
Nikaido Y, Yoshizawa K, Danbara N, Tsujita-Kyutoku M, Yuri T, Uehara N, Tsubura A (2004) Effects of maternal xenoestrogen exposure on development of the reproductive tract and mammary gland in female CD-1 mouse offspring. Reprod Toxicol 18:803–811
National Toxicology Program (2008) NTP-CERHR monograph on the potential human reproductive and developmental effects of Bisphenol A. http://cerhr.niehs.nih.gov/evals/bisphenol/bisphenol.pdf
Olea N, Pulgar R, Perez P, Olea-Serrano F, Rivas A, Novillo-Fertrell A, Pedraza V, Soto AM, Sonnenschein C (1996) Estrogenicity of resin-based composites and sealants used in dentistry. Environ Health Perspect 104:298–305
Palmer JR, Wise LA, Hatch EE, Troisi R, Titus-Ernstoff L, Strohsnitter W, Kaufman R, Herbst AL, Noller KL, Hyer M, Hoover RN (2006) Prenatal diethylstilbestrol exposure and risk of breast cancer. Cancer Epidemiol Biomarkers Prev 15:1509–1514
Potischman N, Troisi R (1999) In-utero and early life exposures in relation to risk of breast cancer. Cancer Causes Control 10:561–573
Rayner JL, Enoch RR, Fenton SE (2005) Adverse effects of prenatal exposure to atrazine during a critical period of mammary gland growth. Toxicol Sci 87:255–266
Robinson GW, Karpf ABC, Kratochwil K (1999) Regulation of mammary gland development by tissue interaction. J Mammary Gland Biol Neoplasia 4:9–19
Rosen PP (2008) Anatomy and physiologic morphology. In: Rosen's breast pathology. Lippincott, Williams, and Wilkins, New York
Rudel RA, Euling SY, Makris SL, Fenton SE (2010) Mammary gland development as a sensitive indicator of early life exposures: recommendations from an interdisciplinary workshop. Society of Toxicology Annual Meeting Abstract #2404
Russo IH, Russo J (1996) Mammary gland neoplasia in long-term rodent studies. Environ Health Perspect 104:938–967
Saji S, Jensen EV, Nilsson S, Rylander T, Warner M, Gustafsson J-A (2000) Estrogen receptors a and b in the rodent mammary gland. Proc Natl Acad Sci U S A 97:337–342
Schweikl H, Schmalz G, Rackebrandt K (1998) The mutagenic activity of unpolymerized resin monomers in *Salmonella typhimurium* and V79 cells. Mutat Res 415:119–130
Shyamala G, Chou Y-C, Louie SG, Guzman RC, Smith GH, Nandi S (2002) Cellular expression of estrogen and progesterone receptors in mammary glands: regulation by hormones, development and aging. J Steroid Biochem Mol Biol 80:137–148
Singh M, McGinley JN, Thompson HJ (2000) A comparison of the histopathology of premalignant and malignant mammary gland lesions induced in sexually immature rats with those occurring in the human. Lab Invest 80:221–231
Sonnenschein C, Soto AM (1999) The enormous complexity of cancer. In: The society of cells: cancer and control of cell proliferation. Springer, New York
Soto AM, Sonnenschein C (2010) Environmental causes of cancer: endocrine disruptors as carcinogens. Nat Rev Endocrinol 6:363–370
Tomooka Y, Bern HA (1982) Growth of mouse mammary glands after neonatal sex hormone treatment. J Natl Cancer Inst 69:1347–1352
Trichopoulos D (1990) Is breast cancer initiated *in utero*? Epidemiology 1:95–96
Tsutsui T, Tamura Y, Yagi E, Hasegawa K, Takahashi M, Maizumi N, Yamaguchi F, Barrett JC (1998) Bisphenol-A induces cellular transformation, aneuploidy and DNA adduct formation in cultured Syrian hamster embryo cells. Int J Cancer 75:290–294

Tyl RW, Myers CB, Marr MC, Sloan CS, Castillo NP, Veselica MM, Seely JC, Dimond SS, Van Miller JP, Shiotsuka RN, Beyer D, Hentges SG, Waechter JM Jr (2008) Two-generation reproductive toxicity study of dietary bisphenol A in CD-1 (Swiss) mice. Toxicol Sci 104:362–384

Vandenberg LN, Chahoud I, Heindel JJ, Padmanabhan V, Paumgartten FJ, Schoenfelder G (2010) Urinary, circulating and tissue biomonitoring studies indicate widespread exposure to bisphenol A. Environ Health Perspect 118:1055–1070

Vandenberg LN, Maffini MV, Schaeberle CM, Ucci AA, Sonnenschein C, Rubin BS, Soto AM (2008) Perinatal exposure to the xenoestrogen bisphenol-A induces mammary intraductal hyperplasias in adult CD-1 mice. Reprod Toxicol 3–4:210–219

Vandenberg LN, Maffini MV, Sonnenschein C, Rubin BS, Soto AM (2009) Bisphenol-A and the great divide: a review of controversies in the field of endocrine disruption. Endocr Rev 30:75–95

Vandenberg LN, Maffini MV, Wadia PR, Sonnenschein C, Rubin BS, Soto AM (2007) Exposure to the xenoestrogen bisphenol-A alters development of the fetal mammary gland. Endocrinology 148:116–127

Vandenberg LN, Wadia PR, Schaeberle CM, Rubin BS, Sonnenschein C, Soto AM (2006) The mammary gland response to estradiol: monotonic at the cellular level, non-monotonic at the tissue-level of organization? J Steroid Biochem Mol Biol 101:263–274

Veltmaat JM, Mailleux AA, Thiery JP, Bellusci S (2003) Mouse embryonic mammogenesis as a model for the molecular regulation of pattern formation. Differentiation 71:1–17

Wadia PR, Vandenberg LN, Schaeberle CM, Rubin BS, Sonnenschein C, Soto AM (2007) Perinatal bisphenol-A exposure increases estrogen sensitivity of the mammary gland in diverse mouse strains. Environ Health Perspect 115:592–598

Warner M, Eskenazi B, Mocarelli P, Gerthoux PM, Samuels S, Needham L, Patterson D, Brambilla P (2002) Serum dioxin concentrations and breast cancer risk in the Seveso Women's Health Study. Environ Health Perspect 110:625–628

Weihua Z, Saji S, Makinen S, Cheng G, Jensen EV, Warner M, Gustafsson J-A (2000) Estrogen receptor (ER) beta, a modulator of ER alpha in the uterus. Proc Natl Acad Sci U S A 97:5936–5941

White SS, Calafat AM, Kuklenyik Z, Villanueva L, Zehr RD, Helfant L, Strynar MJ, Lindstrom AB, Thibodeaux JR, Wood C, Fenton SE (2007) Gestational PFOA exposure of mice is associated with altered mammary gland development in dams and female offspring. Toxicol Sci 96:133–144

Chapter 5
Endocrine Disruptors Affect the Genomic Profile of the Rat Mammary Gland at Different Developmental Stages

Ricardo López de Cicco, Julia Santucci-Pereira, Raquel Moral, Suraj Peri, Michael Slifker, Irma H. Russo, Patrícia A. Russo, Richard Wang, and Jose Russo

Abstract Bisphenol A (BPA), *n*-butyl benzyl phthalate (BBP), and 2,3,7,8-tetrachlorodibenzo-*p*-dioxin (TCDD) are endocrine disruptors that are widely present in the environment. Exposure to these compounds, at different stages of life (prenatal, prepubertal) and dose levels (low, high), affects the global gene expression profile of the rat mammary gland at different ages. Each compound has a specific action on the gene expression of the mammary gland. Moreover, the changes observed also vary with dose administered, stage of life at the time of exposure, and the age studied. It was observed that transcription and DNA-related genes, including estrogen and DNA damage response signaling pathways and developmental genes, were mainly affected upon BPA action. TCDD had the greatest effect on the tumor suppressor genes. Several genes related to the lipid metabolism were regulated by BBP and TCDD treatments, but not by BPA. Immune-related genes were modulated by TCDD at several conditions and were suppressed by BBP in early puberty. Our data demonstrate that each endocrine disruptor induces a set of specific changes in the mammary gland, leading to different biological responses.

Keywords Endocrine disruptors • Mammary cancer • Tumorigenesis • DMBA • Microarrays

5.1 Introduction

The breast is intrinsically a hormone-responsive organ. During its development and throughout the adult life, it is influenced by several hormones and growth factors that account for its degree of differentiation, proliferation, and regression

J. Russo (✉)
Breast Cancer Research Laboratory, Breast Cancer and the Environment Research Center, Fox Chase Cancer Center, 333 Cottman Avenue, Philadelphia, PA 19111, USA
e-mail: jose.russo@fccc.edu

J. Russo (ed.), *Environment and Breast Cancer*, DOI 10.1007/978-1-4419-9896-5_5,

(Russo and Russo 1996, 1998). As a consequence, the breast tissue architecture, behavior, and physiology are modified either temporarily or permanently. Estrogens have an important effect on the breast. It is well known that estrogens are associated with enhanced proliferation of normal and neoplastic breast tissue. Estrogens act locally on the mammary gland, stimulating DNA synthesis and promoting bud formation. This standard paradigm provides a general mechanistic explanation for the association of chronic exposure to high levels of estrogen and breast cancer risk. Proliferating cells are susceptible to genetic errors during DNA replication that, if uncorrected, can ultimately lead to a malignant phenotype. Xenoestrogens are synthetic chemicals that are structurally similar and act as endogenous estrogen and are found in the environment with the ability to bind to estrogen receptors and mimic its actions.

The effect that estrogenic compounds can have on cancer susceptibility depends on the timing of environmental exposure (Shellabarger and Soo 1973; Nagasawa et al. 1974; Boylan and Calhoon 1979; Lamartiniere 2002). Several lines of evidence in both humans and animal models suggest that in utero exposure to an estrogenic environment increases breast cancer risk later in life (Hilakivi-Clarke et al. 2001; Birnbaum and Fenton 2003). Unfortunately, the US Environmental Protection Agency (US EPA) does not regularly evaluate the safety and risks associated with all existing or new chemicals that are released in the domestic market (Guerrero 1994). Herein, we will discuss the impact that three endocrine disruptors – Bisphenol A (BPA), butyl benzyl phthalate (BBP), and 2,3,7,8 tetrachlorodibenzo-*p*-dioxin (TCDD) – have on the genomic profile of the rat mammary gland.

5.1.1 Bisphenol A

BPA is used in the manufacture of polycarbonate plastics and epoxy resins that are found in a wide variety of common products including reusable food and drink containers, baby bottles, protective liners in metal canned foods and beverages, dental composites and sealants, and many other products (Welshons et al. 2006). A large number of in vivo studies have reported adverse effects concerning low-dose exposures to BPA, even below the current reference dose (Welshons et al. 2006). This compound has been found in 95% of urinary samples in a human reference population in the USA (Calafat et al. 2005), in maternal and fetal plasma, in placental tissue at birth (Ikezuki et al. 2002) and in human colostrum (Kuruto-Niwa et al. 2007). Experimental animal models have shown BPA to have an estrogenic effect, and thus an endocrine-disrupting action that may influence tumor development later in life (Birnbaum and Fenton 2003). Prenatal exposure to BPA has been associated with hormonal, morphological, functional, and behavioral anomalies related to reproduction (Adriani et al. 2003), including alterations in the testosterone levels at birth in rats (Tanaka et al. 2006), in the male and female genital tract (Maffini et al. 2006), and in the tissue organization of the rat and mouse mammary gland (Markey et al. 2001; Munoz-de-Toro et al. 2005). Of special interest, recent data have suggested BPA has an effect on mammary transformation (Durando et al. 2007; Murray et al. 2007). Markey et al. (2001) reported a significant increase in the number of ductal and alveolar structures in mice exposed in utero to BPA relative to the control group. Studies in our laboratory showed that prenatal BPA exposure via the dams produced modifications of the mammary gland, mainly in the number of undifferentiated epithelial structures (Moral et al. 2008). Of great relevance is the study carried out by Betancourt et al. (2010) in which they demonstrated that oral prenatal exposure to BPA increases mammary susceptibility in rat offspring and shifts the window of susceptibility for DMBA-induced tumorigenesis. These data indicate possible BPA exposure and accumulation in pregnant women and fetuses, and significant exposure during the prenatal period. Although it is difficult to determine the precise dose of exposure for experimental studies, the doses chosen in our studies (25 and 250 μg BPA/kg body weight (BW) to pregnant rats) were based on reported human exposures, experimental studies in rats, and the US EPA maximum acceptable dose. Within the USA, an exposure of up to 50 μg/kg/day (50 ppb) is considered safe by the US EPA. Based on published pharmacodynamics and distribution data of radioactively labeled BPA, less than 0.01% of the dose administered to the lactating dam would be observed in the offspring carcasses (Snyder et al. 2000). Hence, the offspring are exposed to approximately 10,000-fold less BPA than the dose administered to the dam. Thus, each offspring is exposed to approximately 2.5 ng BPA/kg BW/day at the higher dose, both of which are well below human exposure levels.

5.1.2 Butyl Benzyl Phthalate

BBP is a compound added to polymers such as polyvinyl chloride (PVC) to increase flexibility and softness and is commonly used in pipes, vinyl floor tiles, vinyl foams, and carpet backing, and to a minor extent, in cellulose plastics and polyurethane. It has been estimated that adult BBP intake is 2 μg/kg BW/day and that BBP exposure in infants and children could be up to threefold higher (IPCS 1999). Several animal studies have been carried out in the last decade. It is well accepted that BBP exposure is responsible for developmental and testicular toxicity as well as malformations and embryonic deaths in mice and in rats (Ema et al. 1992a, b, 2003; Gray et al. 2000; Piersma et al. 2000; Agas et al. 2007). More importantly, Swan et al. (2005) have shown that prenatal phthalate exposure at environmental levels can adversely affect male reproductive development in humans. In females, BBP is suggested to have an etiological association with endometriosis (Reddy et al. 2006). A decrease in the weight of the ovaries in females exposed during adulthood, as well as changes in the offspring of exposed rats, including a decrease of BW of males and females at birth, and an increase in the anogenital distance in females have also been reported. Data published by Moral et al. (2007) strongly suggest that BBP has an effect on the gene expression profile of the mammary gland. Although the risks of BBP exposure to human health are controversial, BBP has been banned from toys and child care items by the European Commission (European Commission 2005).

5.1.3 2,3,7,8-Tetrachlorodibenzo-p-Dioxin

TCDD is a member of the chlorinated dioxins and very common in the environment (US Department of Health and Human Services 2005). The main form of TCDD production is through the combustion of organic material in the presence of chlorinated products. The principal route of TCDD exposure is through ingestion of contaminated food, especially foods rich in animal fat (Committee on the Implications of Dioxin in the Food Supply 2003; U.S. Department of Health and Human Services 2005). TCDD has a long half-life of 5–10 years in human beings as a result of its high affinity to fat. Studies have shown that fetuses can be exposed to dioxin through the placenta, and infants are exposed through lactation. In the USA, it is estimated that in the first year of life breast-fed infants are exposed to 35–53 pg/kg BW/day of TCDD equivalents through their mother's milk (U.S. Department of Health and Human Services 2005). TCDD has antiestrogenic effects and is classified as an environmental endocrine disruptor. It causes simple biochemistry alterations, as well as extremely toxic responses, including death. Some of the TCDD hazards to health include immune suppression, gonadal atrophy, chloracne, hepatotoxicity, neurotoxicity, cardiotoxicity, alterations in growth and endocrine factors, teratogenesis and in 1997, the International Agency for Research on Cancer (IARC) classified TCDD as a group 1 carcinogenic compound (IARC 1997). Using a carcinogen induced rat mammary cancer model, Jenkins et al. (2007) have shown that prenatal exposure to TCDD alters mammary gland differentiation and increases susceptibility for mammary cancer. The same group also found that prenatal TCDD treatment resulted in an increased number of chemically induced mammary adenocarcinomas in rats. This susceptibility to mammary cancer from prenatal exposure to TCDD is related to an alteration to mammary gland differentiation. TCDD also delayed time of vaginal opening and caused disruption to the estrous cycle (Brown et al. 1998). It has also been shown that gestational and lactational exposure to TCDD, prior to migration of the mammary bud into the fat pad, permanently alters mammary epithelial development in female rat offspring (Fenton et al. 2002). As an endocrine disruptor, TCDD exposure also has an adverse effect on the male reproductive system. Indeed, Gray et al. have reported changes in the rat male reproductive system after TCDD exposure (Gray and Ostby 1995). Recently, Ding et al. (Ding et al. 2011) reported that developmental exposure of either parent to TCDD is associated with preterm birth in a subsequent adult pregnancy due to altered progesterone receptor expression and placental inflammation. Moreover, the uterine phenotype of toxicant-exposed mice is markedly similar to the endometrial phenotype of women with endometriosis (Nayyar et al. 2007).

It is well described that TCDD binds with high affinity to the cytosolic aromatic hydrocarbon receptor (AhR) (Safe 1995). The newly formed and active TCDD–AhR complex translocates to the nucleus where it binds with the aromatic hydrocarbon receptor nuclear translocator (ARNT). In the nucleus, this heterodimer acts as a nuclear transcription factor, binding to dioxin-responsive elements (DRE) and altering specific gene transcription. While the majority of the observed toxic effects of TCDD are thought to be mediated through the activated AhR, the exact mechanisms are presently unknown. In humans, epidemiological and occupational studies have failed to provide a consistent link between TCDD exposure and the occurrence of breast cancer. In 1976, an accident in a plant near Seveso, Italy, exposed the local population to TCDD. Interestingly, Bertazzi et al. (1993) found lower incidence of breast cancer than expected in the most contaminated zones. Nonetheless, studies performed 25 years after the dioxin catastrophe revealed human milk from mothers in Seveso had high levels of TCDD. This means that breast-fed infants in Seveso still store an appreciable amount of TCDD in their body fat (Weiss et al. 2003). Another epidemiological study was carried out in Chapaevsk, Russia, where The Middle Volga chemical plant produced hexachlorocyclohexane for 20 years. High levels of TCDD were found in the air, soil, drinking water, and in cow's milk. In contrast to the Seveso case, in a study based on the population of the Chapaevsk region, an increased incidence of breast cancer was observed (Revich et al. 2001). This finding was coupled by increased incidences in reproductive difficulties, congenital morphogenetic conditions in children, and spontaneous abortions (Revich et al. 2001). Nonetheless, a meta-analysis of the literature on occupational exposure to TCDD did not yield a statistically different rate ratio of breast cancer incidence between exposed and unexposed women (Adami et al. 1995).

5.2 The Experimental Model

The rat mammary carcinogenesis model is one of the most widely used surrogate models because it closely mimics the human disease. In rats, tumors can be chemically induced by the administration of dimethylbenz[*a*]anthracene (Russo and Russo 1996). It has long been suggested that the sensitivity of the mammary gland to neoplastic transformation depends on the stage of mammary gland differentiation at the time of carcinogenic stimuli (Russo and Russo 1996). To model human exposure in laboratory rats and test the effects on the mammary gland, Russo and Lamartiniere used 8-week-old female Sprague–Dawley CD rats fed on phytoestrogen-free diet.

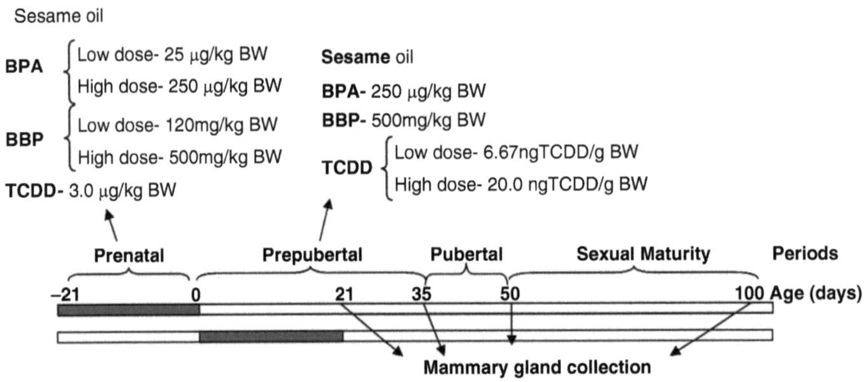

Fig. 5.1 Experimental model: 8-week-old female Sprague–Dawley CD rats were exposed for 21 days to three different compounds (bisphenol A (BPA), butyl benzyl phthalate (BBP), 2,3,7,8 tetrachlorodibenzo-*p*-dioxin (TCDD)), at different stages of development, either prenatally or prepubertally. At 21, 35, 50 and 100 days of age female offspring were sacrificed and mammary gland was collected for morphologic and genomic analysis

The female rats were exposed to three different compounds (BPA, BBP and TCDD) at different stages of development – prenatally or prepubertally (Fig. 5.1). This model allows us to determine whether the exposure to these pollutants at different times during development has a negative impact on mammary gland development and/or its transcriptome.

For prenatal BPA exposure, pregnant female rats were gavaged with 25 and 250 μg BPA/kg BW or an equivalent volume of sesame oil on days 10–21 postconception. For neonatal and prepubertal exposure, lactating dams were gavaged with 250 μg BPA/kg BW or an equivalent volume of sesame oil on days 1–21 postdelivery.

For prenatal BBP exposure, the pregnant female rats received 120 and 500 mg BBP/kg BW or an equivalent volume of the vehicle on days 10–21 postconception. For the BBP prepubertal exposure, the lactating dams received 500 mg BBP/kg BW or an equivalent volume of sesame oil until offspring weaning.

For prenatal TCDD exposure, the pregnant female rats received by gavage a single dose of 3 μg TCDD/kg BW or vehicle on the 15th day of pregnancy. For TCDD prepubertal treatment, the nursing dams were gavaged with 6.67 ng TCDD/g BW, 20 ng TCDD/g, or equivalent volume of sesame oil on days 14 and 17 postconception.

For any treatment, female offspring were weaned at 21 days of age; females were euthanized at 21, 35 ± 1, 50 ± 1, and 100 ± 2 days. For the latter three ages, all females were sacrificed in the estrous phase of estrus; the fourth mammary glands were rapidly dissected and processed for microarray analysis.

5.3 Genomic Analysis of Mammary Glands of Rats Prenatally or Prepubertally Exposed to BPA, BBP, or TCDD Showed That Each Compound Has a Unique Signature That Affects Multiple Genes Relevant to Development and Carcinogenesis

The complete set of RNA transcripts produced by the genome at any one time is called a transcriptome. The transcriptome is dynamic and changes under different circumstances due to different patterns of gene expression. An in-depth knowledge of the changes in the transcriptome due to exposure to any of these compounds is crucial in predicting their possible effects on the mammary gland. The profile of mRNA expression is what is called genomic signature.

For every available combination of compound (BPA, BBP, TCDD), exposure stage (prenatal, prepubertal), dose level (low, high), and age (21, 35, 50, 100), a test of differential expression (relative to untreated age-matched control pool samples) was performed. The resulting lists of genes were tested for overrepresentation in Gene Ontology (GO) terms representing biological processes (BP). The analysis shows that each compound renders a unique signature, or transcriptome, to the mammary gland that affects multiple genes relevant to development and carcinogenesis (Fig. 5.2). These pivotal findings are summarized as follows: (1) The genomic signature in the mammary gland is compound specific (each compound induces a different transcriptome). (2) The transcriptome is determined by the developmental period at the time of exposure, which in turn controls the route of exposure and dose received (i.e., placental circulation in prenatal, oral ingestion in lactation). (3) The effect of prenatal and prepubertal exposures on the mammary gland transcriptome is manifested at different stages of postnatal/postpubertal development of the mammary gland, i.e., prenatal exposure to BPA and BBP induces major transcriptional changes at puberty (35 days of age), whereas TCDD exerts its major transcriptional effect later in the rat life (100 days). (4) The diverse genomic signatures imprinted by these compounds in the mammary gland suggest a differential risk for mammary cancer. The most important discovery from these studies is that each of the compounds, BPA, BBP, and TCDD, defines specific genomic signatures that modulate specific biological process through different pathways and gene interactions.

The most relevant groups of genes related to important biological processes modulated by these compounds are oncogenes, tumor suppressor genes, DNA damage response and repair genes, immunity and inflammation genes, and fatty acid and lipid metabolism genes. To illustrate the specificity of the changes in the transcriptome due to these compounds, immune-related genes are highly dysregulated at 35 days in animals exposed to BPA prenatally. TCDD has a greater effect on the dysregulation of tumor suppressor genes as compared to the other two compounds. Changes in the pattern of fat metabolism-related genes are more evident after TCDD and BBP treatment; BPA does not seem to affect lipid metabolism homeostasis. Also, changes were observed at the proteomic level. Prenatal TCDD exposure can

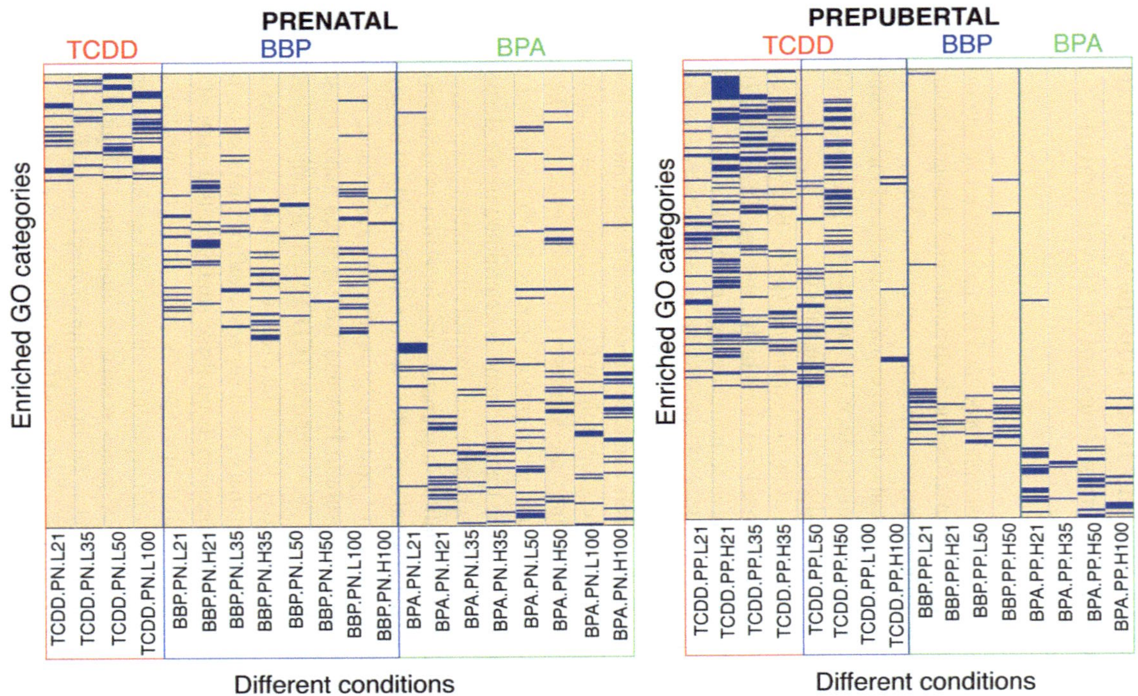

Fig. 5.2 Distribution of enriched GO terms in prenatally or prepubertally exposed animals with every available combination of compound (BPA, BBP, TCDD), dose level (low, high), and age (21, 35, 50, 100 days). *Blue* indicates that specific GO terms (*rows*) were overrepresented among genes differentially expressed at specific conditions (*columns*). Little overlap of GOs was observed for the three compounds, emphasizing that each compound induces a specific genomic signature

predispose for mammary cancer susceptibility in the adult offspring by altering the mammary proteome. Jenkins et al. (2007) have shown seven proteins to be differentially regulated, including a decrease in superoxide dismutase 1 (SOD1). Downregulation of SOD1 could provide an environment ill equipped to deal with subsequent free radical exposure. Also, protein expression in mammary glands of 50-day-old rats exposed prepubertally to BPA was different than that of age-matched control rats. Using Western blot analysis, steroid receptor coactivators (SRCs) 1–3, Akt, phospho-Akt, progesterone receptor A (PR-A), and erbB3 proteins were significantly upregulated at 50 days of age (Jenkins et al. 2009).

5.3.1 Endocrine Disruptors Affect the Expression of Fatty Acid and Lipid Metabolism Genes in the Rat Mammary Gland at Different Developmental Stages

Gene expression analysis of the mammary gland of rats exposed to BPA, BBP and TCDD has shown a large number of fatty acid and lipid metabolism genes modulated by these endocrine disruptors. Each compound has its own effect depending on the developmental stage of exposure, and TCDD was responsible for most changes observed in this class of genes (Fig. 5.3). The effects of BPA and BBP depend on the dose and the age of the animals at the time the mammary glands were studied, while TCDD shows a more consistent effect on this group of genes. Dysregulation in the expression of 28 genes was common for the three compounds (Fig. 5.4); in addition, we observed another 33 genes commonly modulated by BBP and TCDD. Few genes were exclusively modulated by BBP or BPA; however, TCDD dysregulated the expression of 21 genes not affected by BBP nor BPA (Fig. 5.4).

TCDD-exposed mammary glands showed the most dramatic change in the expression of genes related to fatty acid and lipid metabolism (Figs. 5.3 and 5.5). Known effects of TCDD are weight loss caused by alteration in the fatty acid, carbohydrates, and lipid metabolism (Gorski et al. 1988; Weber et al. 1991a, b) and alteration in the insulin levels in the serum (Ebner et al. 1988). Our gene analysis identified several alterations caused by TCDD in this group of genes. The prenatal exposure to TCDD resulted in the modulation of 12 in the younger ages and 45 genes in the 100-day-old group rats. The prepubertal treatment affected a larger number of genes, mainly the higher dose, which induced changes in the expression of around 50 genes in 21-, 35-, and 50-day-old animals, but showed no effect in 100-day-old animals (Fig. 5.5). The most drastic effect in terms of gene expression was observed at 35 days, independent of exposure dose. Noteworthy is the expression behavior of a group of genes that increased as the rats grew older. While downregulated at 21 days, their expression was increased at 35 or 50 days of age (Fig. 5.6). Elovl6 (ELOVL family member 6, elongation of long chain fatty acids), one of the most dysregulated genes, encodes an enzyme that catalyzes the elongation of saturated and monounsaturated fatty acids, and can modulate the insulin resistance (Matsuzaka and Shimano 2009). Other genes – also involved in insulin sensibility – are Fasn

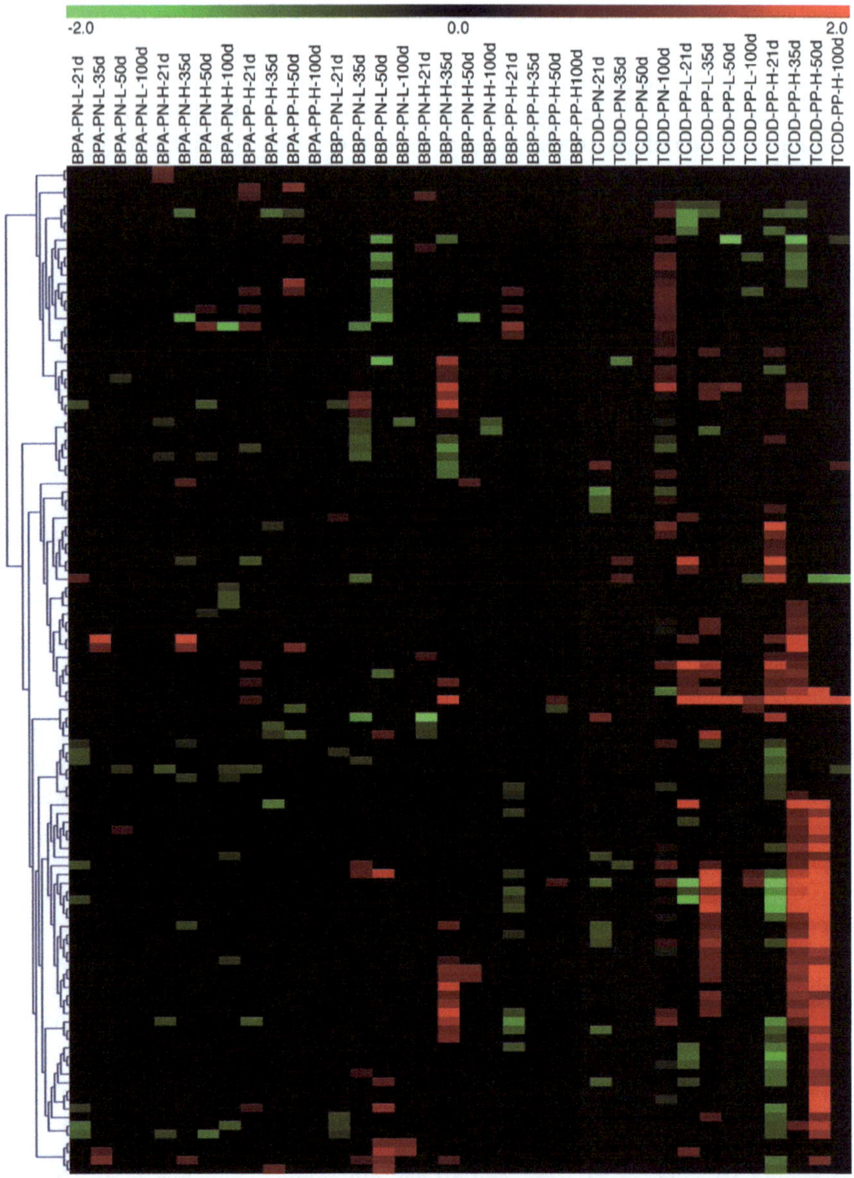

Fig. 5.3 Heatmap of fatty acid and lipid metabolism-related genes that were dysregulated by prenatal or prepubertal BPA, BBP, or TCDD exposure. *Red squares* represent upregulated genes, *green squares* represent downregulated genes and *black* represents no change in expression. As it can be seen in the figure, TCDD exposure resulted in the most drastic effect on gene expression

(fatty acid synthase), Insig 1 (insulin-induced gene 1), Slc25a10 (solute carrier family 25, mitochondrial carrier, dicarboxylate transporter, member 10), while Pparg (peroxisome proliferator-activated receptor gamma), Gcgr (glucagon receptor), and Gpam (glycerol-3-phosphate acyltransferase, mitochondrial) are related to glucose

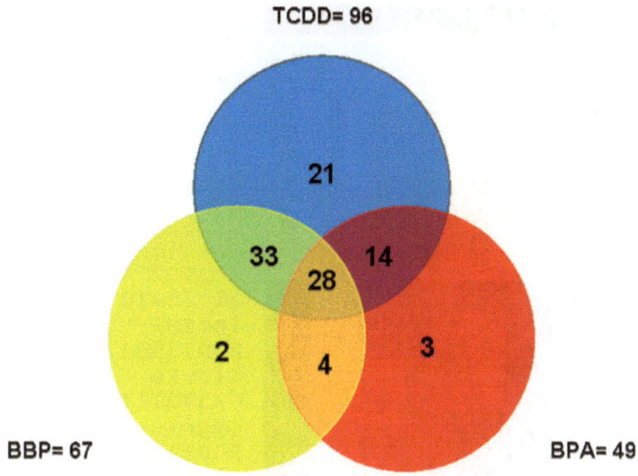

Fig. 5.4 Venn diagram showing the number of genes related to fatty acid and lipid metabolism modulated by each compound. Twenty-eight genes were found to be commonly modulated by BPA, BBP, and TCDD

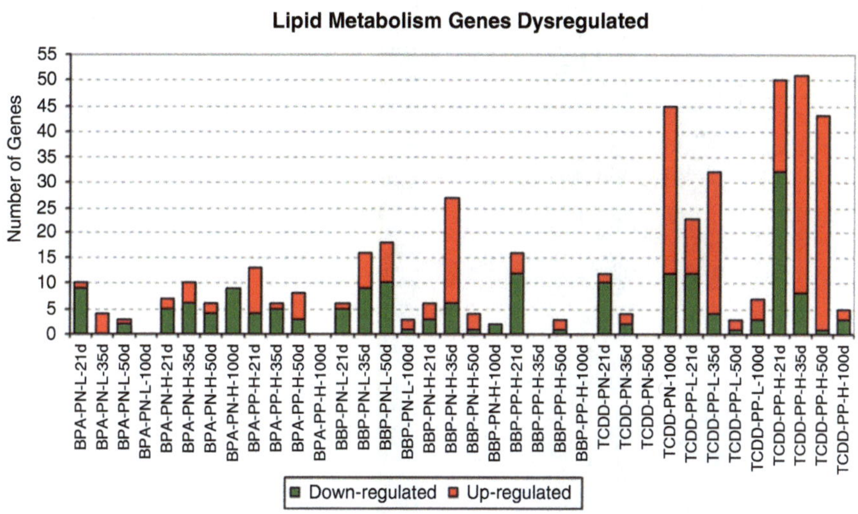

Fig. 5.5 Histogram shows the number of upregulated (*red*) and down-regulated (*green*) genes related to fatty acid and lipid metabolism modulated at each condition after prenatal or prepubertal exposure to BPA, BBP, or TCDD. The more extensive effect on the expression of fatty acid and lipid metabolism genes was observed after prepubertal exposure to high dose of TCDD

tolerance. Correlation between TCDD exposure and increased incidence of diabetes has been demonstrated in veterans exposed to Agent Orange. Indeed, high levels of TCDD in blood can promote insulin resistance (Kern et al. 2004).

The effect of BBP in genes related to fatty acids and lipid metabolism was smaller than those exerted by TCDD. Most of the genes dysregulated by BBP were specific for each condition; thus, there were few changes in the expression of genes among different doses, times of exposure, and ages studied. A larger numbers of genes were

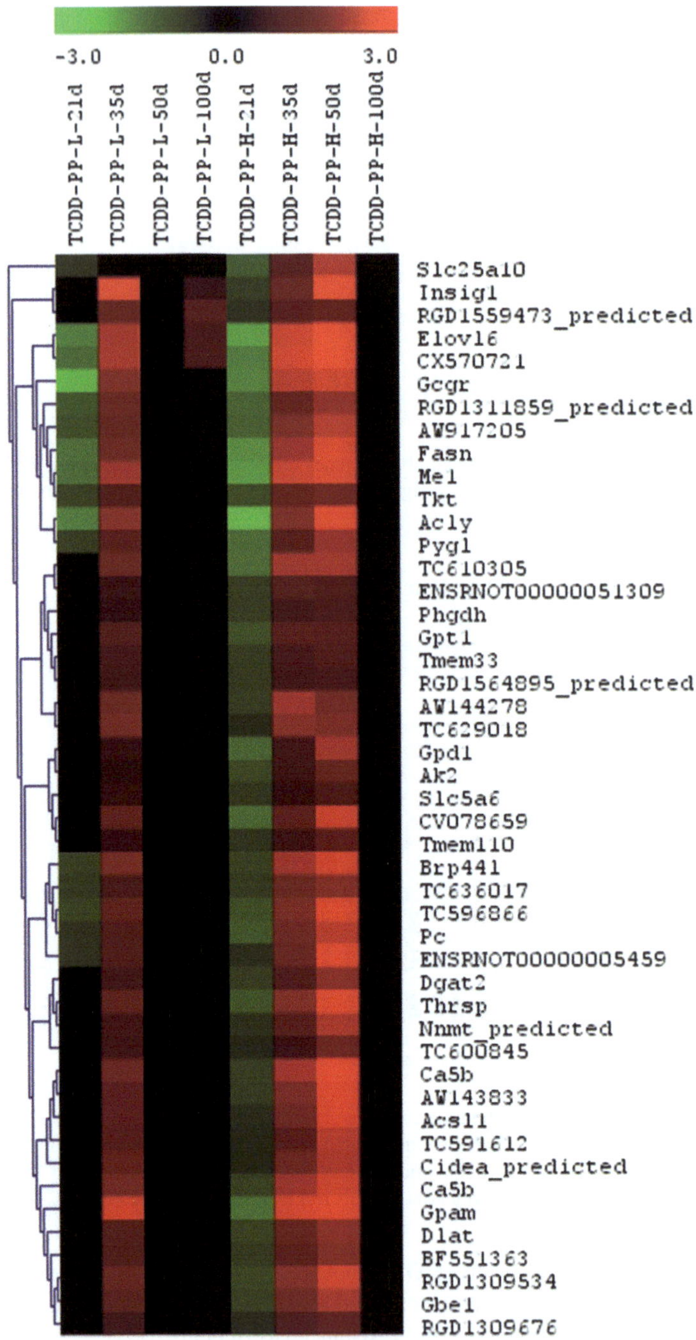

Fig. 5.6 The heatmap shows the expression of genes involved in the lipid metabolism downregulated by TCDD at 21 days but upregulated at later ages. *Red squares* represent upregulated genes, *green squares* represent downregulated genes and *black* represents no change in expression

Table 5.1 Genes related to lipid metabolism commonly regulated by TCDD and BBP

Gene symbol	BBP-PN-H-35d	TCDD-PP-H-35d
Abcd2	3.52	2.52
Adm	1.84	1.77
Cd36	2.36	2.00
Cpt2	1.37	2.20
Cyp1b1	3.29	21.10
Dbi	2.33	2.05
Fabp4	3.08	2.60
Lipe	2.62	1.77
Lpl	3.13	1.82
Pck1	3.01	1.75
Pex7	1.86	2.36
Pparg	2.11	2.45
Hnf4a	0.55	0.32

*Numbers*represent fold change of the genes related to the untreated age-matched animals
PN Prenatal, *PP* prepubertal, *35d* 35 days of age

modulated by prenatal exposure to BBP. Thirty-five day-old animals treated prenatally with a high dose of BBP showed the largest number of dysregulated genes (27 genes). Low-dose treatment affected mainly gene expression of 35- and 50-day-old rats, in which 16 and 18 genes were modulated, respectively. Prepubertal treatment affected mainly young rats (21-days-old) in which 4 genes were upregulated and 12 were downregulated; nonetheless, these effects faded later in life (Fig. 5.5).

Analysis of the interaction among the lipid metabolism genes modulated by prenatal exposure to the high dose of BBP demonstrated that some of these genes were also related to important biological functions or disorders, such as endocrine system disorder, modification of beta-estradiol, glucose tolerance, modification of aldosterone, and biosynthesis of progesterone. These functions could be related to the changes of puberty and body mass observed in girls exposed to this compound. Interestingly, 15 genes were found to be commonly modulated by prenatal BBP and prepubertal TCDD exposure in 35-day-old animals. The pattern of expression for these genes is similar in both treatments (Table 5.1).

BPA is the compound that shows the least changes in the expression of genes associated with fatty acids and lipid metabolism. A total of 49 differentially expressed genes were found, of which only few genes were regulated in more than one condition (Fig. 5.3). The highest effect was found after the prepubertal treatment of BPA in 21-day-old animals, in which 13 genes were modulated (Fig. 5.5).

We conclude from these data that exposure to these compounds, mainly TCDD and BBP, affects genes regulating the endogenous lipid metabolism. Lipogenesis is regulated by the enzyme fatty acid synthase (FASN) and breakdown of fatty acids is regulated by carnitine palmitoyltransferase-I (CPT-I). FASN is highly expressed in breast cancer and most common human carcinomas. In normal cells, FASN expression is tightly regulated by hormonal and nutritional signals, whereas, in cancer cells, FASN overexpression is thought to be the result of inappropriate activation of growth factors such as epidermal growth factor, keratinocyte growth factor, and HER-2 receptor tyrosine kinase. FASN expression is upregulated in animals treated prepubertally with the TCDD high dose (35 days). CPT-I is upregulated in animals treated prepubertally with the TCDD high dose (50 days). FASN is the sole protein in the human genome capable of the reductive de novo synthesis of long-chain fatty acids from acetyl-CoA, malonyl-CoA, and nicotinamide adenine dinucleotide phosphate. Many different enzymes key for lipid synthesis in cancer cells are upregulated by TCDD treatment. The protein encoded by ACSL-1 is an isozyme of the long-chain fatty-acid-coenzyme A ligase family. Although differing in substrate specificity, subcellular localization, and tissue distribution, all isozymes of this family convert free long-chain fatty acids into fatty acyl-CoA esters, and thereby play a key role in lipid biosynthesis and fatty acid degradation. This protein is upregulated in TCDD prepubertal 35 and 50 days. A pathway analysis for TCDD at prepubertal 35 and 50 days treatment shows that many lipid metabolism-related genes are upregulated. Also, pathways such as citric acid cycle, butanoate, propanoate, valine, leucine, and isoleucine degradation pathways are enriched. It is possible that at these stages a lot of lipid homeostasis is driven through PPAR-related pathway for conversion of sugars to adipose, fat, and cholesterol. A set of genes that are mostly common among the above conditions and that are upregulated were analyzed for a functional network they might suggest further clue to their involvement in fat metabolism. Overall, in these treatments lipid metabolism homeostasis is affected, which suggests a disposition toward weight changes and diabetes risk factors. This aggressive pattern of fat metabolism is more evident in the case of TCDD and BBP. BPA does not seem to affect lipid homeostasis.

5.3.2 Immunity- and Inflammation Related Genes Are Dysregulated in the Mammary Gland of Animals Exposed to BPA, BBP, and TCDD at Different Developmental Stages

Microarray gene analysis of the mammary gland showed modulation in the expression of a large number of genes involved in the immune response after exposure of the animals to BPA, BBP or TCDD. Comparing the three compounds, we found that TCDD exposure resulted in most changes among this class of genes. Not only are the effects observed compound dependent, but also specific for each stage of life at which the animal received the treatment, dose and age of the rats when studied. Expression of genes related to immune response was greatly affected after exposure to TCDD (Fig. 5.7) and these genes were mainly involved in antigen presentation, inflammatory response, cell-mediated response, and humoral response. Prenatal exposure to TCDD appears to modulate the highest number of genes (40 genes), which were mainly downregulated in the animals at 100 days of age (Fig. 5.8). The prepubertal treatment appears to affect mainly 35-day-old animals, independently of the dose administered, yet the high dose given during lactation showed to be the

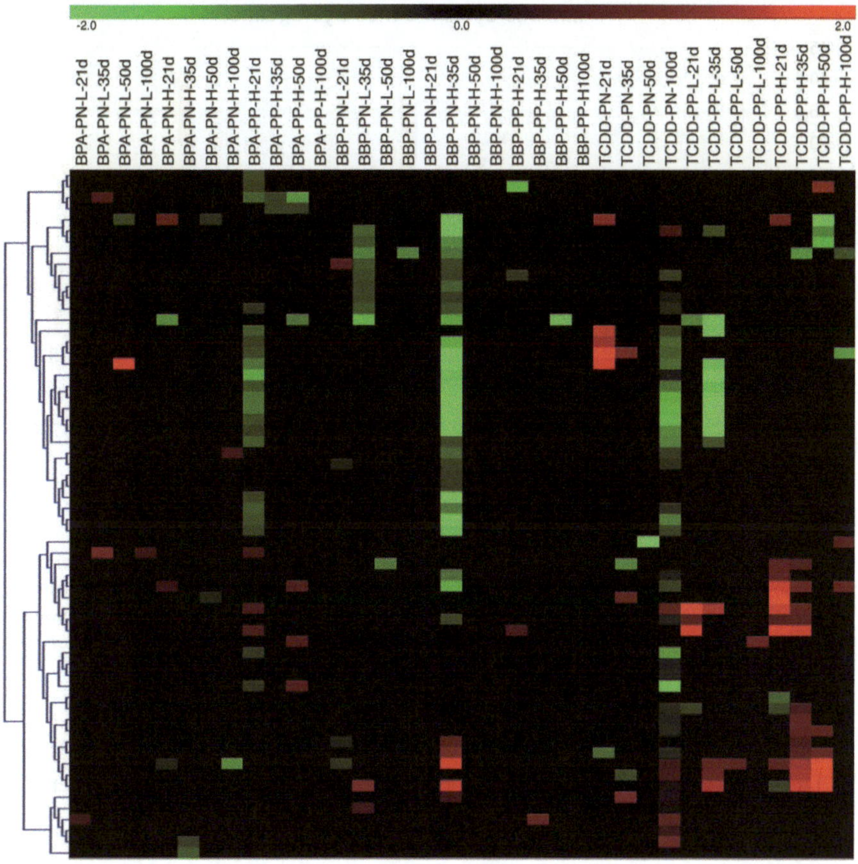

Fig. 5.7 Heatmap of immune system-related genes that were dysregulated by prenatal or prepubertal BPA, BBP, or TCDD exposure. *Red squares* represent upregulated genes, *green squares* represent downregulated genes, and *black* represents no change in expression. As it can be seen in the figure, BBP and TCDD exposure resulted in the most drastic effect on gene expression

treatment that modulated more genes in the other ages (Fig. 5.8). The modulation induced by BBP was age specific: 35-day-old animals showed changes in gene expression (Table 5.2). The low and high dose received prenatally caused the downregulation of several genes, nine of which were common between both doses. Not much effect was observed in the other conditions (Figs. 5.7 and 5.8).

Canonical pathway analysis showed that the genes found downregulated by BBP are part of antigen presentation pathway, B-cell receptor signaling pathways, and natural killer cell signaling. Some of the genes belonging to these pathways are Tap1, Sh2d2a, Hla-dma, Cd74, and Tapbp.

Similar to BBP, BPA's effect was also specific for one condition. The prepubertal treatment with the high dose of BPA was responsible for the changes – mainly downregulation – in the expression of immune-related genes in 21-day-old animals. Very few genes were affected in the other conditions (Figs. 5.7 and 5.8). Twenty-three different probes were commonly dysregulated among the three compounds

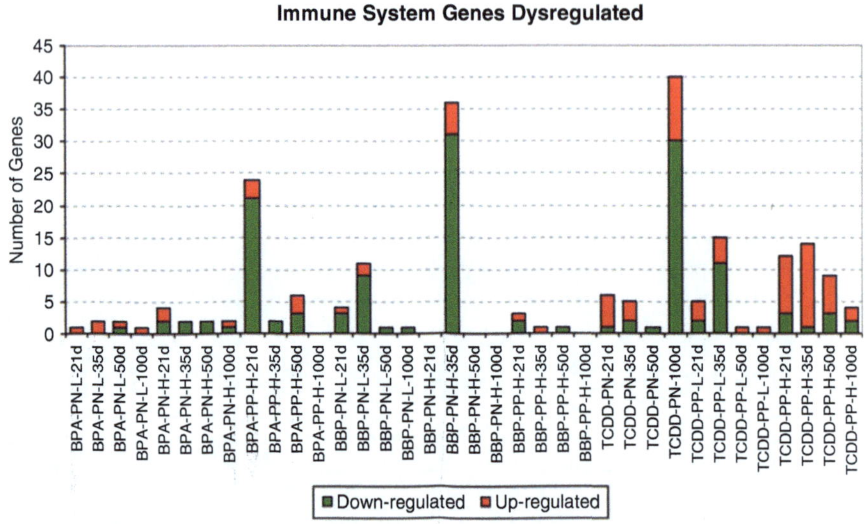

Fig. 5.8 Histogram shows the number of upregulated (*red*) and downregulated (*green*) genes related to immune system modulated at each condition after prenatal or prepubertal exposure to BPA, BBP, or TCDD. Prenatal exposure to BBP and TCDD dysregulated mammary gland gene expression mostly at 35 and 100 days of life, respectively. BPA effects on gene expression were more apparent after prepubertal exposure to this compound at 21-days-old rats

studied (Fig. 5.9; Table 5.3). As observed in the lipid metabolism genes, BBP and TCDD were the compounds that had the largest number of common genes between them (36 genes) (Fig. 5.9).

Tap1, one of the genes downregulated by all three compounds, encodes a protein responsible for the delivery of the antigen peptides to the endoplasmic reticulum. Different polymorphisms on this protein have been correlated to the response to some diseases, allergies and were related to risk of hypertension, as well BMI levels (Shen et al. 2007). Also affected by all three compounds, Bnip3 gene (BNIP3 BCL2/adenovirus E1B 10-kDa interacting protein 3) contains a BH3 domain and a transmembrane domain, which have been associated with proapoptotic function (Boyd 1994). The dimeric mitochondrial protein encoded by this gene is known to induce apoptosis, even in the presence of *BCL2*. Its expression is markedly upregulated in breast and nonsmall cell lung (Sowter et al. 2003; Giatromanolaki et al. 2004).

Also related to cell death and modulated by BBP and TCDD is CD59, a membrane regulatory protein of the complement cascade, where such complement regulatory proteins (CRPs) normally protect against inappropriate immune-mediated cell death (Rushmere et al. 2004). CRPs are commonly elevated in malignancy and during progression allowing tumor cells to escape immune attack. Recent studies by Rushmere et al. (2004) have shown that CRPs are detectable in ER+clinical breast cancer. Overall, these endocrine disruptors change the expression of immune system genes. TCDD is the compound with wider broad effect, affecting several genes

Table 5.2 List of genes modulated by BBP exposure in 35-days-old animals

Gene symbol	Gene name	BBP-PN-H-35d
Cidea_predicted	Cell death-inducing DNA fragmentation factor, alpha subunit-like effector A (predicted)	1.66
Bnip3	BCL2/adenovirus E1B 19-kDa-interacting protein 3	1.71
Cd59	CD59 antigen	1.12
Reg3a	Regenerating islet-derived 3 alpha	0.49
Cebpg	CCAAT/enhancer binding protein (C/EBP), gamma	0.76
Syk	Spleen tyrosine kinase	–0.53
Hla-dma	Major histocompatibility complex, class II, DM alpha	–0.53
Cxcl12	Chemokine (C-X-C motif) ligand 12	–0.61
RT1-Aw2	RT1 class Ib, locus Aw2	–0.64
Cd8b	CD8 antigen, beta chain	–0.66
Hprt	Hypoxanthine guanine phosphoribosyl transferase	–0.59
Prkcd	Protein kinase C, delta	–0.89
Ier3	Immediate early response 3	–0.97
Cd74	CD74 antigen (invariant polypeptide of major histo-compatibility complex, class II antigen-associated)	–1.06
Tapbp	TAP binding protein	–0.57
Fcgr2b	Fc receptor, IgG, low affinity IIb	–1.40
Blnk	B-cell linker	–1.40
Nck2_predicted	Noncatalytic region of tyrosine kinase adaptor protein 2 (predicted)	–0.87
Cd7_predicted	CD7 antigen (predicted)	–0.74
LOC500449	Similar to SHP2-interacting transmembrane adaptor protein	–1.71
Rhoh	Ras homolog gene family, member H	–1.73
Ppt1	Palmitoyl-protein thioesterase 1	–0.56
Lat	Linker for activation of T cells	–1.86
Vav1	Vav 1 oncogene	–1.94
Bat1a	HLA-B-associated transcript 1A	–1.19
Sh2d2a	SH2 domain protein 2A	–2.07
Pap	Pancreatitis-associated protein	–2.18
Il18	Interleukin 18	–2.23
Cd2	CD2 antigen	–2.60
Coro1a	Coronin, actin binding protein 1A	–2.65
Ptpn22_predicted	Protein tyrosine phosphatase, nonreceptor type 22 (lymphoid) (predicted)	–3.06
Egr1	Early growth response 1	–2.26
Ap3d1	Adaptor-related protein complex 3, delta 1 subunit	–1.04
Cd3g	CD3 antigen, gamma polypeptide	–3.99
Cd5	CD5 antigen	–4.15
Tap1	Transporter 1, ATP-binding cassette, subfamily B (MDR/TAP)	–1.33

Expression values (log2) compared to untreated age-matched animals

at different studied ages. BBP and BPA induce more age-specific effects; while BBP induces the suppression of several of these genes at early puberty when the animals are exposed through the placenta, BPA suppresses immune-related genes right after the end of exposure.

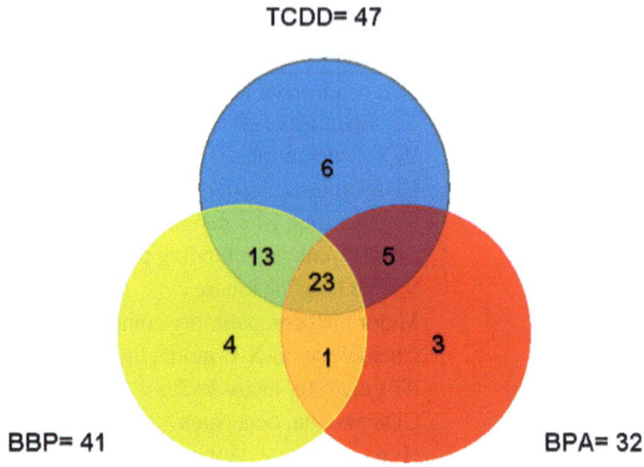

Fig. 5.9 Venn diagram showing the number of genes related to immune system modulated by each compound. Twenty-three genes were found to be commonly modulated by BPA, BBP, and TCDD

Table 5.3 Genes related to immune system dysregulated by BPA, BBP, and TCDD

Target ID	Gene symbol	Gene name
ENSRNOT00000025878	Ap3d1	Adaptor-related protein complex 3, delta 1 subunit
NM_001025767	Blnk	B-cell linker
BM389524	BM389524	BM389524 UI-R-CN1-cjn-b-16-0-UI.s1 UI-R-CN1 *Rattus norvegicus* cDNA clone UI-R-CN1-cjn-b-16-0-UI 3′, mRNA sequence [BM389524]
NM_053420	Bnip3	BCL2/adenovirus E1B 19-kDa-interacting protein 3
NM_001077646	Cd3g	CD3 antigen, gamma polypeptide
NM_019295	Cd5	CD5 antigen
ENSRNOT00000054934	Cd7_predicted	CD7 antigen (predicted)
NM_013069	Cd74	CD74 antigen (invariant polypeptide of major histocompatibility complex, class II antigen-associated)
NM_130411	Coro1a	Coronin, actin binding protein 1A
NM_013097	Dnase1	Deoxyribonuclease I
NM_175756	Fcgr2b	Fc receptor, IgG, low affinity IIb
NM_019165	Il18	Interleukin 18
NM_030853	Lat	Linker for activation of T cells
NM_001024344	LOC500449	Similar to SHP2-interacting transmembrane adaptor protein
NM_012845	Ms4a2	Membrane-spanning 4-domains, subfamily A, member 2
NM_053289	Pap	Pancreatitis-associated protein
NM_133307	Prkcd	Protein kinase C, delta
XM_001068074	Ptpn22_predicted	Protein tyrosine phosphatase, nonreceptor type 22 (lymphoid) (predicted)
NM_001013430	Rhoh	Ras homolog gene family, member H
NM_012645	RT1-Aw2	RT1 class Ib, locus Aw2
NM_207605	Sh2d2a	SH2 domain protein 2A
NM_032055	Tap1	Transporter 1, ATP-binding cassette, subfamily B (MDR/TAP)
NM_012759	Vav1	Vav 1 oncogene

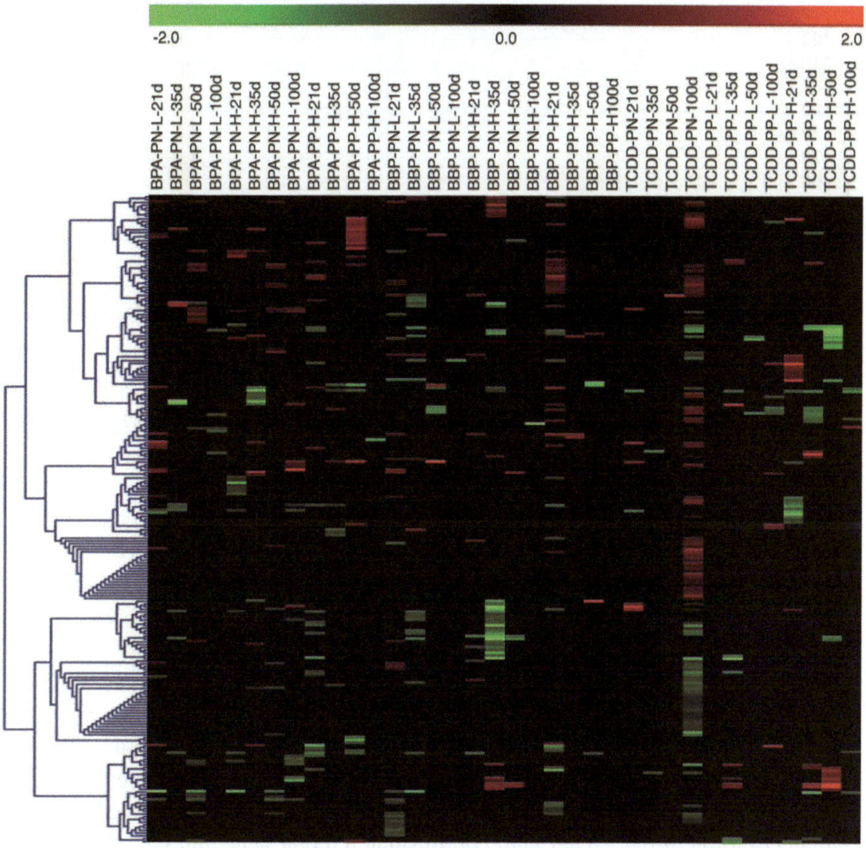

Fig. 5.10 Heatmap of oncogenes that were dysregulated by prenatal or prepubertal BPA, BBP, or TCDD exposure. *Red squares* represent upregulated genes, *green squares* represent downregulated genes, and *black* represents no change in expression

5.3.3 Oncogenes and Tumor Suppressor-Related Genes Are Dysregulated in the Mammary Glands of Animals Exposed to BPA, BBP, and TCDD at Different Developmental Stages

A list of 327 known and novel oncogenes was annotated using GeneRIF information from Gene Database of NCBI (Figs. 5.10 and 5.11). A similar list of over 550 tumor suppressor genes was annotated. Rat homolog were taken and viewed as heatmaps (Fig. 5.12). Particularly, gene expression analysis of the mammary gland at 21 days of age of animals treated with high dose of TCDD at a prepubertal stage of life showed two clusters of up and downregulated genes.

The upregulated tumor suppressor genes included Phf17_predicted, Ppm1d_predicted, Msh2, Wif1, Nr4a3, Ptgs2, Atm, Pik3c3, and Mlh1, whereas the downregulated genes included MLL, RGD1565602_predicted, Lrp12_predicted, Slit2, Gtf2e1, Lzts2, and Nbr1.

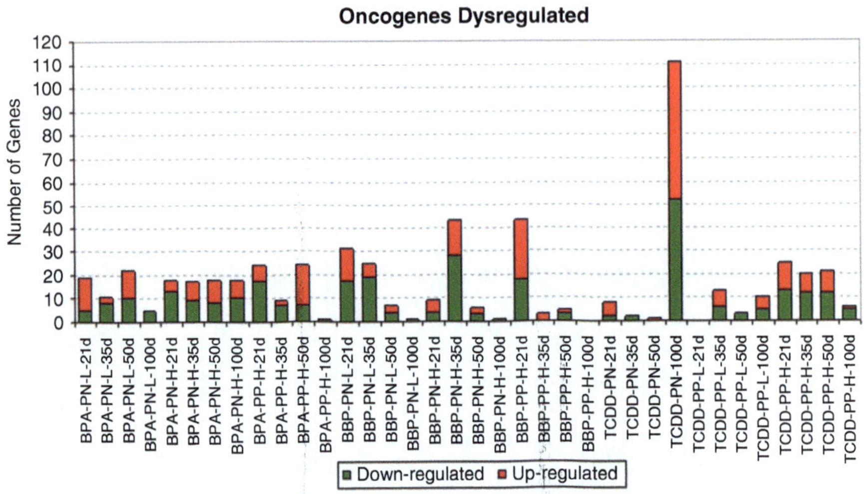

Fig. 5.11 Histogram shows the number of upregulated (*red*) and down-regulated (*green*) oncogenes modulated at each condition after prenatal or prepubertal exposure to BPA, BBP, or TCDD. Prenatal exposure to TCDD dysregulated mammary gland gene expression mostly at 100 days of life

PHF17 or JADE-1 (PHD finger protein 17) was described by Zhou et al. (2005) as a renal tumor suppressor candidate gene. It has been shown to suppress renal cancer cell growth in part by increasing apoptosis. MSH2 (mutS homolog 2, colon cancer, nonpolyposis type 1) was identified as a locus frequently mutated in hereditary nonpolyposis colon cancer (HNPCC). When cloned, it was discovered to be a human homolog of the *Escherichia coli* mismatch repair gene mutS, consistent with the characteristic alterations in microsatellite sequences found in HNPCC. Findings by Jensen et al. (2010) support the hypothesis of a role for defective mismatch repair in breast cancer progression in HNPCC, presumably through accelerated accumulation of mutations in breast cancer-associated genes. WIF1 (WNT inhibitory factor 1) functions as a tumor suppressor gene, and has been found to be epigenetically silenced in various cancers (Wissmann et al. 2003). Specifically, the WIF1 gene, which encodes a secreted protein antagonistic to Wnt-dependent signaling, is targeted for epigenetic silencing in human breast cancer (Ai et al. 2006). Prostaglandin-endoperoxide synthase (PTGS), also known as cyclooxygenase, is the key enzyme in prostaglandin biosynthesis, and acts both as a dioxygenase and as a peroxidase. There are two isozymes of PTGS: a constitutive PTGS1 and an inducible PTGS2, which differ in their regulation of expression and tissue distribution. This gene encodes the inducible isozyme. It is regulated by specific stimulatory events, suggesting that it is responsible for the prostanoid biosynthesis involved in inflammation and mitogenesis. COX-2 contributes to the development of various types of tumors (Juuti et al. 2006; Panel et al. 2006). Expression of PTGS2 or COX-2 in breast cancer varied from 5 to 100% in reviewed papers with significantly higher values in poorly differentiated tumors (Krcova et al. 2008). In breast cancer COX-2 plays role in many

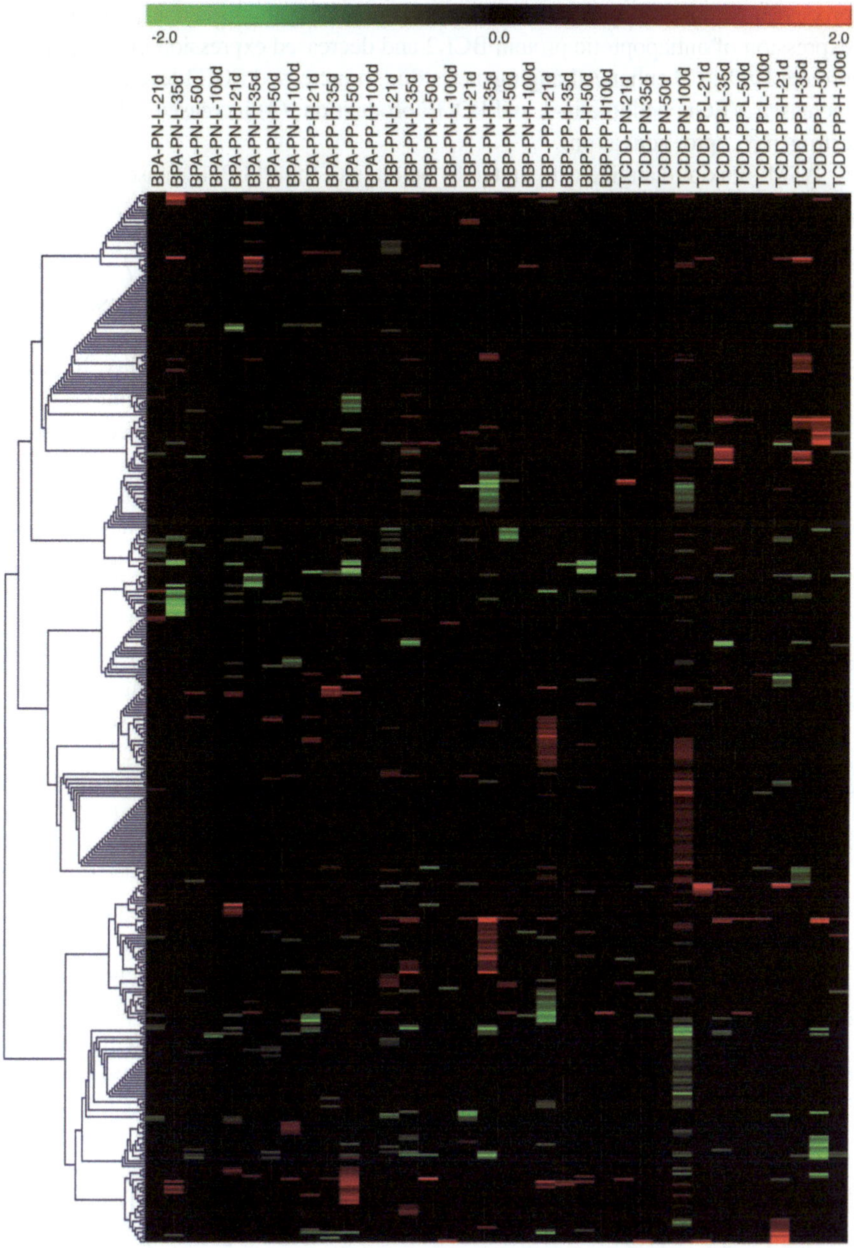

Fig. 5.12 Heatmap of tumor suppressor-related genes that were dysregulated by prenatal or prepubertal BPA, BBP, or TCDD exposure. *Red squares* represent upregulated genes, *green squares* represent downregulated genes, and *black* represents no change in expression

processes. Among those we can cite are: (1) apoptosis inhibition due to an increased expression of antiapoptotic protein BCL2 and decreased expression of proapoptotic protein BAX; (2) enhanced angiogenesis due to increased PGE2 level, followed by increased VEGF, endothelin-1 and PDGF production; (3) increased cell growth via estrogen receptor activation.

ATM (ataxia telangiectasia mutated) belongs to the PI3/PI4-kinase family. This protein is an important cell cycle checkpoint kinase and it functions as a regulator of a wide variety of downstream proteins, including tumor suppressor proteins p53 and BRCA1, checkpoint kinase CHK2, checkpoint proteins RAD17 and RAD9, and DNA repair protein NBS1. This protein and the closely related kinase ATR are thought to be master controllers of cell cycle checkpoint signaling pathways, which are required for cell response to DNA damage and for genome stability. Recently, Oka et al. (2010) found that ATM was significantly expressed during tumor progression in advanced human colon carcinoma. The etiology of breast cancer is associated with several factors, one of the most important being genetic susceptibility. Both BRCA1/2 and ATM/ATR play a role in DNA repair pathways and breast cancer. Several studies found that the frequencies of mutations in ATM were many times greater for cases with a strong family history than for controls.

Oncogenes and tumor suppressor genes that are differentially expressed by TCDD were subjected to pathway analysis. Erythropoietin and IGF-1 signaling pathways were enriched. For instance in IGF-1 signaling, PI3K, 14-3-3, PKC, and Jun were all upregulated (while AKT was downregulated) suggesting cell growth and proliferation. In the case of EPO signaling, the downstream NFKB expression was downregulated. NFKB is a transcription regulator that is activated by various intra- and extracellular stimuli such as cytokines, oxidant-free radicals, ultraviolet irradiation, and bacterial or viral products. Inappropriate activation of NFKB has been associated with a number of inflammatory diseases, while persistent inhibition of NFKB leads to inappropriate immune cell development or delayed cell growth (Sun and Zhang 2007). Mycn, a viral oncogene, was downregulated.

Tumor suppressor genes and oncogenes down- or upregulated in prepubertal BPA at high dose at 50 days were enriched in the following canonical pathways: erythropoietin signaling, IGF-1 signaling, B-cell receptor, GM-CSF signaling, PI3K/Akt, 14-3-3 mediated signaling, inositol phosphate metabolism, and p53 signaling. Figures 5.11 and 5.13 show histograms depicting the number of up- and downregulated oncogenes and tumor suppressor genes in all treatments and at all ages. It is noteworthy that prenatal exposure to TCDD at 100 days showed the highest amount of downregulated and upregulated genes. On the other hand, exposure at 21 days showed almost no change in gene expression. The other two treatments (BPA and BBP) did not show such a change in gene expression at 100 days. However, both BBP and BPA showed the highest change in gene expression at 35 and 50 days for both oncogenes and tumor suppressor genes. In conclusion, these endocrine disruptors change the expression of oncogenes and tumor suppressor genes for any combination of compound, dose, time of exposure, and age. Noteworthy, it is evident the changes that prenatal exposure to TCDD exerts at 100 days suppress immune-related genes right after the end of exposure.

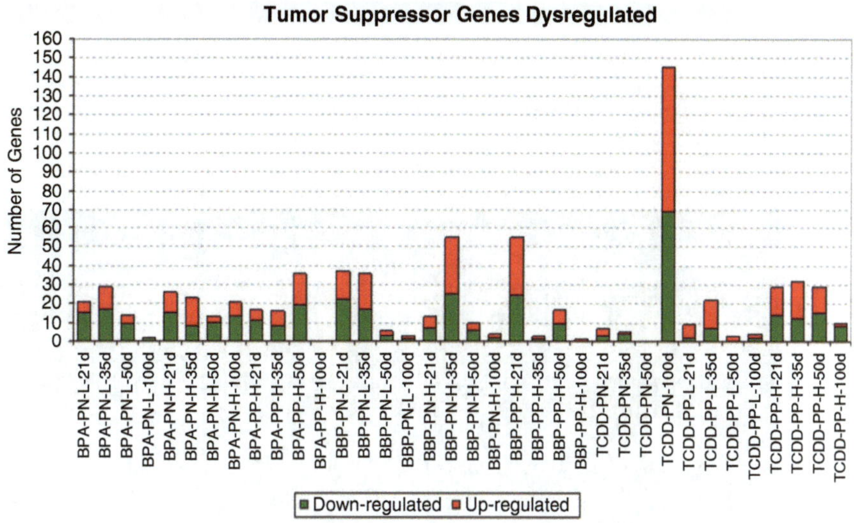

Fig. 5.13 Histogram shows the number of upregulated (*red*) and downregulated (*green*) tumor suppressor genes modulated at each condition after prenatal or prepubertal exposure to BPA, BBP, or TCDD. Prenatal exposure to TCDD dysregulated mammary gland gene expression mostly at 100 days of life

5.3.4 DNA Damage Response and Repair Genes

DNA mismatch repair is an evolutionarily conserved process that corrects mismatches generated during DNA replication and escape proofreading. The integrity of genetic information depends on the fidelity of DNA replication and on the efficiency of several different DNA repair processes. It is responsible for correcting base substitution mismatches and insertion–deletion mismatches generated during DNA replication in all existing organisms. Epidemiological and experimental data link estrogen with the pathogenesis of breast cancer. Hormones stimulate cell proliferation and thus increased exposure to these hormones promotes the opportunity to develop and accumulate random genetic errors. It is valid then to hypothesize that any estrogen-mimicking compound could potentially increase the rate of DNA mutation and/or decrease the cell's DNA repair ability. Balogh et al. have previously reported a premature protein truncation due to a nonsense mutation in the hPMS2 gene in 55% of the breast tumor tissues studied. These results suggest that the hPMS2 mismatch repair gene could be involved in DNA repair defect in human breast tumors (Balogh et al. 2006).

In our experimental studies with animals exposed to xenobiotic agents, we observed a large number of genes related to DNA damage response and repair regulated by the BBP exposure (Fig. 5.14). Genes were dysregulated at 21 days of age

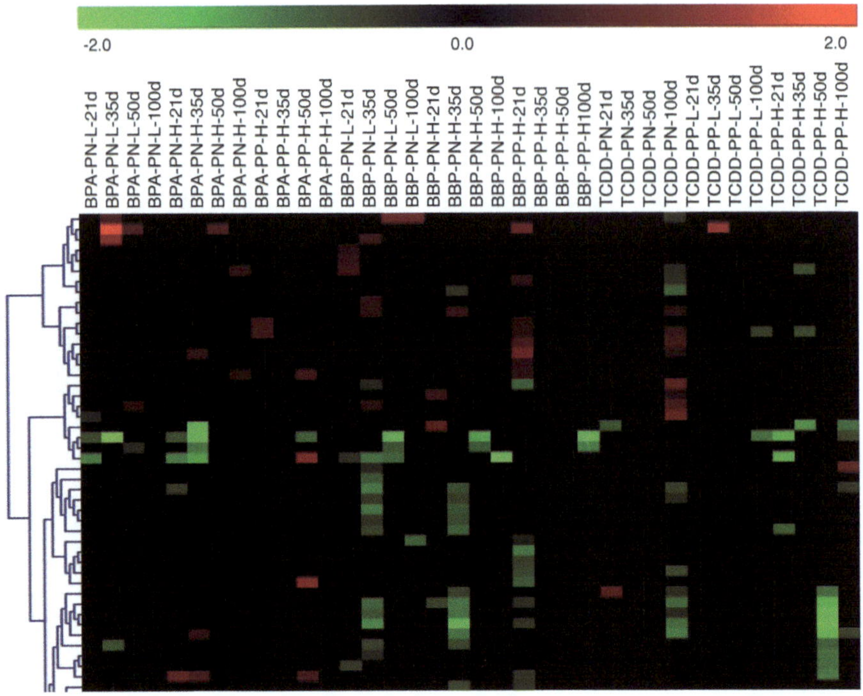

Fig. 5.14 Heatmap of DNA repair-related genes that were dysregulated by prenatal or prepubertal BPA, BBP, or TCDD exposure. *Red squares* represent upregulated genes, *green squares* represent downregulated genes, and *black* represents no change in expression

when exposed prepubertally but not in older animals. In animals prenatally treated with BBP, gene dysregulation was evident at an early age (day 21) and it was maintained at 35 and 50 days of age with no significant changes at 100 days (Fig. 5.14). As depicted in Fig. 5.15, the largest number of modulated genes was observed at 35 days of age. Among these, eight genes were common for both doses at this age. FANCA_predicted was increased by low and high doses. In humans, the FANCA gene belongs to the Fanconi anemia complementation group (FANC). Mutations of members of this group can lead to Fanconi anemia, a genetically heterogeneous recessive disorder characterized by cytogenetic instability, hypersensitivity to DNA crosslinking agents, increased chromosomal breakage, and defective DNA repair. Fanconi anemia (FA) family of proteins participates in the DNA repair pathway by homologous recombination. Some of these proteins also confer susceptibility to hereditary breast and ovarian cancer (HBOC). Barroso et al. (2009) demonstrated a significant correlation between FA and BRCA pathways. Significantly downregulated genes are Ube2a, Gtf2h3, Gtf2h2_predicted, Pole, RGD1566119_predicted, Pnkp, and RGD1304924_predicted. Ube2a (ubiquitin-conjugating enzyme E2A) is one of the cellular proteins involved in the process of ubiquitination. The modification of proteins with ubiquitin is an important cellular mechanism for targeting

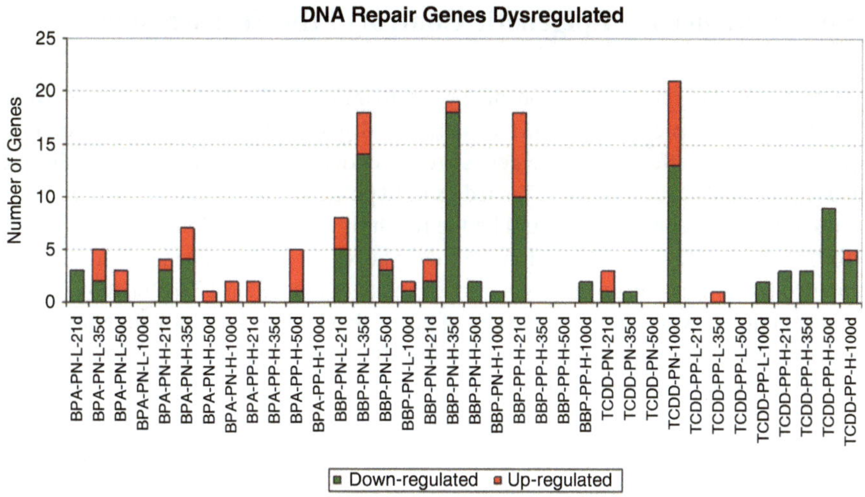

Fig. 5.15 Histogram shows the number of upregulated (*red*) and downregulated (*green*) DNA repair-related genes modulated at each condition after prenatal or prepubertal exposure to BPA, BBP, or TCDD. BBP is the compound that shows the most striking changes in gene expression

abnormal or short-lived proteins for degradation. Ubiquitination involves at least three classes of enzymes: ubiquitin-activating enzymes, or E1s, ubiquitin-conjugating enzymes, or E2s, and ubiquitin-protein ligases, or E3s. This gene encodes a member of the E2 ubiquitin-conjugating enzyme family. This enzyme is required for postreplicative DNA damage repair. Although there are no current data in the literature linking Ube2a and breast cancer, Yang et al. (2005) found this gene to be upregulated in the metastatic 5–8 F cell line when compared to the nonmetastatic nasopharyngeal carcinoma cell line counterparts.

The efficient repair of double-strand breaks (DSBs) in DNA is critical for the maintenance of genome stability. The PNKP gene encodes for a polynucleotide kinase 3′ phosphatase, which catalyzes the 5′ phosphorylation of nucleic acids and also has an associated 3′ phosphatase activity, predictive of an important function in DNA repair following ionizing radiation or oxidative damage. Chappell et al. (2002) demonstrated a direct, specific role for human PNK in DSB repair. There is not yet a direct correlation between PNKP levels and breast cancer. POLE polymerase (DNA directed) epsilon is a member of the family of DNA polymerases, which represent potential candidates for cancer genes because of their pivotal roles in DNA metabolism. Defects of some DNA Pols have shown cancer associations; however, the first report to link this enzyme with breast cancer is only recent. In 2008, Zhou et al. found an AATT deletion in the 55-kDa small subunit DNA sequence of DNA polymerase epsilon is associated with breast cancer (Zhou et al. 2008). This compelling data may not affect the protein code, but could potentially influence splicing efficiency and expression levels, possibly impairing the function of Pol epsilon DNA. In summary, these xenobiotics change the expression of DNA damage response and repair genes. Interestingly, BBP induced the major changes in gene expression of this class of genes.

5.4 Evidence for Epigenetic Control of the Transcriptome

Analysis of the gene expression of the rat mammary gland after receiving BPA, BBP, or TCDD prenatally showed that several genes are affected by these compounds, and the effects on these genes are dependent on the doses used and the age that the animals were studied. This led us to hypothesize that some of the regulation caused by these compounds could be the result of the methylation of certain genes. To find the list of genes that might be methylated, through *k*-means clustering, we divided the expression profiles of all doses and ages studied in 12 patterns of expression and in this way, observed clusters of genes that had peaks of downregulation by one of the compounds at certain time points after which their expression returned to normal or it became upregulated.

Prenatally BBP-exposed animals had two clusters of genes (Fig. 5.16) which were downregulated at 35 days, independently of the doses. A list of 38 genes that

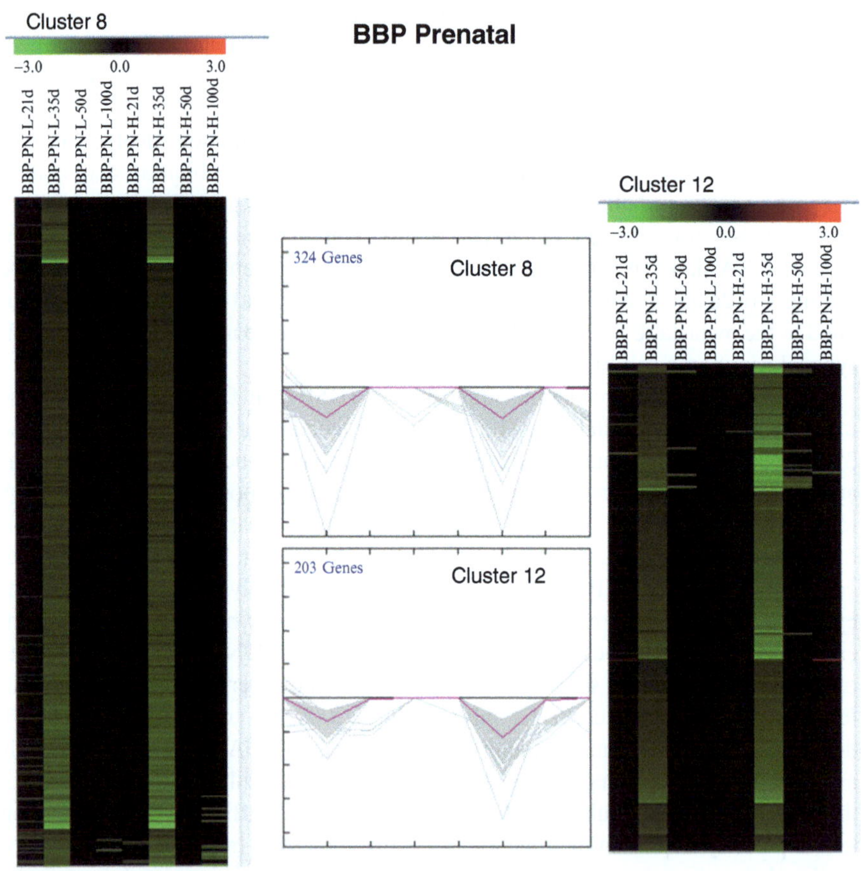

Fig. 5.16 Clusters of genes downregulated at 35 days of age after prenatal exposure to BBP. The *pink line* represents the average expression and *gray lines* represent the expression of each selected gene

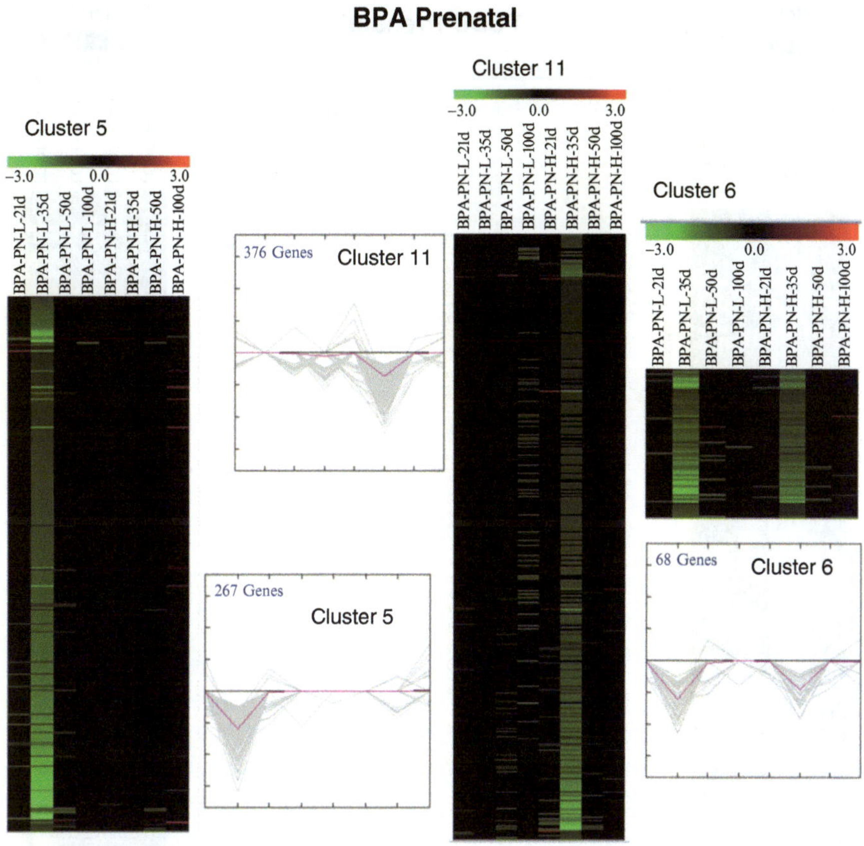

Fig. 5.17 Clusters of genes downregulated at 35 days of age after prenatal exposure to BPA. The *pink line* represents the average expression and *gray lines* represent the expression of each selected gene

were at least twofold downregulated compared to the control group was identified with methylation sites in their promoter or exon 1. Among the patterns of expression found after the prenatal treatment with BPA, three clusters were considered to have potential methylated genes (Fig. 5.17). TCDD-prenatally exposed animals induced the downregulation of 83 genes clustered at 35 days of age and other cluster of 85 genes at 100 days of age (Fig. 5.18). In summary, these findings suggest that the compounds – when administered prenatally – induced at the time of puberty (35 days of age) downregulation of genes that are specific to BBP and BPA. The fact that this effect disappears at 50 and 100 days of age and returns to the same values observed at 21 days indicates that at puberty a series of events not yet identified regulate the transcriptional pattern of the mammary gland. The same effect is observed with TCDD-prenatally treated animals, in which a different cluster of downregulated genes appears at 100 days. We postulate that this transcription pattern could be epigenetically controlled.

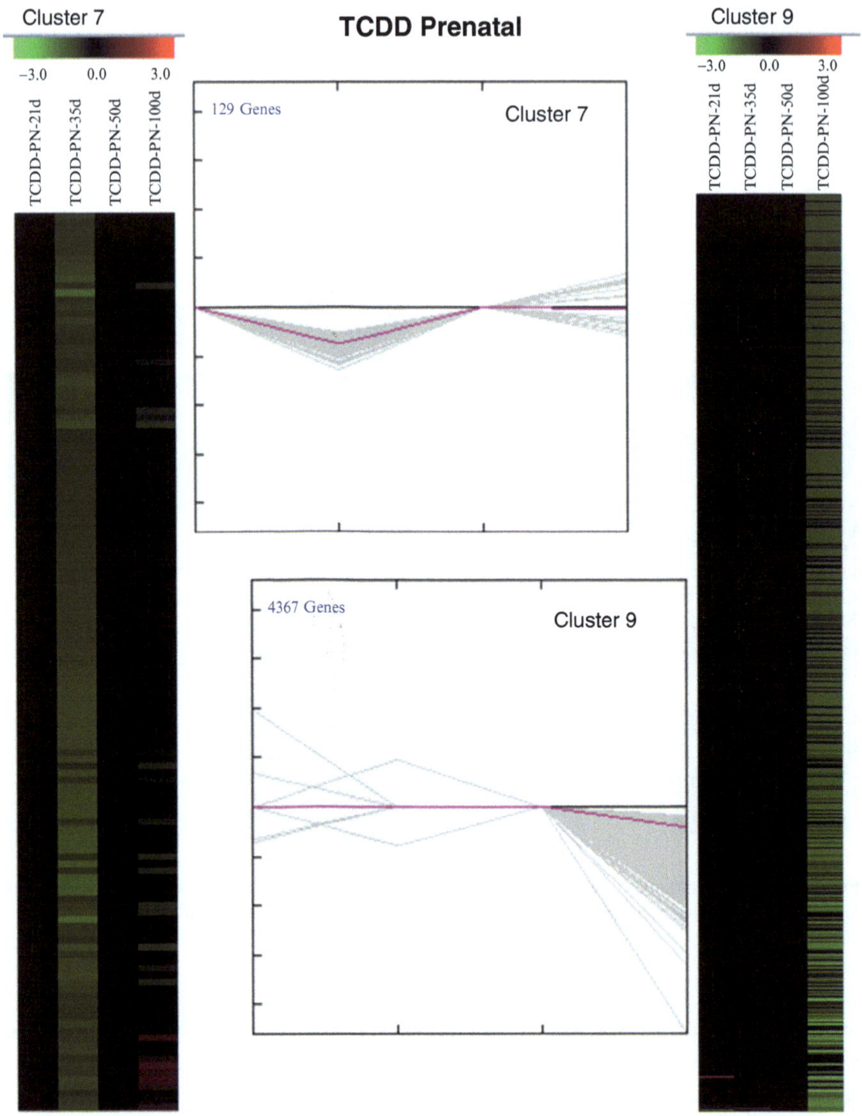

Fig. 5.18 Pattern of expression of two clusters of genes after prenatal exposure to TCDD. The *pink line* represents the average expression and *gray lines* represent the expression of each selected gene

5.5 Tumorigenesis as an End Point

To perform the tumorigenesis studies, female offspring that had been exposed to these compounds were challenged with a single dose of 30 mg DMBA/kg BW.

5.5.1 *Tumorigenesis Effects of BPA in Rats*

It has been described in the literature that exposure to BPA during the prenatal period produces an increased proliferation/apoptosis ratio in both the epithelial and stromal compartments at puberty. During adulthood, BPA-exposed animals showed an increased number of hyperplastic ducts and an increased number of mast cells, suggesting a heightened risk of neoplastic transformation (Durando et al. 2007). Terminal end buds (TEBs) are the structures most susceptible to carcinogenesis in the rat mammary gland (Russo and Russo 1978). In animals lactationally exposed to BPA 250, a significantly increased cell proliferation in TEBs of 50-day-old but not 21-day-old rats was observed. Interestingly, apoptosis was significantly decreased in the mammary gland of 50-day-old but not 21-day-old BPA 250 rats (Jenkins et al. 2009). The data clearly indicate that genomic and proteomic changes detected in the mammary glands of prepubertally exposed animals show signatures that predict the response to a carcinogen challenge. Indeed, this assumption is supported by experimental data published by Jenkins et al. They reported that rats exposed prepubertally to BPA and then at day 50 to the mammary carcinogen DMBA showed a dose-dependent increase in mammary tumor multiplicity and reduced tumor latency compared to controls (Jenkins et al. 2009). Recently, Betancourt et al. reported that oral prenatal exposure to BPA increases mammary cancer susceptibility in offspring and shifts the window of susceptibility for DMBA-induced tumorigenesis in the rat mammary gland from 50 to 100 days. These changes are accompanied by differential effects of prenatal BPA exposure on the expression of key proteins involved in cell proliferation (Betancourt et al. 2010). Thus, effects of BPA in rats, including a dose dependent increase in mammary tumor multiplicity and reduced tumor latency, have been observed at exceedingly low exposure levels that are well below environmental human exposure.

5.5.2 *Tumorigenesis Effects of TCDD in Rats*

Brown et al. (1998) reported that prenatal TCDD treatment resulted in an increased number of chemically induced mammary adenocarcinomas in rats. Also, TCDD delayed time of vaginal opening and caused disruption to the estrous cycle.

Prenatal exposure to TCDD was investigated for its potential to predispose to breast cancer. Analysis of mammary gland differentiation and cell proliferation were used as biomarkers. Timed pregnant Sprague–Dawley CD rats were gavaged with 1 μg TCDD/kg on day 15 postconception. Control animals were treated with the same volume of vehicle (sesame oil) on the same schedule. Mammary gland differentiation studies revealed that prenatal TCDD treatment, as compared to sesame oil treatment, resulted in significantly more TEBs and fewer lobules II in 50-day-old offspring, but no significant alterations to mammary gland differentiation in 21-day-old offspring. TEBs are the most susceptible terminal ductal structures and lobules the least susceptible to carcinogenesis. Prenatal TCDD treatment did not alter the labeling index in the mammary terminal ductal structures of 21- and 50-day-old rats, but the total proliferative compartment in TEBs of 50-day-old rats was larger. In summary, TCDD-induced alteration of the mammary gland differentiation (increased number of TEBs) is correlated with increased susceptibility to mammary cancer after prenatal exposure to TCDD (Brown et al. 1998).

5.6 Concluding Remarks

Breast cancer is a complex, multifactorial disease. It is well known that estrogen and estrogen-like compounds can exert profound changes in the mammary gland. These changes can happen at any time during the mammary gland development and will depend on many different factors. Among them, we can consider: type of xenobiotic, window of exposure, time of exposure, doses, and method of exposure. For many years, research has been geared toward the study of the phenotypical manifestations of the interaction of the mammary tissue with these compounds. In this chapter, we summarized the current knowledge of the impact these ubiquitous compounds produce on the transcriptome of the mammary gland. Noteworthy, genomic changes can alter the susceptibility of the breast tissue to cancer. In the near future this knowledge can be used to regulate the use of these xenobiotics in our society to lessen the burden of breast cancer.

References

Adami HO, Lipworth L et al (1995) Organochlorine compounds and estrogen-related cancers in women. Cancer Causes Control 6(6):551–566

Adriani W, Seta DD et al (2003) Altered profiles of spontaneous novelty seeking, impulsive behavior, and response to D-amphetamine in rats perinatally exposed to bisphenol A. Environ Health Perspect 111(4):395–401

Agas D, Sabbieti MG et al (2007) Benzyl butyl phthalate influences actin distribution and cell proliferation in rat Py1a osteoblasts. J Cell Biochem 101(3):543–551

Ai L, Tao Q et al (2006) Inactivation of Wnt inhibitory factor-1 (WIF1) expression by epigenetic silencing is a common event in breast cancer. Carcinogenesis 27(7):1341–1348

Balogh GA, Heulings RC et al (2006) The mismatch repair gene hPMS2 is mutated in primary breast cancer. Int J Mol Med 18(5):853–857

Barroso E, Pita G et al (2009) The Fanconi anemia family of genes and its correlation with breast cancer susceptibility and breast cancer features. Breast Cancer Res Treat 118(3):655–660

Bertazzi A, Pesatori AC et al (1993) Cancer incidence in a population accidentally exposed to 2,3,7,8-tetrachlorodibenzo-para-dioxin. Epidemiology 4(5):398–406

Betancourt AM, Eltoum IA et al (2010) In utero exposure to bisphenol a shifts the window of susceptibility for mammary carcinogenesis in the rat. Environ Health Perspect 118(11):1614–1619

Birnbaum LS, Fenton SE (2003) Cancer and developmental exposure to endocrine disruptors. Environ Health Perspect 111(4):389–394

Boyd JM (1994) Adenovirus E1B 19 kDa and Bcl-2 proteins interact with a common set of cellular proteins. Cell 79(6):1121

Boylan ES, Calhoon RE (1979) Mammary tumorigenesis in the rat following prenatal exposure to diethylstilbestrol and postnatal treatment with 7,12-dimethylbenz[a]anthracene. J Toxicol Environ Health 5(6):1059–1071

Brown NM, Manzolillo PA et al (1998) Prenatal TCDD and predisposition to mammary cancer in the rat. Carcinogenesis 19(9):1623–1629

Calafat AM, Kuklenyik Z et al (2005) Urinary concentrations of bisphenol A and 4-nonylphenol in a human reference population. Environ Health Perspect 113(4):391–395

Chappell C, Hanakahi LA et al (2002) Involvement of human polynucleotide kinase in double-strand break repair by non-homologous end joining. EMBO J 21(11):2827–2832

Committee on the Implications of Dioxin in the Food Supply, N. R. C (2003) Dioxins and dioxin-like compounds in the food supply: strategies to decrease exposure. National Academy Press, Washington, DC

Ding T, McConaha M et al (2011) Developmental dioxin exposure of either parent is associated with an increased risk of preterm birth in adult mice. Reprod Toxicol 31(3):351–358

Durando M, Kass L et al (2007) Prenatal bisphenol A exposure induces preneoplastic lesions in the mammary gland in Wistar rats. Environ Health Perspect 115(1):80–86

Ebner K, Brewster DW et al (1988) Effects of 2,3,7,8-tetrachlorodibenzo-p-dioxin on serum insulin and glucose levels in the rabbit. J Environ Sci Health B 23(5):427–438

Ema M, Itami T et al (1992a) Embryolethality and teratogenicity of butyl benzyl phthalate in rats. J Appl Toxicol 12(3):179–183

Ema M, Itami T et al (1992b) Teratogenic evaluation of butyl benzyl phthalate in rats by gastric intubation. Toxicol Lett 61(1):1–7

Ema M, Miyawaki E et al (2003) Decreased anogenital distance and increased incidence of undescended testes in fetuses of rats given monobenzyl phthalate, a major metabolite of butyl benzyl phthalate. Reprod Toxicol 17(4):407–412

European Commission (2005) Directive 2005/84/EC of the European Parliament and of the Council of 14 December 2005. Official J Eur Union 344:40–43

Fenton SE, Hamm JT et al (2002) Persistent abnormalities in the rat mammary gland following gestational and lactational exposure to 2,3,7,8-tetrachlorodibenzo-p-dioxin (TCDD). Toxicol Sci 67(1):63–74

Giatromanolaki A, Koukourakis MI et al (2004) BNIP3 expression is linked with hypoxia-regulated protein expression and with poor prognosis in non-small cell lung cancer. Clin Cancer Res 10(16):5566–5571

Gorski JR, Weber LW et al (1988) Tissue-specific alterations of de novo fatty acid synthesis in 2,3,7,8-tetrachlorodibenzo-p-dioxin (TCDD)-treated rats. Arch Toxicol 62(2–3):146–151

Gray LE Jr, Ostby JS (1995) In utero 2,3,7,8-tetrachlorodibenzo-p-dioxin (TCDD) alters reproductive morphology and function in female rat offspring. Toxicol Appl Pharmacol 133(2):285–294

Gray LE Jr, Ostby J et al (2000) Perinatal exposure to the phthalates DEHP, BBP, and DINP, but not DEP, DMP, or DOTP, alters sexual differentiation of the male rat. Toxicol Sci 58(2):350–365

Guerrero PF (1994) U.S. General Accounting Office, “Toxic Substances Control Act: EPA’s Limited Progress in Regulating Toxic Chemicals,” testimony at hearings before the Senate Subcommittee on Toxic Substances, Research and Development, GAO/T-RCED-94-212

Hilakivi-Clarke L, Cho E et al (2001) Maternal and prepubertal diet, mammary development and breast cancer risk. J Nutr 131(1):154S–157S

IARC (1997) Polychlorinated dibenzo-para-dioxins and polychlorinated dibenzofurans. IARC monographs on the evaluation of carcinogenic risks to humans. W. H. Organization. Lyon, France, International Agency for Research on Cancer. IARC Monogr Eval Carcinog Risks Hum 69:1–666

Ikezuki Y, Tsutsumi O et al (2002) Determination of bisphenol A concentrations in human biological fluids reveals significant early prenatal exposure. Hum Reprod 17(11):2839–2841

IPCS (1999) Concise International Chemical Assessment Document 17 – butyl benzyl phthalate. World Health Organization, Geneva
Jenkins S, Rowell C et al (2007) Prenatal TCDD exposure predisposes for mammary cancer in rats. Reprod Toxicol 23(3):391–396
Jenkins S, Raghuraman N et al (2009) Oral exposure to bisphenol a increases dimethylbenzanthracene-induced mammary cancer in rats. Environ Health Perspect 117(6):910–915
Jensen UB, Sunde L et al (2010) Mismatch repair defective breast cancer in the hereditary nonpolyposis colorectal cancer syndrome. Breast Cancer Res Treat 120(3):777–782
Juuti A, Louhimo J et al (2006) Cyclooxygenase-2 expression correlates with poor prognosis in pancreatic cancer. J Clin Pathol 59(4):382–386
Kern PA, Said S et al (2004) Insulin sensitivity following agent orange exposure in Vietnam veterans with high blood levels of 2,3,7,8-tetrachlorodibenzo-p-dioxin. J Clin Endocrinol Metab 89(9):4665–4672
Krcova Z, Ehrmann J et al (2008) Tpl-2/Cot and COX-2 in breast cancer. Biomed Pap Med Fac Univ Palacky Olomouc Czech Repub 152(1):21–25
Kuruto-Niwa R, Tateoka Y et al (2007) Measurement of bisphenol A concentrations in human colostrum. Chemosphere 66(6):1160–1164
Lamartiniere CA (2002) Timing of exposure and mammary cancer risk. J Mammary Gland Biol Neoplasia 7(1):67–76
Maffini MV, Rubin BS et al (2006) Endocrine disruptors and reproductive health: the case of bisphenol-A. Mol Cell Endocrinol 254–255:179–186
Markey CM, Luque EH et al (2001) In utero exposure to bisphenol A alters the development and tissue organization of the mouse mammary gland. Biol Reprod 65(4):1215–1223
Matsuzaka T, Shimano H (2009) Elovl6: a new player in fatty acid metabolism and insulin sensitivity. J Mol Med 87(4):379–384
Moral R, Wang R et al (2007) The plasticizer butyl benzyl phthalate induces genomic changes in rat mammary gland after neonatal/prepubertal exposure. BMC Genomics 8:453
Moral R, Wang R et al (2008) Effect of prenatal exposure to the endocrine disruptor bisphenol A on mammary gland morphology and gene expression signature. J Endocrinol 196(1):101–112
Munoz-de-Toro M, Markey CM et al (2005) Perinatal exposure to bisphenol-A alters peripubertal mammary gland development in mice. Endocrinology 146(9):4138–4147
Murray TJ, Maffini MV et al (2007) Induction of mammary gland ductal hyperplasias and carcinoma in situ following fetal bisphenol A exposure. Reprod Toxicol 23(3):383–390
Nagasawa H, Yanai R et al (1974) Effect of neonatally administered estrogen or prolactin on normal and neoplastic mammary growth and serum estradiol-17 beta level in rats. Cancer Res 34(10):2643–2646
Nayyar T, Bruner-Tran KL et al (2007) Developmental exposure of mice to TCDD elicits a similar uterine phenotype in adult animals as observed in women with endometriosis. Reprod Toxicol 23(3):326–336
Oka K, Tanaka T et al (2010) DNA damage signaling is activated during cancer progression in human colorectal carcinoma. Cancer Biol Ther 9(3):246–252
Panel V, Boelle PY et al (2006) Cytoplasmic phospholipase A2 expression in human colon adenocarcinoma is correlated with cyclooxygenase-2 expression and contributes to prostaglandin E2 production. Cancer Lett 243(2):255–263
Piersma AH, Verhoef A et al (2000) Developmental toxicity of butyl benzyl phthalate in the rat using a multiple dose study design. Reprod Toxicol 14(5):417–425
Reddy BS, Rozati R et al (2006) Association of phthalate esters with endometriosis in Indian women. BJOG 113(5):515–520
Revich B, Aksel E et al (2001) Dioxin exposure and public health in Chapaevsk, Russia. Chemosphere 43(4–7):951–966
Rushmere NK, Knowlden JM et al (2004) Analysis of the level of mRNA expression of the membrane regulators of complement, CD59, CD55 and CD46, in breast cancer. Int J Cancer 108(6):930–936

Russo IH, Russo J (1978) Developmental stage of the rat mammary gland as determinant of its susceptibility to 7,12-dimethylbenz[a]anthracene. J Natl Cancer Inst 61(6):1439–1449
Russo IH, Russo J (1996) Mammary gland neoplasia in long-term rodent studies. Environ Health Perspect 104(9):938–967
Russo IH, Russo J (1998) Role of hormones in mammary cancer initiation and progression. J Mammary Gland Biol Neoplasia 3(1):49–61
Safe SH (1995) Modulation of gene expression and endocrine response pathways by 2,3,7,8-tetrachlorodibenzo-p-dioxin and related compounds. Pharmacol Ther 67(2):247–281
Shellabarger CJ, Soo VA (1973) Effects of neonatally administered sex steroids on 7,12-dimethylbenz(a)anthracene-induced mammary neoplasia in rats. Cancer Res 33(7):1567–1569
Shen C, Guo Z et al (2007) Association study between hypertension and A/G polymorphism at codon 637 of the transporter associated with antigen processing 1 gene. Hypertens Res 30(8):683–690
Snyder RW, Maness SC et al (2000) Metabolism and disposition of bisphenol A in female rats. Toxicol Appl Pharmacol 168(3):225–234
Sowter HM, Ferguson M et al (2003) Expression of the cell death genes BNip3 and NIX in ductal carcinoma in situ of the breast; correlation of BNip3 levels with necrosis and grade. J Pathol 201(4):573–580
Sun XF, Zhang H (2007) NFKB and NFKBI polymorphisms in relation to susceptibility of tumour and other diseases. Histol Histopathol 22(12):1387–1398
Swan SH, Main KM et al (2005) Decrease in anogenital distance among male infants with prenatal phthalate exposure. Environ Health Perspect 113(8):1056–1061
Tanaka M, Nakaya S et al (2006) Effect of prenatal exposure to bisphenol A on the serum testosterone concentration of rats at birth. Hum Exp Toxicol 25(7):369–373
U.S. Department of Health and Human Services (2005) Report on carcinogens, 11th edn. U.S. Department of Health and Human Services, Public Health Service, National Toxicology Program, Washington, DC
Weber LW, Lebofsky M et al (1991a) Key enzymes of gluconeogenesis are dose-dependently reduced in 2,3,7,8-tetrachlorodibenzo-p-dioxin (TCDD)-treated rats. Arch Toxicol 65(2):119–123
Weber LW, Lebofsky M et al (1991b) Reduced activities of key enzymes of gluconeogenesis as possible cause of acute toxicity of 2,3,7,8-tetrachlorodibenzo-p-dioxin (TCDD) in rats. Toxicology 66(2):133–144
Weiss J, Papke O et al (2003) Concentrations of dioxins and other organochlorines (PCBs, DDTs, HCHs) in human milk from Seveso, Milan and a Lombardian rural area in Italy: a study performed 25 years after the heavy dioxin exposure in Seveso. Acta Paediatr 92(4):467–472
Welshons WV, Nagel SC et al (2006) Large effects from small exposures. III. Endocrine mechanisms mediating effects of bisphenol A at levels of human exposure. Endocrinology 147(6 suppl):S56–S69
Wissmann C, Wild PJ et al (2003) WIF1, a component of the Wnt pathway, is down-regulated in prostate, breast, lung, and bladder cancer. J Pathol 201(2):204–212
Yang XY, Ren CP et al (2005) Identification of differentially expressed genes in metastatic and non-metastatic nasopharyngeal carcinoma cells by suppression subtractive hybridization. Cell Oncol 27(4):215–223
Zhou MI, Foy RL et al (2005) Jade-1, a candidate renal tumor suppressor that promotes apoptosis. Proc Natl Acad Sci U S A 102(31):11035–11040
Zhou Q, Effati R et al (2008) Genomic changes of the 55 kDa subunit of DNA polymerase epsilon in human breast cancer. Cancer Genomics Proteomics 5(5):287–292

Chapter 6
Proteomic Basis for the Increased Susceptibility of the Mammary Gland to Carcinogenesis After Perinatal Exposure to Bisphenol A

Sarah Jenkins, Angela M. Betancourt, Jun Wang, James A. Mobley, and Coral A. Lamartiniere

Abstract Bisphenol A (BPA) is a compound used to produce a myriad of popular consumer goods, such as food and beverage containers, the lacquer lining of canned food, infant formula bottles, and some dental sealants. Recent studies have shown BPA to leach from these products in appreciable amounts, resulting in nearly ubiquitous exposure to humans. In this chapter, we review two key studies performed in our laboratory which investigate the ability of early life exposure to BPA to alter susceptibility to mammary cancer during adulthood. Prepubertal exposure to BPA (2–20 days of age only) increased mammary carcinogenesis and altered cell proliferation and apoptosis in the mammary gland in a classical model of chemically induced rodent mammary carcinogenesis (dimethylbenz(a)anthracene [DMBA] administered at 50 days of age). However, prenatal exposure to BPA (gestational days 10–21) failed to significantly alter tumorigenesis. However, genomic and proteomic data indicated that 100 days of age, as opposed to 50 days of age, represented a time in which the mammary gland had the most changes to gene and protein expressions. Accordingly, when the DMBA was administered at 100 days of age, prenatal BPA significantly altered mammary tumorigenesis.

However, purely descriptive studies of chemical carcinogens do little to further our understanding into the molecular functions underpinning these deleterious effects. Thus, using prenatal exposure to BPA as a model, we utilized discovery proteomics technology in order to identify novel targets of the latent molecular action of BPA. Using bioinformatics software, these novel protein identifications allowed us to perform targeted analysis of the activation and expression of interconnected, downstream

C.A. Lamartiniere (✉)
Department of Pharmacology and Toxicology, University of Alabama at Birmingham, University Blvd, Volker Hall L-106D, Birmingham, AL 35294, USA

Division of Urology, Department of Surgery, University of Alabama at Birmingham, Birmingham, AL 35294, USA
e-mail: coral@uab.edu

J. Russo (ed.), *Environment and Breast Cancer*, DOI 10.1007/978-1-4419-9896-5_6,

signaling pathways. These studies suggest potential adverse health effects to low concentrations of exposure during early life exist. Further, our work emphasizes the emerging role of new technology, such as proteomics, in prompting hypothesis-generating research which can be utilized in deciphering the molecular mechanisms causing these deleterious effects.

Keywords Bisphenol A • Mammary cancer • Proteomics

6.1 Environmental Contaminants and Breast Cancer Development

Breast cancer etiology attributed to hereditary causes is low, only accounting for an estimated 5–15% of all diagnosed cases (American Cancer Society 2009). This is suggestive of other causative factors being involved. Extrinsic factors, such as the environment, diet, and lifestyle, therefore, may play substantial roles in the high incidence of breast cancer. The myriad of chemical contaminants present in the environment represents one potentially contributing factor. One specific group of environmental chemicals, termed endocrine disruptors, is capable of altering endocrine signaling. Because normal endocrine signaling, especially that of the sex steroid hormones, has been shown to play a vital role in the development and progression of breast cancer, chemicals found to disrupt these signaling pathways may present the most obvious threat. For this reason, environmental contaminants with endocrine disrupting properties are currently being scrutinized for their potential role in breast cancer causation and progression.

One of the best known examples of an environmental endocrine disruptor influencing the development of human pathology is found in the case of the synthetic estrogen, diethylstilbestrol (DES). Women were prescribed DES from 1947 until 1971 to prevent spontaneous abortions. However, not only was the drug therapeutically ineffective in reducing the incidence of miscarriages, but research has revealed other, unintended side effects. Women exposed *in utero* to DES have shown an increased incidence of a rare type of vaginal cancer during adolescence (Herbst et al. 1999). As this population of women prenatally exposed to DES has aged, it has become increasingly apparent that they are also more susceptible to developing breast cancer than their unexposed, age-matched counterparts. Indeed, a recent study found that DES-exposed women greater than 40 years of age exhibited a significant increase in the relative risk of developing breast cancer (Palmer et al. 2006). This increased susceptibility toward developing breast cancer was even more pronounced in prenatally DES-exposed women older than 50 years of age, though the small sample size limited statistical significance (Palmer et al. 2006). Importantly, these effects, occurring more than a decade after the original exposure, have caused greater public awareness of the role that early life exposure to endocrine disruptors can play in lifetime breast cancer risk. Likewise, recent media attention has focused on another common environmental contaminant, Bisphenol A (BPA), as a potentially harmful agent due to its classification as an endocrine disruptor and its widespread exposure to humans. This has led to extensive research into the potential adverse health effects elicited by early life BPA exposure and the molecular origin of these latent actions in the mammary gland.

6.2 Bisphenol A: The Widespread Environmental Contaminant

6.2.1 Human Exposure to Bisphenol A

BPA is a synthetically made chemical used in the production of polycarbonate plastics and epoxy resins. These products are used to manufacture a plethora of commonly used consumer goods, such as plastic food and beverage containers, the lacquer lining of canned foods and drinks, infant formula bottles, office water coolers, laboratory supplies, intravenous tubing, and some dental sealants, among other uses. The primary route of human exposure is believed to occur through the oral route due to the leaching of BPA from incomplete polymerization or polymer bond degradation. Detectable concentrations of BPA have been found to leach from canned fruits, vegetables, and meat products, condensed and infant formula milk, canned sodas and juice, infant formula bottles, cardboard milk and juice containers, plastic food wrap, and polycarbonate plastic food and beverage containers (Brede et al. 2003; Joskow et al. 2006; Kang et al. 2003; Kang and Kondo 2002; Lopez-Cervantes and Paseiro-Losada 2003; Lopez-Espinosa et al. 2007; Munguia-Lopez et al. 2005; Olea et al. 1996; Thomson and Grounds 2005; Yoshida et al. 2001). As such, the scope of BPA exposure in the general public extends far beyond that of DES. Indeed, BPA has been routinely detected in human biofluids and tissues, including urine, serum, maternal and fetal plasma, amniotic fluid, breast milk and colostrum, mammary adipose tissue, and placental tissue (Ikezuki et al. 2002; Schonfelder et al. 2002; Takeuchi and Tsutsumi 2002). In the United States, studies have consistently reported that greater than 90% of the populations under study have detectable concentrations of BPA metabolites in the urine, indicating widespread exposure (Calafat et al. 2005, 2008; Wolff et al. 2007). However, it is the detection of BPA in biofluids and tissues accessible to the developing fetus and infant which present a special concern, as limited hepatic capacity for BPA metabolism exists in early life.

6.2.2 The Effects of Early Life Exposure to Bisphenol A In Vivo

A number of studies have linked early life exposure to low concentrations of BPA with a host of reproductive and developmental abnormalities in both sexes (reviewed in Richter et al. 2007). BPA has been shown to alter body weight (BW), fat composition and distribution, estrous cyclicity, oogenesis, the timing of puberty, behavior (aggression, hyperactivity, learning, etc.), and circulating levels of lipids and leptin, among other effects (Richter et al. 2007). Early exposure to BPA has been shown to increase the susceptibility of male rodents to prostate cancer, decrease serum testosterone concentrations, and increase prostate gland weights (Akingbemi et al. 2004; Gupta 2000; Ho et al. 2006; Kawai et al. 2003; Nagel et al. 1997; Prins et al. 2008; Timms et al. 2005). A number of effects have also been reported on metabolism, including alterations in blood glucose homeostasis and cellular glucose uptake (Alonso-Magdalena et al. 2006; Sakurai et al. 2004).

Because the mammary gland is a complex organ whose development spans from *in utero* to adulthood, it was hypothesized that early life exposure to BPA may alter normal patterns of development or induce pathology. Indeed, several studies have found effects of BPA related specifically to the mammary gland. Perinatal exposure to 250 ng BPA/kg BW per day through a subcutaneously implanted pump was observed to cause significant alterations in the mammary glands, including increased number of terminal end buds (TEBs), decreased index of apoptosis in the TEBs, increased percentage of cells expressing the progesterone receptor in the mammary gland, and increased mammary gland ductal tree branching (Munoz-de-Toro et al. 2005). With gestational exposure alone, BPA has been reported to increase the number of terminal ducts, TEBs, alveolar buds, and preneoplastic lesions in the mammary gland (Markey et al. 2001; Murray et al. 2007). Further, Durando et al. (2007) have shown that prenatal exposure to BPA (via subcutaneously implanted osmotic pumps) coupled to a subcarcinogenic dose of *N*-nitroso-*N*-methylurea (NMU) (Durando et al. 2007) resulted in an increased incidence of preneoplastic lesions in the mammary gland. However, despite this, the actual molecular actions of BPA that initiate these alterations remain largely unknown.

6.3 Proteomics as a Method to Determine Complex and Novel Mechanisms of Action

6.3.1 Introduction to Proteomics

The use of traditional laboratory techniques, such as immunoblotting and immunohistochemical staining, in attempts to elucidate novel pathways altered by pathological states or chemical exposure can largely result in unsuccessful guesswork. This approach tends to rely solely on logical, familiar, and previously identified protein signaling pathways, thus limiting its usefulness in identifying novel regulated pathways. The use of relatively new, high throughput technologies, such as genomic and proteomic screening tools, has become an attractive alternatives. Broadly, these tools allow one to determine global changes in mRNA or protein expression for use in hypothesis generating research. While genomic tools provide a more developed, standardized methodology, it is undercut by the lack of consistency in mRNA expression predicting protein expression. For this reason, we have recently explored proteomic technologies.

6.3.2 *Two-Dimensional Gel Electrophoresis*

Since its advent in the 1970s, two-dimensional (2D) gel electrophoresis has been one of the most utilized methods for multidimensional protein fractionation. Two-dimensional gel electrophoresis functions by harnessing the chemical and structural differences inherent in proteins, namely the isoelectric point and molecular weight. Beginning from a crude protein mixture derived from lysed cells or whole tissue, proteins are absorbed, passively or actively, into dehydrated immobilized pH gradient (IPG) strips. The first dimension, termed isoelectric focusing, causes the protein mixture to separate according to each individual protein's isoelectric point, the pH at which a protein becomes electrically neutral. Briefly, proteins not at their designated isoelectric point along the pH gradient are charged. The application of an electrical current to the IPG strips causes the charged proteins to migrate along the pH gradient until they arrive at their specific isoelectric point. The focused IPG strips are then coupled to polyacrylamide gels, and the proteins are separated in a second dimension according to molecular weight. The resultant gel is populated with distinct protein spots that are visualized using various stains, such as SyproRuby and Silver Stain. Gel images are converted into digital images using laser scanners, and these gels are compared using computer software.

Software programs align and match protein spots between gels, making it possible to detect changes in protein expression and/or shifts in placement (due to degradation, posttranslational modifications, etc.). Statistical analysis identifies differentially regulated spots of interest, which are manually excised and subjected to trypsin digestion. Utilizing mass spectrometry, these peptides are used for protein identification. Thus, coupling 2D gels with mass spectrometry allows for a robust and well-developed method for the global analysis of a large subsection of the proteome. This method can be used to identify novel pathways of altered protein expression for a given set of cells or whole tissues. Indeed, we have previously used this method to successfully determine changes in protein expression patterns in the mammary gland that can serve as possible biomarkers. This has included identifying novel pathways altered by environmental or dietary xenoestrogen exposure (Betancourt et al. 2010a; Rowell et al. 2005). For this reason, we utilized 2D gel electrophoresis and mass spectrometry in order to identify novel alterations in protein expression in the mammary gland caused by early life exposure to BPA.

6.4 The Case of Early Bisphenol A Exposure

Given the complexity of mammary gland development, we first investigated whether early life exposure to BPA could alter mammary cancer susceptibility in the well-established model of mammary cancer, dimethylbenz(a)anthracene (DMBA)-induced carcinogenesis in Sprague Dawley rats (Betancourt et al. 2010b; Jenkins et al. 2009). This modeling system provides an acceptable method of inducing mammary carcinogenesis in an animal model that closely mimics human mammary gland development (Russo and Russo 1978). Furthermore, in order to mimic human exposure we chose to administer BPA through the oral route only, since that is the primary route by which humans are exposed to BPA. We selected two discrete early life exposure schemes to investigate the effects of BPA on two potentially critical windows of mammary gland development, prenatal and early postnatal life. The following sections describe our efforts to determine the carcinogenic properties of early life BPA exposure in an *in vivo* model system and the application of proteomics and traditional immunologic lab techniques to aid in identifying novel protein alterations.

6.4.1 Prepubertal Exposure of Rats to Bisphenol A

We first examined the impact of BPA exposure during the prepubertal period, which for our purpose was defined as the time frame shortly following birth (2 days of age) until weaning (21 days of age) (Jenkins et al. 2009). Briefly, female Sprague Dawley rats were bred and allowed to give birth. Beginning on 2 days of age and continuing through 20 days of age, the lactating dam of each litter was intragastrically gavaged with 0 or 250 μg BPA/kg BW per day. This exposure protocol resulted in an indirect, oral exposure of the offspring to BPA through the dam's milk. At 21 days of age, the female offspring were weaned from the lactating dam, thus concluding the window of BPA exposure. It is worth emphasizing that while we continued to monitor these rats postpubertally, they were exposed to BPA during the prepubertal (2–20 days of age) period only.

These animals were sacrificed at select time points in order to determine and differentiate between direct and latent effects of BPA exposure. For this reason, we selected time points of 21 days of age (immediately following BPA treatment) and 50 days of age (~4 weeks following the last BPA treatment). Interestingly, no direct effects were observed for any of the end points investigated, such as protein expression and indices of cell proliferation and apoptosis, in the mammary glands of 21-day old rats (Jenkins et al. 2009). However, latent effects were observed. At 50 days of age, 4 weeks after discontinuing BPA treatment, we observed a significantly increased proportion of cells undergoing cell proliferation in the mammary glands of rodents prepubertally exposed to BPA (Fig. 6.1) (Jenkins et al. 2009). This was coupled to a significant decrease in the proportion of cells undergoing apoptosis in the mammary glands of rats prepubertally exposed to BPA (Fig. 6.1). When these two indices were combined to produce a cell proliferation-to-apoptosis ratio, prepubertal exposure to BPA resulted in a ratio that was twofold greater than the ratio of control-treated rodents.

Using the traditional DMBA model of rodent mammary carcinogenesis, exposure to BPA during the prepubertal period followed by 30 mg DMBA/kg BW at 50 days of age resulted in increased carcinogenesis during adulthood (Jenkins et al. 2009).

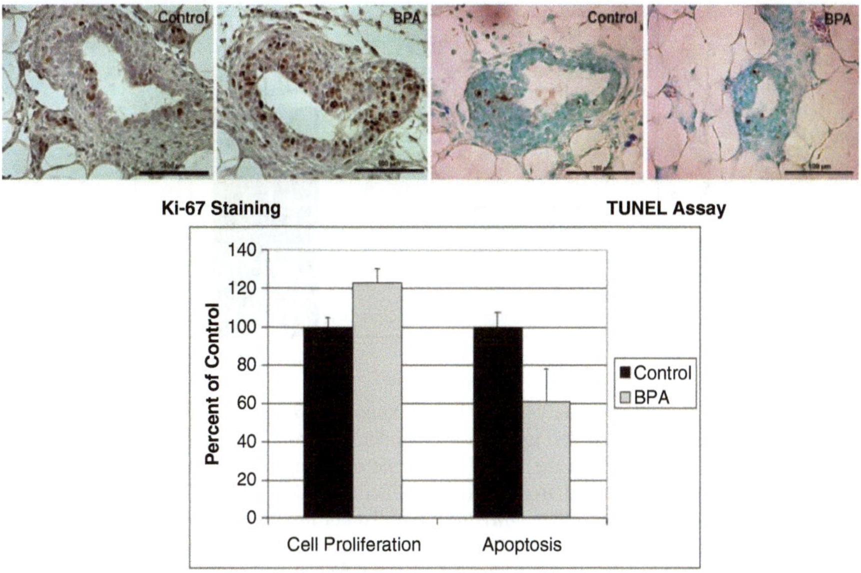

Proliferation			
Treatment (n)	**Stained**	**Not Stained**	**p-value**
Control (5)	432 (13.00%)	2890	<0.001
BPA (5)	526 (16.98%)	2572	
Apoptosis			
Treatment (n)	**Stained**	**Not Stained**	**p-value**
Control (5)	107 (2.52%)	4136	0.001
BPA (5)	95 (1.60%)	5851	

Fig. 6.1 Cell proliferation and apoptosis in mammary glands of 50 day old rats exposed lactationally to dams treated with 250 mg Bisphenol A (BPA)/kg BW per day. The upper panel depicts Ki-67 expression as an indicator of cell proliferation and the TUNEL assay as measure of apoptosis. Terminal end buds from five biologically distinct samples ($n=5$) were analyzed per treatment. The graph illustrates mean index values ± SEM as a percent of the control group. The resulting numbers were used to construct a contingency table. All images were taken at 40× magnification. The scale bar represents 100 mm. Adapted from Jenkins et al. (2009)

This caused a significant increase in the average number of tumors per rat, with prepubertal BPA exposure increasing the average number of tumors by nearly two-fold (Fig. 6.2). Latency (time-to-first-tumor formation) was also significantly reduced by prepubertal BPA treatment. These data provided the first evidence that maternal exposure to BPA during lactation (prepubertal period) decreased tumor latency and increased mammary tumor multiplicity in the female offspring (Jenkins et al. 2009). We concluded that increased cell proliferation and decreased apoptosis indices in the mammary gland at the time of DMBA administration play a vital role in the latent adverse effects caused by prepubertal BPA exposure.

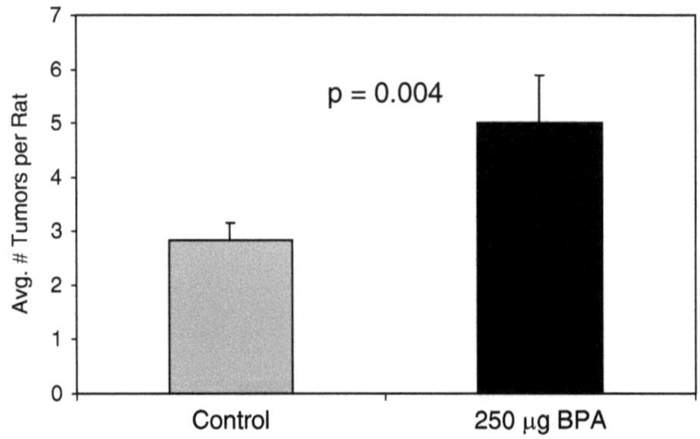

Fig. 6.2 DMBA-induced mammary tumors in rats exposed lactationally to Bisphenol A. Lactating dams were gavaged with 0 or 250 μg BPA/kg BW per day from days 2 through 20 postpartum (Monday–Friday only). There were 32 and 24 female offspring in the control- and BPA-treated groups, respectively, all derived from individual litters. At day 50, all female offspring were gavaged with a single dose of 30 mg DMBA/kg BW. Tumor multiplicity data ware analyzed with the GENMOD procedures in SAS using Poisson regression on the tumor appearance rates. *p*-Values are provided for mean number ± SEM of tumors per rat. *p*-Values greater than or equal to 0.05 were considered significant. Adapted from Jenkins et al. (2009)

6.4.2 Prenatal Exposure of Rats to Bisphenol A

The initial formation of the mammary gland begins in mid- to late-gestation. For this reason, we also investigated whether exposure to BPA during *in utero* development could alter later life mammary gland development and cancer susceptibility (Betancourt et al. 2010b). For this series of experiments, timed pregnant Sprague Dawley rats were intragastrically gavaged with 0 or 250 μg BPA/kg BW during mid- to late-gestation, from gestational days 10 through 21. In this manner, the developing offspring were exposed indirectly to BPA during organogenesis. Following birth, the female offspring were evaluated for alterations in BW, the onset of puberty, patterns of estrous cyclicity, and the circulating concentrations of estradiol-17β and progesterone (Betancourt et al. 2010b). No significant alterations in early or adult BWs were observed. Likewise, no significant differences were found in the onset of puberty, estrous cyclicity, or in the circulating concentrations of estradiol-17β or progesterone. When prenatal exposure to BPA was coupled to the traditional DMBA model of rodent mammary carcinogenesis (wherein DMBA is administered at 50 days of age), no significant effects on tumorigenesis were observed. There were no significant changes in tumor incidence, tumor latency (median time to tumor onset), multiplicity (average number of tumors per rat), or the grade of the developing tumors (Betancourt et al. 2010b). However, we had previously observed that prenatal exposure to BPA (in the absence of DMBA) resulted in a greater disruption to gene expression in the mammary gland of female rats at 100 days of age than at 50 days of age. For this reason, we investigated whether this age-dependent disruption to mRNA expression in the mammary gland translated to differences in the susceptibility of the mammary gland to carcinogenesis at 100 days of age (Moral et al. 2008; Betancourt et al. 2010b).

Female Sprague Dawley rats were prenatally exposed to BPA as previously described. However, instead of administering DMBA on 50 days of age, as in the previous tumorigenesis studies described here, DMBA was administered (30 mg DMBA/kg BW) at 100 days of age. The timeline to palpable tumor onset and multiplicity was recorded. Upon necropsy, tumors were excised to confirm incidence and paraffin blocked for histopathological grading. When prenatal exposure to BPA was followed by DMBA administration at 100 days of age, mammary carcinogenesis was significantly increased (Betancourt et al. 2010b). This was unlike the lack of significant differences observed when prenatal BPA exposure was paired to the traditional model of chemically induced carcinogenesis wherein DMBA was administered at 50 days of age. Tumor incidence was significantly increased from a 54% incidence in control-treated rats to an 83% increase for BPA-treated females (Fig. 6.3a) (Betancourt et al. 2010b). Prenatal BPA exposure caused a stark and significant reduction in tumor latency (time-to-first tumor development), with BPA treatment accelerating the median time to development by 78 days (Fig. 6.3b). Furthermore, prenatal exposure to BPA trended toward increased tumor multiplicity and significantly increased the grade of tumors that developed (Fig. 6.3c, d). Thus, in a model of chemically induced mammary carcinogenesis, prenatal exposure to BPA shifted the window of mammary cancer susceptibility and increased mammary carcinogenesis.

While direct comparisons cannot be made between the results of the prenatal and prepubertal BPA tumorigenesis studies, it seems as if BPA exposure occurring during the prenatal window results in the greatest changes for mammary cancer susceptibility. For this reason, we selected the prenatal BPA exposure protocol for further investigation into the molecular mechanisms responsible for increased mammary cancer susceptibility.

6.4.3 Proteomics

In order to gain insight into the molecular mechanisms responsible for prenatal BPA exposure predisposing rodents for chemically induced mammary carcinogenesis, we used 2D gel electrophoresis and mass spectrometry to identify novel protein targets of BPA action. We focused our attention at 50 and 100 days of age because these ages are the most relevant to our tumorigenesis studies involving prenatal BPA exposure in a model of chemically induced mammary cancer. For these studies, whole mammary glands were homogenized and prepared for 2D gel electrophoresis. The resultant gels were scanned and analyzed as previously described (Fig. 6.4) (Betancourt et al. 2010a). Prenatal exposure to BPA resulted in the identification of 13 unique proteins being differentially regulated in the mammary gland at 50 and 100 days of age (Tables 6.1 and 6.2).

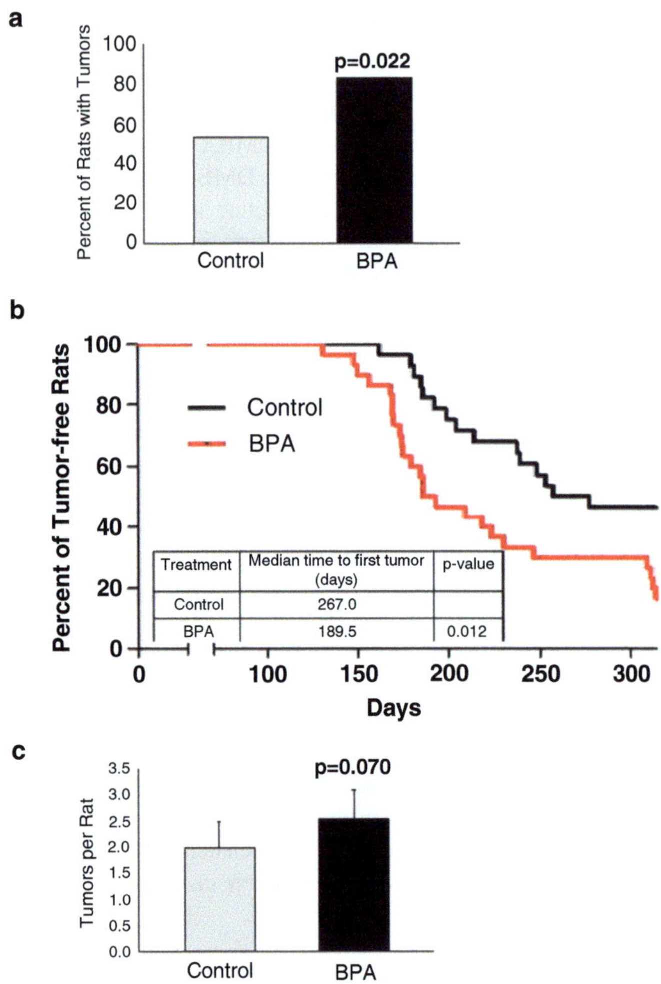

d

Treatment	Tumor Grade			Percent of Grade II Tumors
	0	1	2	
Control	14	10	3	23%
BPA	10	11	9	45%*

Fig. 6.3 Chemically induced mammary tumorigenesis in adult rats exposed prenatally to Bisphenol A. (**a**) Tumor incidence (proportion of rats that developed at least one tumor), (**b**) Kaplan-Meier survival curve with median time (days) to first tumor development, (**c**) tumor multiplicity (number of tumors per rat), and (**d**) tumor grade in adult female rats whose mothers were exposed prenatally to 0 or 250 μg BPA/kg body weight (BW) per day. The 100-day old female offspring were subsequently gavaged with a single dose of 30 mg DMBA/kg BW. Adapted from Betancourt et al. (2010b)

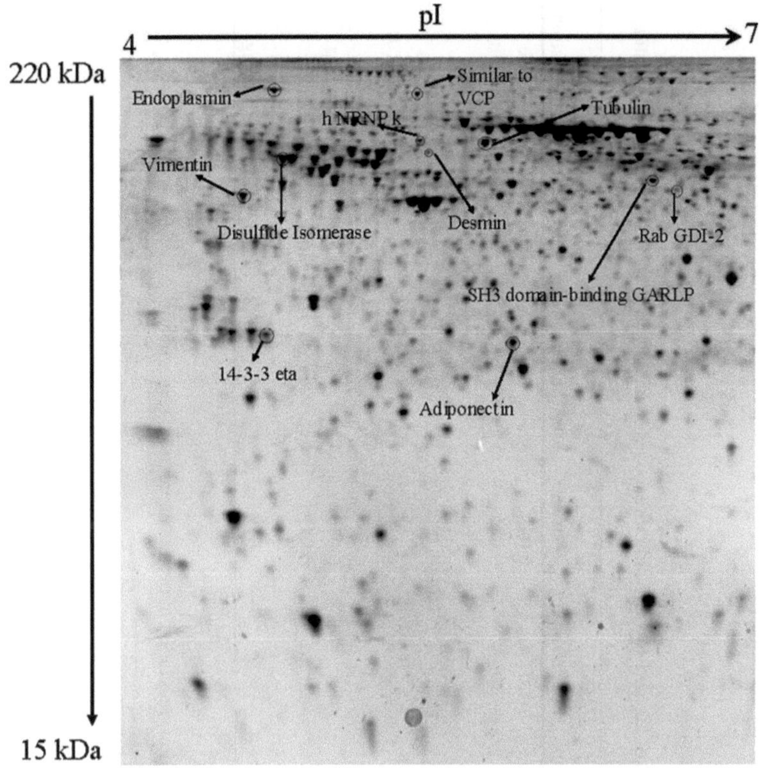

Fig. 6.4 Representative proteomic profile of postnatal rat mammary glands after prenatal exposure to BPA. 2-DE was performed on 150 μg of protein using 18 cm isoelectric focusing strips with a pH range of 4–7 in the first dimension and SDS-PAGE (12.5% polyacrylamide) in the second dimension. The gel was stained with SYPRO Ruby protein stain. Protein spots that were differentially regulated were analyzed with SameSpots software and identified by either MALDI-TOF-TOF or LC-MS/MS analysis. Adapted from Betancourt et al. (2010a)

Some of the proteins identified as being regulated by 2D gel electrophoresis, such as heat shock cognate 71 kDa protein, have been previously identified as potential targets of BPA (Papaconstantinou et al. 2001). However, the majority of the proteins identified were novel, previously unreported potential targets of BPA's actions (Betancourt et al. 2010a). In order to solidify the robustness of this initial discovery technique, we performed immunoblotting for a subset of these proteins using a separate set of identically treated rodents. This provided an independent method of validating differentially regulated protein identifications obtained via 2D gel electrophoresis. Our efforts focused on proteins which were reported to play key roles in mammary gland development and/or cancer pathology and for which we were able to obtain commercially available antibodies. Two of the proteins identified by 2D gel electrophoresis and mass spectrometry that were found to be significantly different in abundance following prenatal exposure to BPA were vimentin and 14-3-3 protein eta. These were validated by immunoblotting as being differentially regulated (Fig. 6.5) (Betancourt et al. 2010a).

Table 6.1 List of differentially expressed proteins from mammary glands of 50- and 100-day old rats exposed prenatally to BPA and sesame oil as identified by MALDI-TOF/TOF analysis

ID no.	Protein identification	Accession no.	Mascot score	Sequence coverage[a]	Fold change[b]	p-Value	MW (kDa)[c]	Age	pI[d]	Molecular function
1	Aldose reductase	P07943	148	43	−2.0	0.040	36	50	6.3	Oxidoreductase
2	Alpha 1B-glycoprotein	P04217	189	18	−2.6	0.025	57	50	7.0	Immunoglobulin receptor
3	Heat shock cognate 71 kDa protein	P19378	194	34	1.3	0.035	71	50	5.1	Chaperone
4	Peroxiredoxin-2	Q61171	184	35	1.2	0.042	22	50	5.1	Oxidoreductase/ peroxidase
5	Actin, cytoplasmic 1	P60710	152	36	−1.5	0.043	42	100	5.2	Protein binding
6	Creatine kinase B type	Q04447	261	42	−3.1	0.042	43	100	6.5	Kinase/protein binding
7	Hemopexin precursor	P02790	123	25	1.8	0.032	52	100	6.5	Iron ion binding

Adapted from Betancourt et al. (2010a, b)

[a]Percent of identified sequence of the known protein

[b]Positive and negative fold change in protein expression indicates up- and downregulation of protein expression, respectively

[c]Molecular weight of the matching protein in kDa

[d]Isoelectric point of the matching protein

Table 6.2 List of differentially expressed proteins from mammary glands of 50- and 100-day old rats exposed prenatally to BPA and sesame oil as identified by LC-MS/MS analysis

ID no.	Protein identification	Accession no.	Xcorr score	Matching peptides[a]	Fold change[b]	*p*-Value	MW (kDa)[c]	Age	pI[d]	Molecular function
8	Fibrinogen gamma	Q8VCM7	4.2	4	−1.4	0.033	40	50	5.6	Protein binding
9	SPARC	P07214	3.4	3	−1.8	0.032	35	50	4.7	Extracellular matrix binding
10	ATP synthase subunit delta	Q9D3D9	5.0	2	−1.7	0.022	17	50	6.5	Hydrogen transporter
11	Coronin 1A	O89053	3.29	2	−2.3	0.025	51	100	6.2	Actin-binding protein
12	14-3-3 eta	P68510	4.8	3	1.9	0.012	28	100	4.7	Protein domain specific binding
13	Vimentin	P20152	4.3	5	1.8	0.035	54	100	4.9	Structural protein/protein binding

Adapted from Betancourt et al. (2010a, b)

[a]Number of matching peptides

[b]Positive and negative fold change in protein expression indicates up- and downregulation of protein expression, respectively

[c]Molecular weight of the matching protein in kDa

[d]Isoelectric point of the matching protein

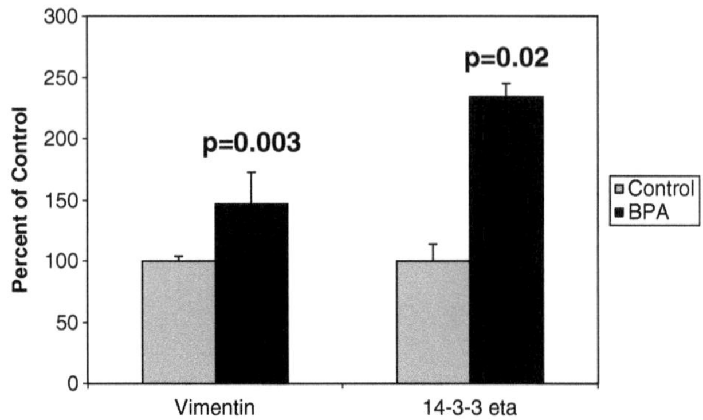

Fig. 6.5 Western blot analysis of vimentin and 14-3-3 eta in the mammary glands of 100-day old rats exposed prenatally to 250 μg BPA/kg BW or an equal volume of sesame oil. Quantitation is reported as percentage of control. Densitometry values for controls were set to 100. Value represents mean density ± SEM as a percent of the control group. $N = 6–8$ per group. Statistical significance was defined as a p-value ≤ 0.05. Adapted from Betancourt et al. (2010a)

Vimentin is a structural cytoskeletal protein that belongs to a family of intermediate filaments. In cancer, vimentin expression is associated with a dedifferentiated malignant phenotype, increased motility and invasiveness, drug resistance, and poor clinical outcome (Heatley et al. 1997; Sommers et al. 1994). An important process involved in the development of breast cancer is the concomitant loss of epithelial phenotype while gaining a mesenchymal phenotype. During development, the cell's intermediate filament status changes from a keratin-rich network to a vimentin-rich network in the epithelial-to-mesenchymal transition. At 100 days of age, we found significantly increased protein expression of vimentin. This change suggests the possibility of prenatal BPA inducing an epithelial-to-mesenchymal transition. This change is consistent with cancer development, a conjecture supported by vimentin expression being upregulated in breast cancer cells (Sousa et al. 2010).

14-3-3 is a family of highly conserved proteins (alpha, beta, delta, sigma, epsilon, eta, and zeta) expressed in all eukaryotic cells. These proteins play a crucial role in regulating multiple cellular processes, including the maintenance of cell cycle checkpoints and DNA repair, the onset of cell differentiation and senescence, and the coordination of cell adhesion and motility. For this reason, disruption of normal expression patterns of 14-3-3 could contribute to a pathological phenotype. Indeed, prenatal BPA exposure increased the expression of 14-3-3 eta in the mammary glands of 100-day old rats. This increase in protein expression suggests that the actions of 14-3-3, specifically 14-3-3 eta, could be playing a role in BPA causing increased susceptibility for mammary cancer.

Using bioinformatics data performed on the collective group of differentially regulated proteins identified by 2D gel electrophoresis, we began targeted investigations into highlighted protein signaling pathways which are known to play roles in the development of cancer, epithelial-to-mesenchymal transition, signal transduction, cell proliferation, and cell motility. These types of proteins are historically absent from 2D gels because they are present in low abundance or are too hydrophobic for solubilization. These proteins include the growth factor receptors, epithelial growth factor receptor (EGFR), erbB2, and insulin-like growth factor 1 (IGF-1) receptor, and downstream proteins involved in the Akt and Ras signaling pathways.

Via immunoblots, we began with the EGFR family of receptor tyrosine kinases as this pathway was identified as being highly connected to the proteins (including Vimentin and 14-3-3), which we found to be differentially regulated by 2D gel electrophoresis. The EGFR (erbB1/HER1) is one member of a closely related family of receptor tyrosine kinases which includes erbB2 (nu/HER2), erbB3 (HER3), and erbB4 (HER4). Except for erbB2, which has no known ligand and exists in a constitutively active conformation, ligand binding to the EGFR family of receptor tyrosine kinases induces activation via the generation of homo- or heterodimers. In the activated form, these proteins function as the initiating kinase in several different protein signaling cascades which control global cell activities such as DNA synthesis, cell proliferation, and apoptosis (DiAugustine et al. 1997; Boonstra et al. 1995). For this reason, the overexpression of several of these family members has been associated with a number of cancers, especially breast cancer. Overexpression of EGFR and erbB2 occurs in approximately 50 and 15–30% of all breast cancer cases, respectively, and is generally associated with an unfavorable outcome.

Another protein tyrosine kinase closely linked to breast cancer is the IGF-1 receptor. The IGF-1 receptor has been reported to cross-talk with both EGFR (erbB1/HER1) and erbB2 (nu/HER2) (Jones et al. 2004). It has been reported to play roles in the formation of cancer, the development of chemoresistance, insulin signaling, and the aging process (reviewed in Jones et al. 2004; Santen et al. 2009; Frasca et al. 2008; Chitnis et al. 2008; Richardson et al. 2004; Narasimhan et al. 2009). Specific to the mammary gland, the IGF-1 receptor has been shown to play important roles in mammary gland development, differentiation, and in the development of carcinogenesis (reviewed in Jones and Moorehead 2008).

The Akt pathway represents one of the major signaling pathways modulated by the EGFR, erbB2, and IGF-1 receptor. These growth factor receptors function by phosphorylating, and thus activating, Akt. Phosphorylation of Akt is associated with a loss of cell adhesion, a decrease in cell-matrix adhesion, a loss of apicobasolateral cell polarization, and induction of cell motility (Bellacosa et al. 2005; Grille et al. 2003). The Akt pathway is also capable of feeding into the Ras signaling pathway through the activation (phosphorylation) of c-Raf.

The Raf-1 protein functions in the mitogen-activated protein kinases (MAPK) signal transduction pathway as part of a protein kinase cascade, functioning downstream of the Ras family of membrane-associated GTPases (Downward 2003). The terminal result of this pathway causes the activation (phosphorylation) of the extracellular signal-regulated kinases (ERKs). Activated ERKs, ERK 1 and ERK 2, are pleiotropic effectors of cell physiology which play an important role in the control of gene expression involved in the cell cycle, apoptosis, differentiation, and migration (Betancourt et al. 2010a). They function by regulating the activities of several transcription factors that are involved in cell proliferation.

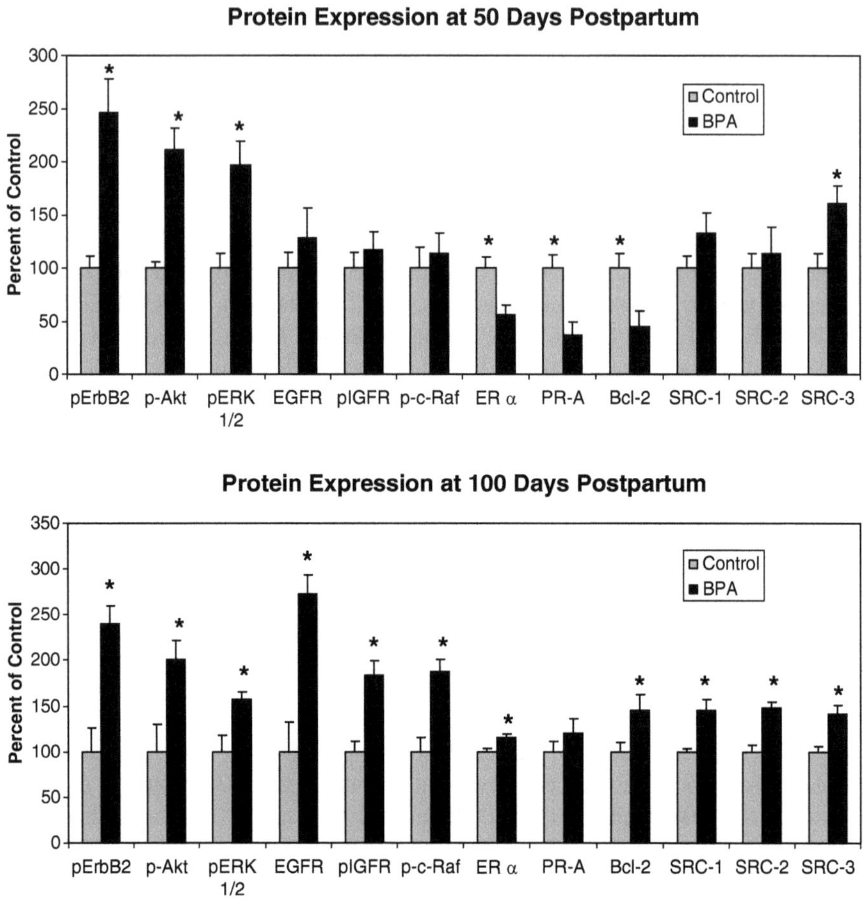

Fig. 6.6 Western blot analysis of phospho-erbB2, phospho-Akt, phospho-ERKs 1/2, EGF receptor, phospho-IGF-1 receptor, phospho-c-Raf, ER alpha, PR-A, Bcl-2, SRC-1, SRC-2, and SRC-3 in mammary glands of 50 and 100 day old rats exposed prenatally to 250 μg BPA/kg BW or an equal volume of sesame oil (controls). Quantitation is reported as percentage change from control. Densitometry values for controls were set to 100. Values represent mean density ± SEM as a percent of the control group. $n = 6$–8 samples per group. *Asterisk* indicates statistically significant difference in detected protein abundance compared to corresponding controls ($p < 0.05$). Adapted from Betancourt et al. (2010b)

Investigating these signaling pathways at both 50 and 100 days of age following prenatal exposure to BPA, we found that phospho-erbB2, phospho-Akt, phospho-ERK 1, and phospho-ERK 2 were upregulated at both 50 and 100 days of age (Fig. 6.6). Further investigation showed that EGFR, phospho-c-Raf, and phospho-IGF-1 receptor were upregulated in mammary glands of 100, but not 50, day old rats prenatally exposed to BPA (Fig. 6.6) (Betancourt et al. 2010b). As noted above, all three of these proteins have been reported to play a role in cell proliferation and could account for the shift in susceptibility to chemically induced mammary cancer. This illustrates that while downstream proteins, such as c-Raf, ERK 1, and ERK 2, were also upregulated at 50 days of age, a greater number of growth factor receptors and downstream targets were upregulated or phosphorylated at 100 days of age by prenatal exposure to BPA (Betancourt et al. 2010a, b).

We also found that prenatal BPA exposure upregulated the expression of estrogen receptor alpha (ER α) at 100 days of age and downregulated it at 50 days of age (Fig. 6.6) (Betancourt et al. 2010b). Since ER regulates the expression of several genes and corresponding proteins, including progesterone receptor A (PR-A) and Bcl-2, we investigated their expression. The expression of downstream targets of ER (PR-A and Bcl-2) in the mammary glands on 50 and 100 days of age followed a similar expression pattern to ER at each age (Fig. 6.6) (Betancourt et al. 2010b). This suggests that ER may play an active role in increased tumorigenesis caused by prenatal BPA exposure. This becomes a concern because DMBA-induced mammary cancer in rats is initially estrogen dependent. Greater expression of ER α at the age of carcinogen administration in this model could lead to an increased opportunity for carcinogenesis. The steroid receptor coactivators, which primarily function to mediate the transcriptional function of nuclear receptors, were all upregulated at 100 days of age (Fig. 6.6) (Betancourt et al. 2010b). This is in contrast to 50 days of age, where only SRC-3 was significantly upregulated (Betancourt et al. 2010b). This demonstrates how the ontology of ER alpha and the sex steroid coregulator expression changed and may explain the shift in the window of mammary cancer susceptibility.

Our results, using a combination of proteomics and traditional laboratory immunotechniques, provide a plausible mechanism of action of how prenatal BPA exposure could alter protein signaling pathways in the mammary gland which in turn could contribute to an increased susceptibility for mammary cancer. In response to prenatal exposure to BPA, initial alterations in proteins such as vimentin and 14-3-3 could lead to alterations to cellular architecture and increased expression and/or activation of the EGFR, erbB2, and IGF-1 receptor. These receptors can then initiate the signaling cascade by activating several downstream proteins, such as c-Raf and Akt. In the case of c-Raf, increased activation could lead to increased phosphorylation of the MAPK, ERK 1 and ERK 2. These activated kinases can be imported into the nucleus where they phosphorylate specific transcription factors involved in cell proliferation.

Further, there is an intriguing link between the steroid coregulators and growth factor signaling. While steroid receptor coregulators have been reported to directly influence steroid receptor action, they have also been suggested to serve as transcription factors that can directly enhance steroid-mediated gene transcription by regulating growth factor signaling. Because we found increased expression and/or activation of several growth factor receptors, ER α, and all three members of the p160 steroid receptor coregulator (SRC) family, this could translate to an increased ability for SRC and growth factor receptor cross talk. Future research is needed to confirm this conjecture. Taken together with our tumorigenesis data, these data suggest that while mild disturbances do exist at 50 days of age after prenatal BPA exposure, it is not until 100 days of age that prenatal BPA exposure induces widespread alterations in the expression and activation of proteins known to play vital roles in mammary carcinogenesis.

6.5 Serum Biomarkers of Xenoestrogen Exposure

6.5.1 Introduction to Serum Biomarkers of Exposure

While proteomic technologies often allow researchers to identify novel mechanisms by which biological processes occur, additional applications include the growing need to identify disease-related biomarkers. Ideally, biomarkers of exposure and susceptibility should utilize noninvasive or minimally invasive sample sources and accurately and reproducibly identify susceptible/effected individuals through the use of a panel of differentially abundant molecules. As the data presented above suggest, early life exposure to BPA has the ability to increase mammary cancer susceptibility later in life. Thus, it is our goal to establish a quantitative approach to biomarker discovery that is of sufficient sensitivity to detect BPA-induced alterations in the serum.

The nature of blood makes it poorly suited for the same type of sample preparation and separation platform used in assessing the mammary gland proteome. An extensive dynamic range present in the circulating serum necessitates a more thorough enrichment step. We have opted to use Seppro IgY spin columns, which depletes the top seven highest expression proteins from serum. While this does lessen the dynamic range of protein expression in serum, a large dynamic range still persists. The application of 2D gel electrophoresis combined with even the most sensitive of stains (ex. Sypro Ruby and Cy dyes) would not be adequate to fully explore the depth of the serum proteome. In order to delve deeper into low abundance proteins, we have implemented a multifaceted approach based on peptide tagging with isobaric labels using tandem mass tag (TMT) technology coupled with multidimensional protein identification technology (MudPIT).

The TMT chemistry that we show here is a six-plex isobaric mass tagging system. Isobaric mass tagging enables stoichiometric labeling of complex protein extracts for global "relative" quantification and identification by tandem mass spectrometry. Each TMT has a unique mass and reports sample-specific abundance of a labeled peptide during MS/MS analysis. Each tag is composed of three elements: (1) a protein reactive group, (2) a mass normalizer group, and (3) a mass reporter. The protein reactive group, an amine-reactive NHS-ester group, provides high-efficiency amine-specific labeling of proteins and peptides. The mass normalizer differs from tag to tag; it functions as a balance to the mass reporter, ensuring that each of the mass tags in the six-plex set has the same overall mass. This method of multiplex peptide labeling allows for the comparison of six different samples by their differing signature mass peaks.

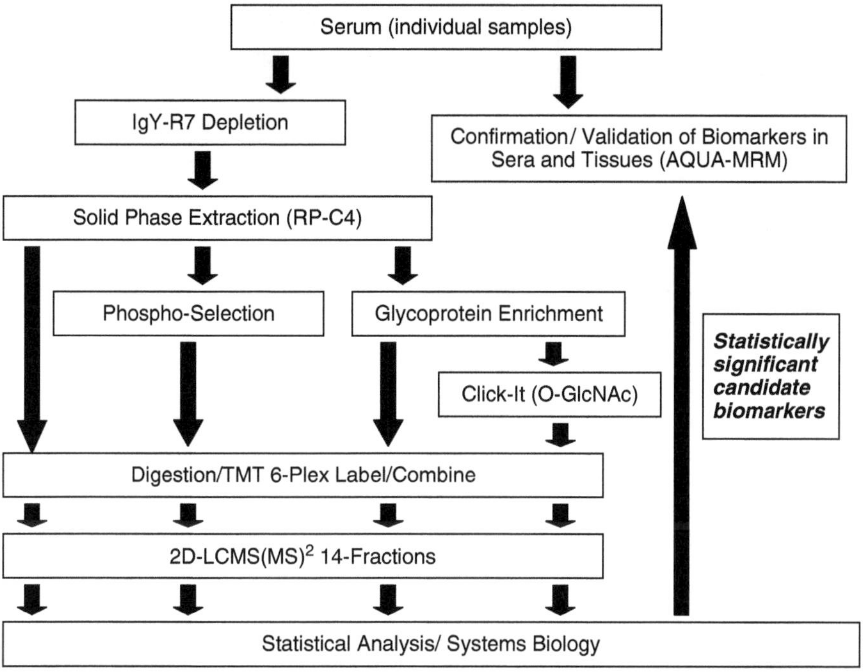

Fig. 6.7 Schematic of sample processing for serum proteomics and confirmation/validation in both sera and tissue. Low abundance proteins are enriched by depleting the top seven highest expressed proteins and selecting for phospho- and glycoproteins. After protein digestion and peptide labeling utilizing the TMT 6-plex labeling system, peptides are analyzed using 2D-LCMS(MS)^2

6.5.2 Preliminary Data and Future Directions

We have completed preliminary studies to establish rigorous parameters of use. An in-depth protocol is shown in Fig. 6.7. Rat sera were pooled, and six 100 μL aliquots were depleted of the seven most abundant serologic proteins as described in the previous section. To test the limit of detection and dynamic range of our methods, purified bovine lactoferrin was added in duplicate (12, 60, and 300 ng/100 μg of depleted rat sera). Each sample was digested, labeled with a unique isobaric tag, and analyzed by 2D LC-ESI-MS/MS (Fig. 6.8a). The resultant data were analyzed with SEQUEST and BioInquire's ProteoIQ software. The reproducibility, limit of detection, and dynamic range were calculated based on the internal bovine lactoferrin controls. As shown in Fig. 6.8b, the 2D LC-ESI-MS/MS analysis of the TMT-labeled samples yielded a concentration-dependent lactoferrin profile, and the lowest concentration of 12 ng/100 μg sample was reproducibly detected.

Our preliminary studies using rat serum show that we were able to identify 3,032 peptides, 774 of which were unique peptides. There were 282 unique protein

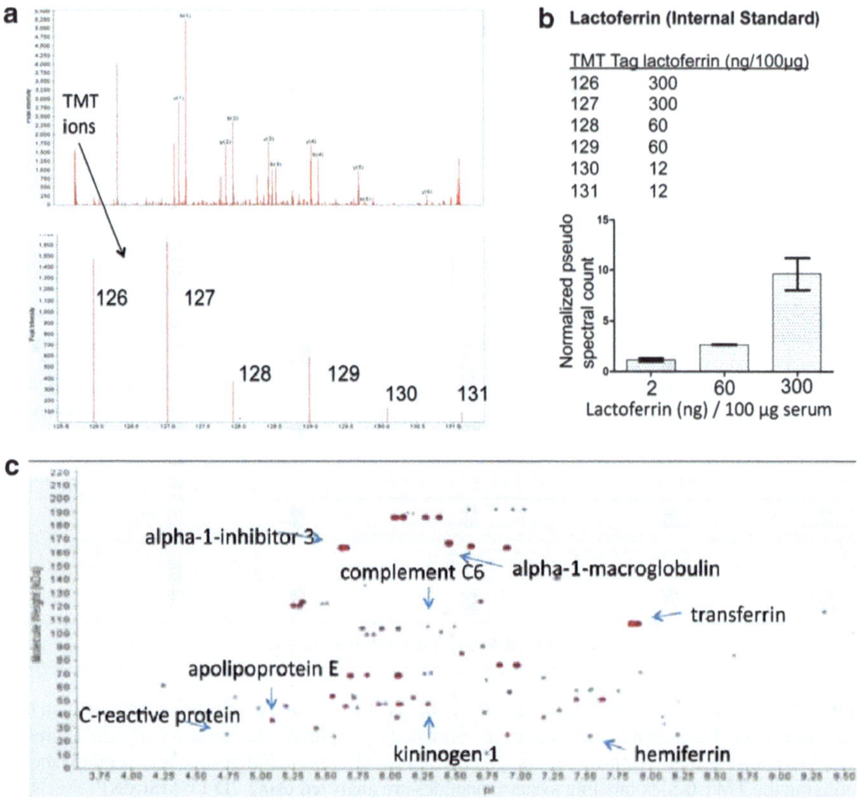

Fig. 6.8 The reproducibility, limit of detection, and dynamic range were calculated based on the internal bovine lactabumin controls. (**a**) To test the limit of detection and dynamic range of 2D LC-ESI-MS/MS, purified bovine lactoferrin was added in duplicate (12, 60, and 300 ng/100 μg of depleted rat sera). Each sample was digested, labeled with a unique isobaric tag, and analyzed by 2D LC-ESI-MS/MS. (**b**) The 2D LC-ESI-MS/MS analysis of the TMT-labeled samples yielded a concentration-dependent lactoferrin profile, and the lowest concentration of 12 ng/100 μg sample was reproducibly detected. (**c**) The in silico generated 2D gel plot of the 87 proteins quantified with high confidence after a 2D LC-ESI-MS run

groups identified, and 126 proteins had more than one unique peptide identified. The number of proteins with unique peptides carrying more than one quantifiable mass tag was 87. Figure 6.8c illustrates the in silico generated 2D view of the proteins from our preliminary studies as identified after a 2D LC-ESI-MS run. Collectively, these data validate this method to quantify serum proteins that may serve as biomarkers of chemical carcinogen exposure. Future work will focus on applying this technology to both rodents and humans in order to identify biomarkers of exposure and susceptibility using an array of environmental chemicals.

6.6 Conclusions

In summary, these studies demonstrate the ability of prenatal and prepubertal exposures to BPA to predispose for chemically induced mammary cancer at 100 and 50 days, respectively. Through discovery proteomics we were able to identify novel putative targets of the latent detrimental effects of perinatal BPA exposures. These novel protein identifications allowed us to perform targeted analysis of downstream signaling transduction pathways that may have been otherwise ignored. While these are purely descriptive studies at this point and differential regulation of proteins does not necessarily imply impaired functionality, these proteins represent novel findings that may provide new directions for determining how the deleterious actions of BPA are mediated. This work demonstrates the value of proteomics in identifying novel protein signaling pathways altered in the mammary gland following early life exposure to environmental chemicals.

Acknowledgments This work was supported by NCI/NIEHS Grants 1UO1 ES012771 and 1UO1 ES016003. SJ is supported through a Department of Defense Pre-Doctoral Traineeship in Breast Cancer Research (W81XWH-08-0777) and has been supported via a stipend from the National Cancer Institute predoctoral fellowship, Cancer Prevention and Control Training Program (R25 CA47888), University of Alabama at Birmingham.

References

Akingbemi BT et al (2004) Inhibition of testicular steroidogenesis by the xenoestrogen Bisphenol A is associated with reduced pituitary luteinizing hormone secretion and decreased steroidogenic enzyme gene expression in rat Leydig cells. Endocrinology 145(2):592–603

Alonso-Magdalena P et al (2006) The estrogenic effect of Bisphenol A disrupts pancreatic beta-cell function in vivo and induces insulin resistance. Environ Health Perspect 114(1):106–112

American Cancer Society (2009) Cancer facts and figures. p 1–72

Bellacosa A et al (2005) Activation of AKT kinases in cancer: implications for therapeutic targeting. Adv Cancer Res 94:29–86

Betancourt AM, Eltoum IA, Desmond RA, Russo J, Lamartiniere CA (2010a) In utero exposure to Bisphenol A shifts the window of susceptibility for mammary carcinogenesis in the rat. Environ Health Perspect 118(11):1614–1619

Betancourt AM, Mobley JA, Russo J, Lamartiniere CA (2010b) Proteomic analysis in mammary glands of rat offspring exposed in utero to Bisphenol A. J Proteomics 73(6):1241–1253

Boonstra J et al (1995) The epidermal growth factor. Cell Biol Int 19(5):413–430

Brede C et al (2003) Increased migration levels of Bisphenol A from polycarbonate baby bottles after dishwashing, boiling and brushing. Food Addit Contam 20(7):684–689

Calafat AM et al (2005) Urinary concentrations of Bisphenol A and 4-nonylphenol in a human reference population. Environ Health Perspect 113(4):391–395

Calafat AM et al (2008) Exposure of the U.S. population to Bisphenol A and 4-tertiary-octylphenol: 2003–2004. Environ Health Perspect 116(1):39–44

Chitnis MM et al (2008) The type 1 insulin-like growth factor receptor pathway. Clin Cancer Res 14(20):6364–6370

DiAugustine RP, Richards RG, Sebastian J (1997) EGF-related peptides and their receptors in mammary gland development. J Mammary Gland Biol Neoplasia 2(2):109–117
Downward J (2003) Targeting RAS signalling pathways in cancer therapy. Nat Rev Cancer 3(1):11–22
Durando M et al (2007) Prenatal Bisphenol A exposure induces preneoplastic lesions in the mammary gland in Wistar rats. Environ Health Perspect 115(1):80–86
Frasca F et al (2008) The role of insulin receptors and IGF-I receptors in cancer and other diseases. Arch Physiol Biochem 114(1):23–37
Grille SJ et al (2003) The protein kinase Akt induces epithelial mesenchymal transition and promotes enhanced motility and invasiveness of squamous cell carcinoma lines. Cancer Res 63(9):2172–2178
Gupta C (2000) Reproductive malformation of the male offspring following maternal exposure to estrogenic chemicals. Proc Soc Exp Biol Med 224(2):61–68
Heatley M et al (1997) Intermediate filament expression of ductal carcinoma cells in fine needle aspirates of the breast. Acta Cytol 41(3):717–720
Herbst AL et al (1999) Adenocarcinoma of the vagina. Association of maternal stilbestrol therapy with tumor appearance in young women. 1971. Am J Obstet Gynecol 181(6):1574–1575
Ho SM et al (2006) Developmental exposure to estradiol and Bisphenol A increases susceptibility to prostate carcinogenesis and epigenetically regulates phosphodiesterase type 4 variant 4. Cancer Res 66(11):5624–5632
Ikezuki Y et al (2002) Determination of Bisphenol A concentrations in human biological fluids reveals significant early prenatal exposure. Hum Reprod 17(11):2839–2841
Jenkins S et al (2009) Oral exposure to Bisphenol a increases dimethylbenzanthracene-induced mammary cancer in rats. Environ Health Perspect 117(6):910–915
Jones RA, Moorehead RA (2008) The impact of transgenic IGF-IR overexpression on mammary development and tumorigenesis. J Mammary Gland Biol Neoplasia 13(4):407–413
Jones HE et al (2004) Insulin-like growth factor-I receptor signalling and acquired resistance to gefitinib (ZD1839; Iressa) in human breast and prostate cancer cells. Endocr Relat Cancer 11(4):793–814
Joskow R et al (2006) Exposure to Bisphenol A from bis-glycidyl dimethacrylate-based dental sealants. J Am Dent Assoc 137(3):353–362
Kang JH, Kondo F (2002) Bisphenol A migration from cans containing coffee and caffeine. Food Addit Contam 19(9):886–890
Kang JH, Kito K, Kondo F (2003) Factors influencing the migration of Bisphenol A from cans. J Food Prot 66(8):1444–1447
Kawai K et al (2003) Aggressive behavior and serum testosterone concentration during the maturation process of male mice: the effects of fetal exposure to Bisphenol A. Environ Health Perspect 111(2):175–178
Lopez-Cervantes J, Paseiro-Losada P (2003) Determination of Bisphenol A in, and its migration from, PVC stretch film used for food packaging. Food Addit Contam 20(6):596–606
Lopez-Espinosa MJ et al (2007) Oestrogenicity of paper and cardboard extracts used as food containers. Food Addit Contam 24(1):95–102
Markey CM et al (2001) In utero exposure to Bisphenol A alters the development and tissue organization of the mouse mammary gland. Biol Reprod 65(4):1215–1223
Moral R et al (2008) Effect of prenatal exposure to the endocrine disruptor Bisphenol A on mammary gland morphology and gene expression signature. J Endocrinol 196(1):101–112
Munguia-Lopez EM et al (2005) Migration of Bisphenol A (BPA) from can coatings into a fatty-food simulant and tuna fish. Food Addit Contam 22(9):892–898
Munoz-de-Toro M et al (2005) Perinatal exposure to bisphenol-A alters peripubertal mammary gland development in mice. Endocrinology 146(9):4138–4147
Murray TJ et al (2007) Induction of mammary gland ductal hyperplasias and carcinoma in situ following fetal Bisphenol A exposure. Reprod Toxicol 23(3):383–390
Nagel SC et al (1997) Relative binding affinity-serum modified access (RBA-SMA) assay predicts the relative in vivo bioactivity of the xenoestrogens Bisphenol A and octylphenol. Environ Health Perspect 105(1):70–76

Narasimhan SD, Yen K, Tissenbaum HA (2009) Converging pathways in lifespan regulation. Curr Biol 19(15):R657–R666
Olea N et al (1996) Estrogenicity of resin-based composites and sealants used in dentistry. Environ Health Perspect 104(3):298–305
Palmer JR et al (2006) Prenatal diethylstilbestrol exposure and risk of breast cancer. Cancer Epidemiol Biomarkers Prev 15(8):1509–1514
Papaconstantinou AD et al (2001) Effects of beta-estradiol and Bisphenol A on heat shock protein levels and localization in the mouse uterus are antagonized by the antiestrogen ICI 182,780. Toxicol Sci 63(2):173–180
Prins GS et al (2008) Developmental exposure to Bisphenol A increases prostate cancer susceptibility in adult rats: epigenetic mode of action is implicated. Fertil Steril 89(2 Suppl):e41
Richardson A et al (2004) The role of insulin and insulin-like growth factor-I in mammalian ageing. Best Pract Res Clin Endocrinol Metab 18(3):393–406
Richter CA et al (2007) In vivo effects of Bisphenol A in laboratory rodent studies. Reprod Toxicol 24(2):199–224
Rowell C, Carpenter M, Lamartiniere CA (2005) Modeling biological variability in 2-D gel proteomic carcinogenesis experiments. J Proteome Res 4(5):1619–1627
Russo IH, Russo J (1978) Developmental stage of the rat mammary gland as determinant of its susceptibility to 7,12-dimethylbenz[a]anthracene. J Natl Cancer Inst 61(6):1439–1449
Sakurai K et al (2004) Bisphenol A affects glucose transport in mouse 3T3-F442A adipocytes. Br J Pharmacol 141(2):209–214
Santen RJ et al (2009) Estrogen signals via an extra-nuclear pathway involving IGF-1R and EGFR in tamoxifen-sensitive and -resistant breast cancer cells. Steroids 74(7):586–594
Schonfelder G et al (2002) In utero exposure to low doses of Bisphenol A lead to long-term deleterious effects in the vagina. Neoplasia 4(2):98–102
Sommers CL et al (1994) Differentiation state and invasiveness of human breast cancer cell lines. Breast Cancer Res Treat 31(2–3):325–335
Sousa B et al (2010) P-cadherin, vimentin and CK14 for identification of basal-like phenotype in breast carcinomas: an immunohistochemical study. Histol Histopathol 25(8):963–974
Takeuchi T, Tsutsumi O (2002) Serum Bisphenol a concentrations showed gender differences, possibly linked to androgen levels. Biochem Biophys Res Commun 291(1):76–78
Thomson BM, Grounds PR (2005) Bisphenol A in canned foods in New Zealand: an exposure assessment. Food Addit Contam 22(1):65–72
Timms BG et al (2005) Estrogenic chemicals in plastic and oral contraceptives disrupt development of the fetal mouse prostate and urethra. Proc Natl Acad Sci U S A 102(19):7014–7019
Wolff MS et al (2007) Pilot study of urinary biomarkers of phytoestrogens, phthalates, and phenols in girls. Environ Health Perspect 115(1):116–121
Yoshida T et al (2001) Determination of Bisphenol A in canned vegetables and fruit by high performance liquid chromatography. Food Addit Contam 18(1):69–75

Chapter 7
Dioxin as an Environmental Pollutant and Its Role in Breast Cancer

Stephen Safe, Kelcey Walker, and Shu Zhang

Abstract 2,3,7,8-Tetrachlorodibenzo-*p*-dioxin (TCDD) and structurally related halogenated aromatics are environmental toxicants that bind and activate the aryl hydrocarbon receptor (AhR) complex. The effects of TCDD and other AhR agonists on mammary gland development and susceptibility to mammary tumor formation in rodent models are dependent on the rodent species/strain, dose and timing of exposure. In contrast, TCDD and selective AhR modulators (SAhRMs) inhibit mammary tumor and cell growth through a complex inhibitory AhR-estrogen receptor α (ERα) cross talk pathway involving multiple general and gene-specific mechanisms. SAhRMs are highly effective chemotherapeutic agents alone and in combination with tamoxifen as inhibitors of ER-positive mammary tumors and show promise as a new class of agents for treating ER-negative breast cancer.

Keywords TCDD • Halogenated aromatics • AhR • SAhRMs • Inhibitory AhR-ERα cross talk • Breast cancer

7.1 Background

Polychlorinated dibenzo-*p*-dioxins (PCDDs), dibenzofurans (PCDFs), and biphenyls (PCBs) are industrial compounds (PCBs) or by-products (Fig. 7.1) that have been widely identified in the environment. Because of their low water solubility and high lipophilicity, these halogenated aromatics (HAs) preferentially

S. Safe (✉)
Department of Veterinary Physiology and Pharmacology, Texas A&M University, 4466 TAMU, College Station, TX 77843-4466, USA

Institute of Biosciences and Technology, Texas A&M Health Sciences Center, 2121 W. Holcombe Blvd, Houston, TX 77030-3303, USA
e-mail: ssafe@cvm.tamu.edu

J. Russo (ed.), *Environment and Breast Cancer*, DOI 10.1007/978-1-4419-9896-5_7,

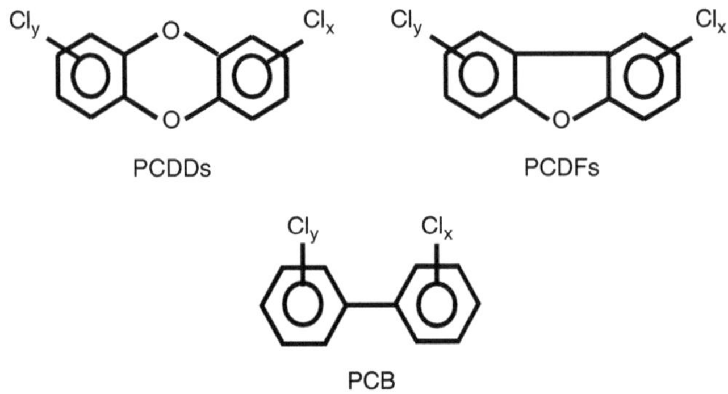

Fig. 7.1 PCDDs, PCDFs, and PCBs. Substitution patterns and the number of substituents are variable

bioaccumulate, and residues have been detected in fish, wildlife, and humans (Patterson et al. 2009; Schecter et al. 2010). There are 75, 135, and 209 possible PCDD, PCDF, and PCB congeners, respectively, and not surprisingly environmental extracts contain complex mixtures of these persistent organic pollutants (POPs). The composition of HAs in these mixtures is variable and dependent on local and regional input sources; however, most mixtures contain relatively higher levels of compounds containing >4 chlorine substituents since many of these congeners are lipophilic and resistant to breakdown in the environment and metabolism in biota. After the initial detection of PCBs in environmental samples, regulatory agencies have banned PCBs and imposed restrictions on emissions of PCDDs and PCDFs so that environmental levels of HAs have been decreasing. Nevertheless, PCBs, PCDDs, and PCDFs are still routinely detected in biota including fish, wildlife, and humans, and there are ongoing studies worldwide that are investigating correlations between exposures to POPs and the incidence of human diseases including cancer (Lee et al. 2007; Wang et al. 2008).

Risk assessment of HA mixtures is a scientific and regulatory challenge, and one approach has been to focus on a subset of these compounds, typified by 2,3,7,8-tetra chlorodibenzo-*p*-dioxin (TCDD, dioxin). TCDD is a by-product formed during the industrial production of the herbicide 2,4,5-trichlorophenoxy acetic acid (2,4,5-T), and initial studies demonstrated that this compound was highly toxic in some species (e.g., guinea pig) (Poland and Knutson 1982; Safe 1986). Subsequent studies have demonstrated that the toxicity of TCDD is age, sex, species, strain and tissue specific, and some of the commonly observed effects include chloracne, immunotoxicity, reproductive and developmental toxicity, hepatotoxicity and porphyria, and a wasting syndrome. TCDD caused hepatic adenocarcinomas in female but not male Sprague-Dawley rats in a lifetime feeding study (Kociba et al. 1978). However, since TCDD is not a genotoxicant, it is presumed that the carcinogenic effects of this compound are due to tumor promotion activity. TCDD also induces many biochemical responses including the induction of CYP1A1 which is observed in most target tissues and is a hallmark response to this compound (Whitlock et al. 1996).

Poland and coworkers first demonstrated that tritiated TCDD bound with high affinity to a mouse hepatic cytosolic protein called the aryl hydrocarbon receptor (AhR) which is widely expressed in most animal and human tissues (Poland et al. 1976; Wilson and Safe 1998). The AhR is a basic helix-loop-helix (b-HLH)/Per-Arnt-Sim (PAS) protein which acts as a ligand-induced transcription factor that forms a nuclear heterodimer with the AhR nuclear translocator (ARNT) protein (Gu et al. 2000). In response to TCDD, the bound nuclear AhR complex interacts with dioxin responsive elements (DREs) in target gene promoters, and after recruitment of other nuclear cofactors, there is an increase in gene transcription. Structure-activity studies among PCDDs, PCDFs, and PCBs identified a series of "TCDD-like" compounds that also bind the AhR and induce many of the same toxic and biochemical responses observed for TCDD but with lower potencies (Safe 1986, 1992). This observation led to the development of the toxic equivalency factor (TEF) and toxic/dioxin equivalent (TEQ) approach for risk assessment of "TCDD-like" AhR agonists that are components of environmental mixtures of HAs (Ahlborg et al. 1992; Van den Berg et al. 1998, 2006). The TEQ for any mixture is defined as follows:

$$\mathrm{TEQ} = \Sigma[\mathrm{PCDD}]_i(\mathrm{TEF})_i + \Sigma[\mathrm{PCDF}]_i(\mathrm{TEF})_i + \Sigma[\mathrm{PCB}]_i(\mathrm{TEF})_i,$$

where the TEQ of a mixture is the summation of its concentration of each individual (i) congener times its corresponding TEF value which has been assigned for all "TCDD-like" AhR agonists by a World Health Organization (WHO) panel of experts (Ahlborg et al. 1992; Van den Berg et al. 1998, 2006). Any discussion of the carcinogenicity or adverse health effects of "TCDD-like" HAs must include the family of compounds in a mixture represented by the TEQ value since TCDD is usually a minor component and a minor contributor to the TEQs of most environmental mixtures.

7.2 Effects of TCDD on the Rodent Mammary Gland and Mammary Cells

The effects of TCDD exposures on the mammary gland and the subsequent effects on gland development and susceptibility to breast cancer have primarily been investigated in rat and mouse models exposed to TCDD at specific time points (pre- and postnatal) and in immortalized MCF10A human mammary cells. Lawrence and coworkers focused on the effects of TCDD exposure during pregnancy on mammary gland differentiation (Vorderstrasse et al. 2004; Lew et al. 2009; Collins et al. 2009). Initial studies showed that exposure of pregnant C57BL/6 mice to TCDD (5 μg/kg) on days 0, 7, and 14 of pregnancy severely stunted mammary gland growth, impaired formation of tubular structures, and decreased branching. Hormone levels in the animals were minimally altered and, at this high dose of TCDD, all the pups were dead within 24 h after birth. The timing of exposure to TCDD modulated the effects of this compound which had a profound influence on mammary epithelial cell proliferation and differentiation; however, based on the high levels of exposure, it was unclear how these responses affected subsequent mammary tumor development in this animal model. Several studies demonstrated that in utero exposure to TCDD could significantly alter rodent mammary gland development in the female offspring and this was consistent with the effects of TCDD on several other hormone-dependent and -independent responses in males and females exposed in utero (Bjerke and Peterson 1994; Bjerke et al. 1994; Gray and Ostby 1995; Gray et al. 1997). Fenton et al. exposed pregnant Long Evans rats to 1 μg/kg TCDD on gestation day (GD) 15 and examined mammary gland development. Their results showed that mammary glands in the offspring exhibited decreased epithelial cell elongation, decreased primary branches, and fewer alveolar buds and, in mammary tissue transplant experiments, there was evidence for stroma as a major target for TCDD (Fenton et al. 2002). Moreover, results of timing studies showed that exposure to TCDD on GD15 resulted in more dramatic effects on mammary gland development than exposure on GD20 or postnatally. Lewis et al. (2001) used a similar approach with Holtzman rats and also observed impaired mammary gland differentiation; however, the in utero exposure to TCDD did not affect their responsiveness to 17β-estradiol (E2). Interestingly, female Holtzman rats exposed in utero to TCDD exhibited significantly higher expression of mammary gland ER, whereas in the adult or ovariectomized female rat or mouse and in human breast cancer cells, TCDD decreased estrogen receptor α (ERα) expression. In contrast, studies in female Sprague-Dawley rats gave results which were somewhat contradictory to those observed in either Holtzman or Long Evan rats (Brown et al. 1998; Jenkins et al. 2007). Female offspring of Sprague-Dawley rats exposed to 1 μg/kg of TCDD on GD15 did not exhibit alterations in mammary gland differentiation (21 days old) but increased the number of terminal end buds (TEBs). The increased TEBs in these animals were also associated with their higher susceptibility to DMBA-induced mammary tumor formation, and they concluded that TCDD may enhance breast cancer development through enhanced formation of TEBs. In the same Sprague-Dawley rat model, in utero exposure to TCDD did not affect mammary gland expression of ERα or ERβ in 50 day-old rats (Jenkins et al. 2007), whereas ERα expression was increased in offspring of Holtzman rats exposed to TCDD in utero. The differences between studies may be due to several factors; however, it is clear that in utero exposure to TCDD affects development of the mammary gland and this, in turn, modulates susceptibility to mammary tumor development.

3,3′,4,4′,5-Pentachlorobiphenyl (PCB126) binds the AhR and induces many of the same responses observed for TCDD but with a decreased potency (TEF=0.1). The effect of prenatal exposure of Sprague-Dawley rats to different doses of PCB126 (2.5, 250, and 7,500 μg/kg) on GD 13–19 have been investigated in the female offspring (Muto et al. 2002; Wakui et al. 2005, 2006). The effects on the mammary gland in 50-day-old offspring were dose dependent. Mammary gland hypoplasia was observed in the high dose (7,500 ng/kg) group. Differentiation of TEBs into alveolar bud and lobules was decreased in the 250 ng/kg group, and ERα levels were increased in all treatment groups (Muto et al. 2002). The incidence of DMBA-induced mammary tumors in the vehicle control (80%), 2.5 (84%), 250 (92%), and 7,500 (64%) μg/kg treatment groups indicated that at the high dose, there was a significant inhibition of percent incidence of mammary tumors compared to the vehicle control. The total number of mammary tumors was higher (82) and lower (41) in the 250 and 7,500 μg/kg treatment groups, respectively, compared to the vehicle control animals (53), whereas the 2.5 μg/kg dose group (58) was similar to the control. Moreover, in the time-course studies, the temporal development of tumors was similar to the number of tumors, demonstrating that in utero exposure to PCB126, a relatively potent AhR agonist, and subsequent development of DMBA-induced mammary tumors were dose dependent.

Several in vivo studies have demonstrated that TCDD and other AhR agonists exhibit antiestrogenic activity and inhibit mammary tumorigenesis (Kociba et al. 1978; Holcombe and Safe 1994; Tritscher et al. 1995). Dietary administration of TCDD (0.1, 0.01, and 0.001 μg/kg/day) to male and female Sprague-Dawley rats resulted in the formation of hepatocellular carcinomas in female but not male rats (Kociba et al. 1978). There was also evidence of increased levels of squamous cell carcinomas of the lung, tongue, hard palate/nasal turbinates; however, several spontaneous tumors decreased in the pituitary, pancreas, and adrenal gland. Moreover, there was a dose-dependent decrease in the incidence of estrogen-responsive uterine and mammary tumors which form spontaneously in older female Sprague-Dawley rats, and this demonstrates that TCDD exhibits antiestrogenic activity. Subsequent long-term feeding studies with TCDD in female Sprague-Dawley rats induced preneoplastic foci in liver; however, the incidence of spontaneous mammary tumors was decreased (Tritscher et al. 1995). Holcomb and coworkers investigated the effects of a single dose of TCDD (10 μg/kg) administered to female Sprague-Dawley rats on day 50 on DMBA-induced mammary tumor formation and growth where DMBA (20 mg) was administered on day 53 (Holcombe and Safe 1994). The experiment was terminated when the rats were 140 days old; 5/10 (50%) of the corn oil/DMBA-treated animals had developed mammary tumors, whereas only 1/10 (10%) of the TCDD/DMBA-treated rats developed tumors. Thus, there is evidence from studies in Sprague-Dawley rats that TCDD inhibits mammary tumor formation and exhibits antiestrogenic activity.

Studies on the in vitro effects of TCDD on "normal" human mammary cells have primarily been carried out in immortalized (but not transformed) MCF10A cells. Burchiel and coworkers (Tannheimer et al. 1998; Davis et al. 2000, 2001) examined the effects of TCDD and benzo[a]pyrene in MCF10A cells and their results suggest that the activation of the AhR by these ligands induces responses that may enhance mammary carcinogenesis. For example, TCDD activates the insulin-like growth factor signaling pathway in MCF10A cells maintained in insulin-deficient conditions, and in cells grown under insulin or epidermal growth factor-deficient media, TCDD induces cell recovery and inhibits apoptosis (Tannheimer et al. 1998; Davis et al. 2000). In a subsequent study, it was shown that TCDD also activates the epidermal growth factor receptor (EGFR) and induces apoptosis which may be due, in part, to induction of transforming growth factor α (TGFα), an EGFR ligand (Davis et al. 2001). Interestingly, TCDD also induces TGFα in ER-negative MDA-MB-468 breast cancer cells; however, in this cell line TGFα acts as a growth inhibitor (Wang et al. 1997a). Matsumura and coworkers (Mazina et al. 2004; Park et al. 2004; Dong and Matsumura 2008, 2009) also used MCF10A cells as a model for investigating the nongenomic pathways activated by TCDD. Their results indicate that TCDD activates cytosolic phospholipase A2 and Src kinase within 30 min and this results in the downstream activation of multiple activator protein 1 (AP-1) and CCAAT enhancer binding protein (CEBP)-dependent genes. Inhibitors of Src and PKA blocked the TCDD-induced response and similar inhibition was observed with an AhR antagonist. However, RNA interference in which AhR and ARNT were knocked down demonstrated that this nongenomic pathway was AhR dependent but ARNT independent, thus defining a novel TCDD-induced pathway that required only the AhR. These results are intriguing; however, their potential role in the development of mammary cancer requires further investigation.

In summary, there is evidence from both in vivo and in vitro studies that exposure to TCDD affects the mammary gland, and these effects in vivo are dependent on the timing of exposure in which TCDD can both inhibit and enhance mammary carcinogenesis. The role of TCDD alone, or in combination with other environmental contaminants and dietary components in breast cancer, is unclear and will require further investigation.

7.3 TCDD and Related Compounds as Antiestrogens

The antiestrogenic effects of TCDD in long-term feeding studies in Sprague Dawley rats (Kociba et al. 1978) suggested that ligand activation of the AhR may affect estrogen signaling and this was initially investigated in the rodent uterus (Gallo et al. 1986; Romkes et al. 1987; Astroff and Safe 1988, 1990; Romkes and Safe 1988; Umbreit et al. 1989; Astroff et al. 1990, 1991; Gierthy et al. 1993; Chen et al. 1998; Buchanan et al. 2000, 2002; McDougal 2000; Safe et al. 2001; Wu et al. 2003; Watanabe et al. 2004; Walker 2004; Boverhof et al. 2008). The estrogen-responsiveness of the mouse and rat uterus has been extensively investigated and, in the immature (noncycling) or ovariectomized rodent uterus, 17β-estradiol (E2) induces several highly characteristic responses and modulates expression of multiple genes. Microarray studies show that E2 modulates expression of several thousand genes which presumably contribute to the hormone-induced uterine phenotype (Wu et al. 2003; Watanabe et al. 2004; Boverhof et al. 2008). Initial studies in the rodent uterus demonstrated that TCDD inhibits multiple E2-induced responses including increased uterine wet weight, uterine epithelial mitogenesis, peroxidase activity, and several hormone-responsive genes including the EGFR, progesterone receptor, and c-fos (Gallo et al. 1986; Romkes et al. 1987; Astroff and Safe 1988, 1990; Romkes and Safe 1988; Umbreit et al. 1989;

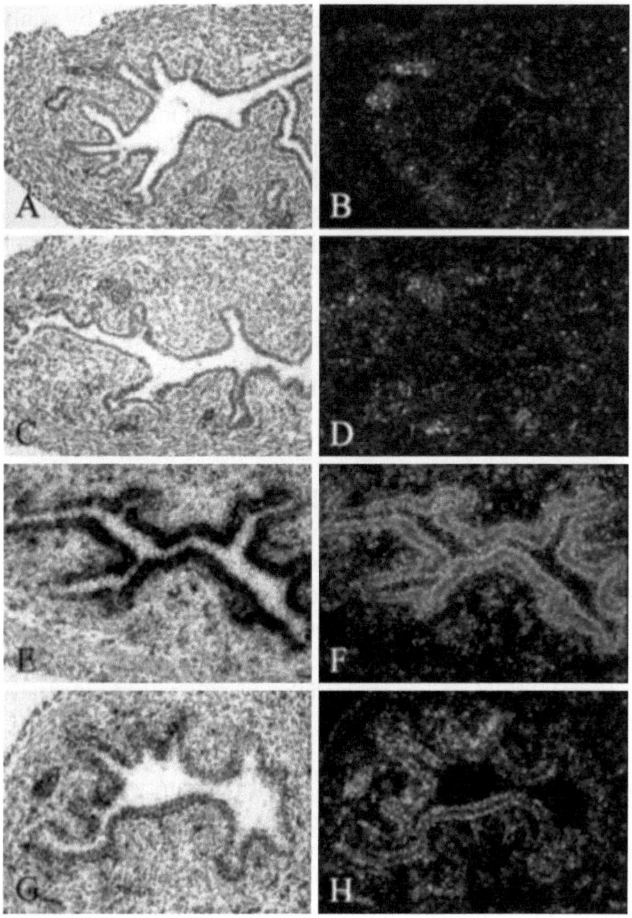

Fig. 7.2 Expression of cyclin D2 mRNA 12 h after treatment with E2 and TCDD in B6C3F1 mice

Astroff et al. 1990, 1991). The antiestrogenic effects of TCDD in wild-type and AhR$^{-/-}$ mice were also investigated using uterine stroma and epithelium in tissue recombination studies in nude mice (Buchanan et al. 2000, 2002) and the results suggest that TCDD primarily targets stromal cells. We also compared the uterine effects of E2 alone and in combination with TCDD in 25 day-old B6C3F1 mice, and the immunostaining results illustrated in Fig. 7.2 clearly show that TCDD significantly inhibits E2-induced cyclin D1 expression in animals treated for 12 h (similar results were observed after 6 h) (Walker 2004). Moreover, in AhR$^{-/-}$ mice, we also observed induction of cyclin D1 after treatment for 14 h; however, TCDD did not inhibit the induction response, demonstrating a role for the AhR in mediating inhibitory cross talk with ER signaling. The effects of TCDD on hormone-responsive gene expression in the mouse uterus were also investigated using ethinyl estradiol (EE) ± TCDD followed by analysis of gene expression 4, 12, 24, and 72 h after administration using microarrays and bioinformatics (Boverhof et al. 2008). In this study, TCDD inhibited EE-induced uterine hypertrophy, hyperplasia, and stromal edema; however, inhibition of induced genes was both time dependent and limited to only a fraction of the induced genes. TCDD inhibited only 133 of the 2,753 EE-mediated (induction/repression) genes, demonstrating the gene selectivity of the inhibitory pathway. Moreover, in this study, genes responsible for the antiestrogenic physiological responses were also identified.

7.4 In Vivo Studies: AhR Agonists as Potential Chemotherapeutic Agents

Exposure of rodents to TCDD can result in both protection and enhancement of breast cancer and this is dependent on the dose of TCDD, timing, and duration of exposure (Holcombe and Safe 1994; Tritscher et al. 1995; Brown et al. 1998; Muto et al. 2002; Wakui et al. 2005, 2006; Jenkins et al. 2007). Several studies have investigated the effects of TCDD and other AhR agonists as inhibitors of mammary tumor growth in rodent models used for screening compounds as chemotherapeutic agents. Initial studies showed that weekly i.p. administration of TCDD (5 μg/kg) transiently inhibited tumor growth in nude mice bearing MCF-7 cells as xenografts and similar results were obtained as a p.o. route of administration (Gierthy et al. 1993). In contrast, studies in this laboratory using the selective AhR modulator (SAhRM) MCDF show that this compound significantly inhibited E2-dependent tumor growth in female nude mice bearing MCF-7 cells as xenografts (McDougal 2000). Studies in this laboratory have used the DMBA-induced Sprague-Dawley rat mammary tumor model to investigate the antitumorigenic activity of TCDD and other AhR agonists (Holcombe and Safe 1994; McDougal et al. 1997; Chen et al. 1998; Ramamoorthy et al. 1999; McDougal 2000; McDougal et al. 2000, 2001; Safe et al. 2001). Administration of a single dose of TCDD (10 μg/kg) after initial tumor formation in female Sprague-Dawley mice decreased tumor growth, whereas in corn oil-treated animals, there was a 3.5-fold increase in tumor volume (Fig. 7.3) (Holcombe and Safe 1994). A similar experiment was carried out with 3,3′,4,4′-tetrachlorobiphenyl (25 mg/kg × 2/week), an AhR agonist with estrogenic activity, and this compound also inhibited mammary tumor growth (Fig. 7.3) (Ramamoorthy et al. 1999).

Initial screening of several alternate-substituted (1,3,6,8- or 2,4,6,8-)PCDFs containing at least one alkyl substituent (McDougal 2000) showed that many of these compounds inhibited DMBA-induced mammary tumor growth in rats and the 6-methyl analog (MCDF) was one of the more active compounds (Fig. 7.4). This compound was used as a model to investigate the comparative effects of MCDF and tamoxifen (alone and in combination) as inhibitors of mammary cancer growth and also their interactions in terms of bone growth and uterine responses

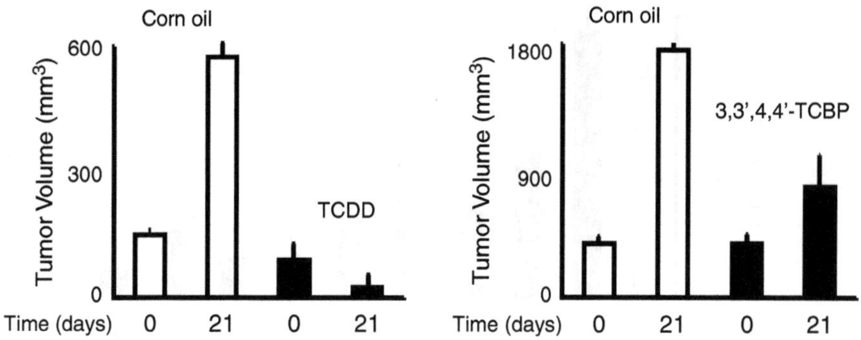

Fig. 7.3 Effects of TCDD (10 μg/kg) and 3,3′,4,4′-TCBP (25 mg/kg × 2/week) on mammary tumor growth in DMBA-induced female Sprague-Dawley rats (Holcombe and Safe 1994; Ramamoorthy et al. 1999)

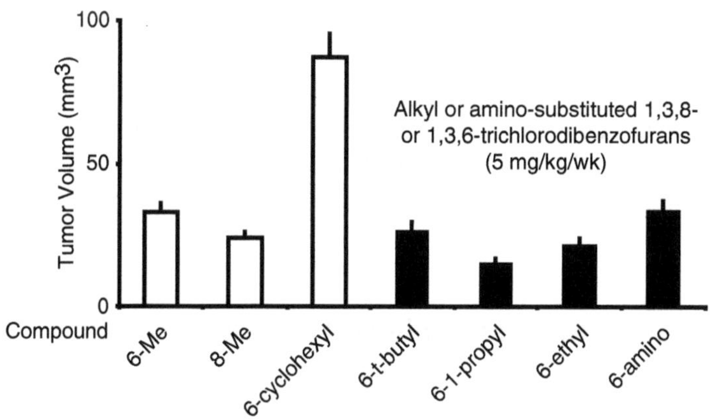

Fig. 7.4 Mammary tumor volumes in DMBA-induced female Sprague-Dawley rats treated with 6- or 8-substituted 1,3,8- or 2,4,6-trichlorodibenzofurans (5 mg/kg/week)

(McDougal et al. 2001). Treatment of DMBA-induced mammary tumors in female Sprague-Dawley rats with tamoxifen or MCDF at doses of 25, 50, and 100 μg/kg/day inhibited tumor growth only at the highest dose of tamoxifen (100 μg/kg) and the two higher doses of MCDF (50 and 100 μg/kg). In contrast, tumor growth was inhibited in animals treated with equal combined doses of tamoxifen plus MCDF (100/100, 50/50, and 25/25 μg/kg) and the low dose (25 μg/kg) combination was synergistic (Fig. 7.5). Since the harmful side effects of tamoxifen are associated with its ER agonist activity in the uterus and the increased risk for endometrial cancer after prolonged use (Fisher et al. 1994), we hypothesized that MCDF may inhibit tamoxifen-induced estrogenic effects in the uterus. At effective doses, MCDF inhibited tamoxifen-induced uterine wet weight increase, progesterone receptor binding, and peroxidase activity, whereas the effects of tamoxifen on

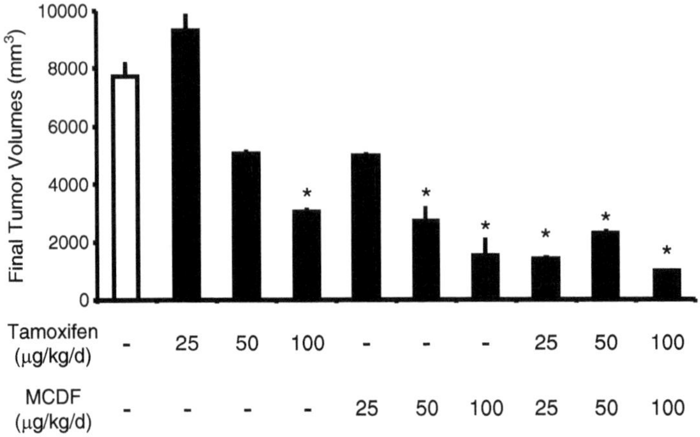

Fig. 7.5 Tamoxifen, MCDF, and their combination inhibit DMBA-induced mammary tumor growth in female Sprague-Dawley rats. * Significant ($p < 0.05$) decreases (McDougal et al. 2001)

increased bone length and weight were not affected by MCDF. These results clearly demonstrate the clinical potential for treatment of ER-positive cancer with a SAhRM (e.g., MCDF) in combination with a selective ER modulator (SERM) such as tamoxifen.

7.5 In Vitro Studies: Inhibitory AhR-ERα Cross Talk

ER-positive breast cancer cells (MCF-7, ZR-75, T47D) have been extensively used to investigate the effects of TCDD and other AhR agonists on these cell lines, particularly with respect to E2-induced physiological responses such as growth and gene expression (Safe et al. 2000, 2001; Safe and McDougal 2002; Safe and Wormke 2003; Safe 2005). TCDD and related compounds inhibit E2-induced post-confluent focus formation, cell growth, and related responses in MCF-7 and other breast cancer cell lines (Gierthy et al. 1987; Gierthy and Lincoln 1988; Biegel and Safe 1990; Fernandez and Safe 1992; Liu et al. 1992; Moore et al. 1994). RNA interference studies in MCF-7 cells showed that AhR knockdown decreased the percentage of cells in G_0G_1 and increased the percentage of cells in S and G_2/M phases (Abdelrahim et al. 2003). Activation of the AhR by TCDD had minimal effects on distribution of MCF-7 cells in G_0/G_1, S, and G_2/M phases (compared to DMSO); however, E2 induced accumulation of cells in S-phase and cotreatment with TCDD inhibited the G_0/G_1 to S phase progression. A recent paper reported the effects of TCDD on breast cancer cell invasion and metastatic features using ER-positive and ER-negative cell lines (Hall et al. 2010) and a modified Boyden chamber assay. Their results showed that TCDD and other AhR agonists inhibit basal (serum) and E2-induced invasiveness and anchorage-independent growth and promoted differentiation; moreover, Ah-responsiveness was blocked by AhR antagonists. We have used benzo[a]pyrene as a selecting agent to isolate hormone-responsive MCF-7 and T47D cell lines in which the AhR expression and Ah-responsiveness (CYP1A1-dependent activity) were significantly decreased (Moore et al. 1994, 1996). In the variant MCF-7 cell line, TCDD did not inhibit E2-induced cell proliferation and similar results were observed in the C10 variant T47D cell line that expressed low AhR levels (Moore et al. 1996). These results clearly demonstrate functional components of inhibitory AhR-ERα cross talk and a role for the AhR.

The effects of TCDD and other AhR agonists on expression of several hormone-induced genes have also been investigated. For example, TCDD and related compounds inhibited E2-induced cathepsin D, prolactin receptor, c-fos, cyclin D1, phosphorylation of Rb, cdk2, and cdk4, heat shock protein-27, pS2, BRCA-1, carbamoylphosphate synthetase/aspartate transcarbamylase/dihydroorotase (CAD), plasminogen activator, and glucose metabolism (Gierthy et al. 1987; Biegel and Safe 1990; Narasimhan et al. 1991; Krishnan et al. 1992, 1995; Krishnan and Safe 1993; Harper et al. 1994; Zacharewski et al. 1994; Lu et al. 1996; Gillesby et al. 1997; Nodland et al. 1997; Sun and Safe 1997; Wang et al. 1998; Duan et al. 1999; Porter et al. 2001; Khan et al. 2006; Hockings et al. 2006; Augereau et al. 2006). TCDD also inhibited E2-induced luciferase activity in cells transfected with constructs containing estrogen responsive elements (EREs), AP-1 motifs, or GC-rich motifs that bind Sp transcription factors (Nodland et al. 1997; Khan et al. 2006; Hockings et al. 2006). The results show that hormone-induced genes and reporter genes (transfected) are inhibited; however, a detailed genomic analysis of ligand-activated AhR-ER interactions and the list of genes that are involved in this pathway have not been determined. TCDD and other AhR agonists also activate two different but related responses that affect E2-responsiveness, namely activation of proteasome-dependent degradation of ERα (Harris et al. 1990; Wang et al. 1993; Wormke et al. 2000, 2003; Ohtake et al. 2007) and induction of CYP1A1 isoforms which catalyze oxidative metabolism of E2, resulting in lower hormone concentrations (Spink et al. 1990, 1992, 1994). Not unexpectedly, the simultaneous activation of these two pathways directly contributes to inhibitory AhR-ERα cross talk through depletion of both E2 and its receptor.

7.6 Molecular Mechanisms of Inhibitor AhR-ER Cross Talk

Studies on the molecular mechanisms of inhibitory AhR-ER cross talk in breast cancer cells have been useful as models for demonstrating the complexity of interactions between two receptor-mediated signaling pathways and includes both "general" and "gene-specific" pathways. As indicated above, TCDD and related compounds decrease expression of both the AhR and ERα and this "general" pathway has been extensively investigated (Harris et al. 1990; Wang et al. 1993;

Wormke et al. 2000, 2003; Ohtake et al. 2007). In MCF-7 cells, treatment with TCDD results in direct interactions between the AhR and ERα in the presence or absence of E2, whereas E2 does not induce ERα-AhR interactions (Wormke et al. 2003). These TCDD-dependent interactions result in increased ubiquitination of ERα and enhanced proteasome degradation which can be attenuated by proteasome inhibitors. An important component of this pathway is the activity of the AhR as an E3 ubiquitin ligase which facilitates ubiquitination of ERα and results in an overall decrease in ERα-dependent transactivation (Ohtake et al. 2007). Another "general" pathway that may play a role in some cell lines involves competition of the ligand-bound AhR and ERα for common cofactors/coactivators required for receptor-mediated transactivation (Kumar et al. 1999; Taylor et al. 2009). There is also some evidence that TCDD may induce inhibitory factors that may block E2-induced gene expression; however, the identity of these factors and their roles have not been determined (Rogers and Denison 2002).

A number of hormone-responsive genes are activated by ERα/Sp1 (or other Sp proteins) in breast cancer cells and this involves interactions with GC-rich promoter sequences where Sp1 binds DNA (Safe and Kim 2004). The CAD gene is typical of an ERα/Sp1-regulated gene and hormone-induced activation of CAD is inhibited after cotreatment with TCDD in MCF-7 or ZR-75 cells (Khan et al. 2006). Fluorescence resonance energy transfer (FRET) was used to investigate the effect of the TCDD-bound AhR and activation of ERα/Sp1 using different fluorescent protein tags (Khan et al. 2006). Treatment of the cells with E2, TCDD, or their combination enhanced FRET efficiency in cells transfected with the AhR and ERα and this was consistent with the known interactions of these proteins. In cells transfected with ERα and Sp1, E2 enhanced FRET efficiency but TCDD decreased this response, suggesting that inhibition of ERα/Sp1-mediated transactivation by TCDD was due to inhibition of ERα/Sp1 binding. Thus, the bound AhR blocks ERα-Sp1 interactions and this could be due, in part, to competition for ERα by Sp1 and AhR (Khan et al. 2006).

Several studies show that AhR-dependent inhibition of hormone-induced gene expression is also gene-specific (Krishnan et al. 1995; Gillesby et al. 1997; Duan et al. 1999; Porter et al. 2001; Khan et al. 2006; Hockings et al. 2006; Augereau et al. 2006). Initial studies in this laboratory characterized core DRE sequences (GCGTG) in E2-responsive pS2, cathepsin D, Hsp27, and c-fos gene promoters that were required for AhR-dependent inhibitory responses and these were called inhibitory DREs (iDREs). The location of iDREs with respect to hormone-responsive elements and transcription start sites was variable but it was likely that the functional role of these sites and the AhR involved disruption of transcription factor/polII complex formation. Augereau et al. (2006) identified an iDRE in the receptor-interacting protein 140 (RIP140) promoter and this sequence overlapped with an ERE motif. This was comparable to an iDRE overlap with a GC-rich sequence in the distal region of the fos gene promoter targeted by ERα/Sp1. Figure 7.6 summarizes the "general" and "gene-specific" mechanisms of inhibitory AhR-ERα cross talk in breast cancer cells and demonstrates the complexities associated with interactions between two signaling pathways.

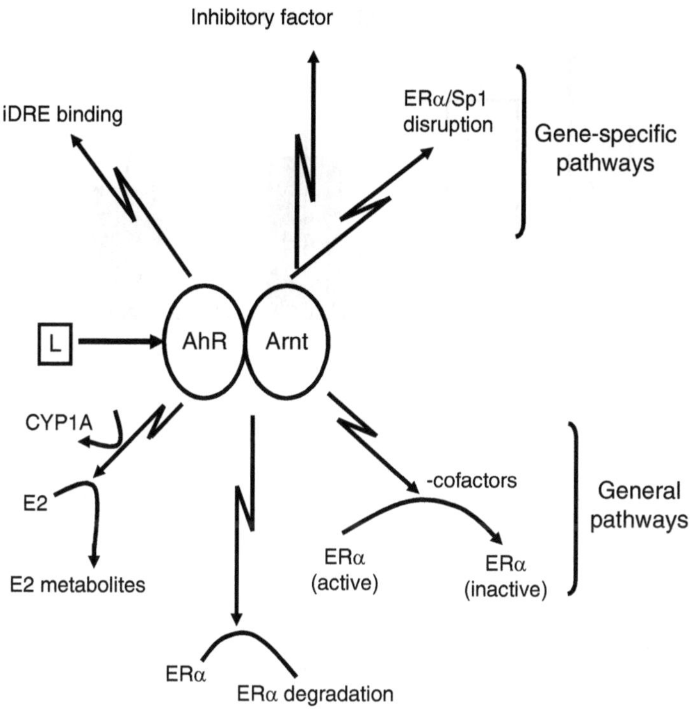

Fig. 7.6 Mechanisms of inhibition of AhR-ERα cross talk involve both gene-specific and general inhibitory pathways (Safe and Wormke 2003)

7.7 Is the AhR a Target for Treatment of ER-Negative Breast Cancer?

Although the AhR is widely expressed in ER-positive and ER-negative breast cancer cells, studies on the Ah-responsiveness of these cell lines have not been extensive. ER-negative MDA-MB-468 cells express the AhR, and TCDD inhibits cell proliferation through induction of TGFα which is a growth inhibitory factor in MDA-MB-468 cells (Wang et al. 1997b). Recent studies in this laboratory have demonstrated that the AhR is expressed in multiple ER-negative breast cancer cell lines, and TCDD also induced CYP1A1 gene expression. The fold induction responses observed in these studies were lower than observed in ER-positive breast cancer cells; however, both TCDD and MCDF decreased cell proliferation (Zhang et al. 2009). These results correlated with studies showing that TCDD induced differentiation responses in ER-negative breast cancer cells and inhibited invasion in a Boyden chamber assay (Hall et al. 2010), and the responses in both assays were abrogated by AhR knockdown by RNA interference. We have also observed similar effects in the Boyden chamber assay using the SAhRM MCDF (Fig. 7.7). Ongoing studies in this laboratory have linked the effects of TCDD and

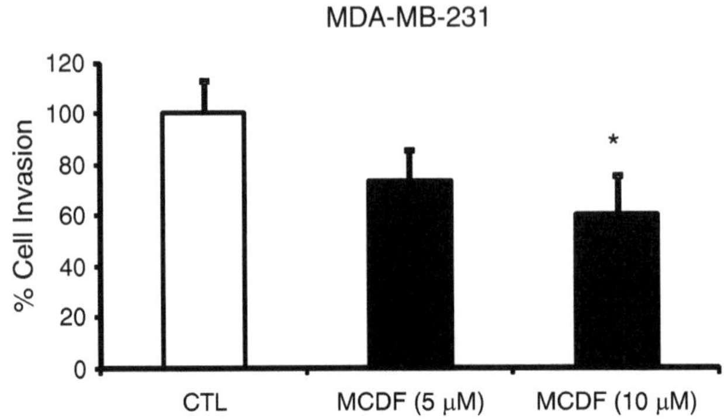

Fig. 7.7 MCDF inhibits MDA-MB-231 cell invasion and migration in the Boyden chamber assay

MCDF to Ah-responsive antimetastatic microRNAs, and AhR-microRNA interactions are currently being investigated.

7.8 Summary

TCDD and other AhR agonists have profound effects on the mammary gland and development of breast cancer, and the effects are dependent on multiple factors including the magnitude and timing of the dose, rodent species/strain, and interactions with other factors including the carcinogen DMBA. Human exposure to TCDD and related HAs is relatively low, and epidemiological studies in a high exposure group in Seveso, Italy, are ongoing but are limited by the low number of highly exposed individuals. A recent report on the Seveso population showed a higher incidence of breast cancer in the most highly exposed women 15 years or more after initial exposure; however, results between high, medium, and low exposure groups are variable and not dose dependent (Pesatori et al. 2009). Moreover, it is difficult to assess overall exposure to AhR-active compounds since the human diet contains relatively high levels of phytochemical compounds that exhibit both AhR agonist and antagonist activities (Casper et al. 1999; Adachi et al. 2001; Amakura et al. 2003; Zhang et al. 2003; Palermo et al. 2003; Jeuken et al. 2003; Nishiumi et al. 2007; Jang et al. 2008; Van der Heiden et al. 2009). Moreover, several endogenous biochemicals including heme breakdown products, prostaglandin 7-ketocholesterol, and other compounds are also AhR agonists or antagonists (Phelan et al. 1998; Seidel et al. 2001; Chiaro et al. 2008). Several pharmaceutical agents are also AhR-active (Hu et al. 2007) and a recent study showed that hydroxy-tamoxifen, the active metabolite of tamoxifen, one of the most widely used drugs for breast cancer therapy, is also an AhR agonist (Dusell et al. 2010). Thus, the role of AhR activation in breast cancer in humans must account for the dietary/pharmaceutical exposures to diverse AhR agonists and antagonists. However, the recent reports that AhR agonists inhibit ER-negative breast cancer cell growth and invasion suggest a promising new approach for treating patients who have limited treatment options and a poor prognosis.

Acknowledgments The financial assistance of the National Institutes of Health (R01-CA142697) and the technical assistance of Dr. Chadalapaka and Dr. Jutooru are gratefully acknowledged.

References

Abdelrahim M, Smith R III, Safe S (2003) Aryl hydrocarbon receptor gene silencing with small inhibitory RNA differentially modulates Ah-responsiveness in MCF-7 and HepG2 cancer cells. Mol Pharmacol 63:1373–1381

Adachi J et al (2001) Indirubin and indigo are potent aryl hydrocarbon receptor ligands present in human urine. J Biol Chem 276:31475–31478

Ahlborg UG et al (1992) Impact of polychlorinated dibenzo-*p*-dioxins, dibenzofurans, and biphenyls on human and environmental health with special emphasis on application of the toxic equivalence factor concept. Eur J Pharmacol 228:179–199

Amakura Y et al (2003) Screening of the inhibitory effect of vegetable constituents on the aryl hydrocarbon receptor-mediated activity induced by 2,3,7,8-tetrachlorodibenzo-p-dioxin. Biol Pharm Bull 26:1754–1760

Astroff B, Safe S (1988) Comparative antiestrogenic activities of 2,3,7,8- tetrachlorodibenzo-*p*-dioxin and 6-methyl-1,3,8- trichlorodibenzofuran in the female rat. Toxicol Appl Pharmacol 95:435–443

Astroff B, Safe S (1990) 2,3,7,8-Tetrachlorodibenzo-*p*-dioxin as an antiestrogen: effect on rat uterine peroxidase activity. Biochem Pharmacol 39:485–488

Astroff B et al (1990) 2,3,7,8-Tetrachlorodibenzo-*p*-dioxin inhibition of 17β-estradiol-induced increases in rat uterine EGF receptor binding activity and gene expression. Mol Cell Endocrinol 72:247–252

Astroff B, Eldridge B, Safe S (1991) Inhibition of 17β-estradiol-induced and constitutive expression of the cellular protooncogene c-*fos* by 2,3,7,8- tetrachlorodibenzo-*p*-dioxin (TCDD) in the female uterus. Toxicol Lett 56:305–315

Augereau P et al (2006) Transcriptional regulation of the human NRIP1/RIP140 gene by estrogen is modulated by dioxin signalling. Mol Pharmacol 69:1338–1346

Biegel L, Safe S (1990) Effects of 2,3,7,8-tetrachlorodibenzo-*p*-dioxin (TCDD) on cell growth and the secretion of the estrogen-induced 34-, 52- and 160- kDa proteins in human breast cancer cells. J Steroid Biochem Mol Biol 37:725–732

Bjerke DL, Peterson RE (1994) Reproductive toxicity of 2,3,7,8-tetrachlorodibenzo-p-dioxin in male rats: different effects of in utero versus lactational exposure. Toxicol Appl Pharmacol 127:241–249

Bjerke DL et al (1994) Effects of in utero and lactational 2,3,7,8-tetrachlorodibenzo-p-dioxin exposure on responsiveness of the male rat reproductive system to testosterone stimulation in adulthood. Toxicol Appl Pharmacol 127:250–257

Boverhof DR et al (2008) Inhibition of estrogen-mediated uterine gene expression responses by dioxin. Mol Pharmacol 73:82–93

Brown NM et al (1998) Prenatal TCDD and predisposition to mammary cancer in the rat. Carcinogenesis 19:1623–1629

Buchanan DL et al (2000) Antiestrogenic effects of 2,3,7,8-tetrachlorodibenzo-*p*-dioxin in mouse uterus: critical role of the aryl hydrocarbon receptor in stromal tissue. Toxicol Sci 57:302–311

Buchanan DL et al (2002) Dioxin inhibition of estrogen-induced mouse uterine epithelial mitogenesis involves changes in cyclin and transforming growth factor-β expression. Toxicol Sci 66:62–68

Casper RF et al (1999) Resveratrol has antagonist activity on the aryl hydrocarbon receptor: implications for prevention of dioxin toxicity. Mol Pharmacol 56:784–790
Chen I et al (1998) Aryl hydrocarbon receptor-mediated antiestrogenic and antitumorigenic activity of diindolylmethane. Carcinogenesis 19:1631–1639
Chiaro CR, Patel RD, Perdew GH (2008) 12(R)-Hydroxy-5(Z),8(Z),10(E),14(Z)-eicosatetraenoic acid [12(R)-HETE], an arachidonic acid derivative, is an activator of the aryl hydrocarbon receptor. Mol Pharmacol 74:1649–1656
Collins LL, Lew BJ, Lawrence BP (2009) TCDD exposure disrupts mammary epithelial cell differentiation and function. Reprod Toxicol 28:11–17
Davis JW et al (2000) 2,3,7,8-Tetrachlorodibenzo-p-dioxin (TCDD) inhibits growth factor withdrawal-induced apoptosis in the human mammary epithelial cell line, MCF-10A. Carcinogenesis 21:881–886
Davis JW et al (2001) Prevention of apoptosis by 2,3,7,8-tetrachlorodibenzo-p-dioxin (TCDD) in the MCF-10A cell line: correlation with increased transforming growth factor alpha production. Cancer Res 61:3314–3320
Dong B, Matsumura F (2008) Roles of cytosolic phospholipase A2 and Src kinase in the early action of 2,3,7,8-tetrachlorodibenzo-p-dioxin through a nongenomic pathway in MCF10A cells. Mol Pharmacol 74:255–263
Dong B, Matsumura F (2009) The conversion of rapid TCCD nongenomic signals to persistent inflammatory effects via select protein kinases in MCF10A cells. Mol Endocrinol 23:549–558
Duan R et al (1999) Transcriptional activation of c-fos protooncogene by 17β-estradiol: mechanism of aryl hydrocarbon receptor-mediated inhibition. Mol Endocrinol 13:1511–1521
Dusell CD et al (2010) Regulation of aryl hydrocarbon receptor function by selective estrogen receptor modulators. Mol Endocrinol 24:33–46
Fenton SE et al (2002) Persistent abnormalities in the rat mammary gland following gestational and lactational exposure to 2,3,7,8-tetrachlorodibenzo-p-dioxin (TCDD). Toxicol Sci 67:63–74
Fernandez P, Safe S (1992) Growth inhibitory and antimitogenic activity of 2,3,7,8-tetrachlorodibenzo-*p*-dioxin (TCDD) in T47D human breast cancer cells. Toxicol Lett 61:185–197
Fisher B et al (1994) Endometrial cancer in tamoxifen-treated breast cancer patients: findings from the National Surgical Adjuvant Breast and Bowel Project (NSABP) B-14. J Natl Cancer Inst 86:527–537
Gallo MA et al (1986) Interactive effects of estradiol and 2,3,7,8-tetrachlorodibenzo- *p*-dioxin on hepatic cytochrome P-450 and mouse uterus. Toxicol Lett 32:123–132
Gierthy JF, Lincoln DW (1988) Inhibition of postconfluent focus production in cultures of MCF- 7 breast cancer cells by 2,3,7,8-tetrachlorodibenzo-*p*-dioxin. Breast Cancer Res 12:227–233
Gierthy JF et al (1987) Suppression of estrogen-regulated extracellular plasminogen activator activity of MCF-7 cells by 2,3,7,8-tetrachlorodibenzo- *p*-dioxin. Cancer Res 47:6198–6203
Gierthy JF et al (1993) Correlation of in vitro and in vivo growth suppression of MCF-7 human breast cancer by 2,3,7,8-tetrachlorodibenzo-*p*-dioxin. Cancer Res 53:3149–3153
Gillesby B et al (1997) Identification of a motif within the 5′-regulatory region on pS2 which is responsible for Ap1 binding and TCDD-mediated suppression. Biochemistry 36:6080–6089
Gray LE Jr, Ostby JS (1995) In utero 2,3,7,8-tetrachlorodibenzo-p-dioxin (TCDD) alters reproductive morphology and function in female rat offspring. Toxicol Appl Pharmacol 133:285–294
Gray LE et al (1997) In utero exposure to low doses of 2,3,7,8-tetrachlorodibenzo-p-dioxin alters reproductive development of female Long Evans hooded rat offspring. Toxicol Appl Pharmacol 146:237–244
Gu YZ, Hogenesch JB, Bradfield CA (2000) The PAS superfamily: sensors of environmental and developmental signals. Annu Rev Pharmacol Toxicol 40:519–561
Hall JM et al (2010) Activation of the aryl-hydrocarbon receptor inhibits invasive and metastatic features of human breast cancer cells and promotes breast cancer cell differentiation. Mol Endocrinol 24:359–369
Harper N et al (1994) Inhibition of estrogen-induced progesterone receptor in MCF-7 human breast cancer cells by aryl hydrocarbon (Ah) receptor agonists. Mol Cell Endocrinol 104:47–55

Harris M, Zacharewski T, Safe S (1990) Effects of 2,3,7,8-tetrachlorodibenzo-*p*-dioxin and related compounds on the occupied nuclear estrogen receptor in MCF-7 human breast cancer cells. Cancer Res 50:3579–3584

Hockings JK et al (2006) The ligand status of the aromatic hydrocarbon receptor modulates transcriptional activation of BRCA-1 promoter by estrogen. Cancer Res 66:2224–2232

Holcombe M, Safe S (1994) Inhibition of 7,12-dimethylbenzanthracene-induced rat mammary tumor growth by 2,3,7,8-tetrachlorodibenzo-*p*-dioxin. Cancer Lett 82:43–47

Hu W et al (2007) Induction of cyp1a1 is a nonspecific biomarker of aryl hydrocarbon receptor activation: results of large scale screening of pharmaceuticals and toxicants in vivo and in vitro. Mol Pharmacol 71:1475–1486

Jang JY et al (2008) Antiteratogenic effect of resveratrol in mice exposed in utero to 2,3,7,8-tetrachlorodibenzo-p-dioxin. Eur J Pharmacol 591:280–283

Jenkins S et al (2007) Prenatal TCDD exposure predisposes for mammary cancer in rats. Reprod Toxicol 23:391–396

Jeuken A et al (2003) Activation of the Ah receptor by extracts of dietary herbal supplements, vegetables, and fruits. J Agric Food Chem 51:5478–5487

Khan S et al (2006) Molecular mechanisms of inhibitory aryl hydrocarbon receptor-estrogen receptor α/Sp1 crosstalk in breast cancer cells. Mol Endocrinol 20:2199–2214

Kociba RJ et al (1978) Results of a 2-year chronic toxicity and oncogenicity study of 2,3,7,8-tetrachlorodibenzo-*p*-dioxin (TCDD) in rats. Toxicol Appl Pharmacol 46:279–303

Krishnan V, Safe S (1993) Polychlorinated biphenyls (PCBs), dibenzo-*p*-dioxins (PCDDs) and dibenzofurans (PCDFs) as antiestrogens in MCF-7 human breast cancer cells: quantitative structure-activity relationships. Toxicol Appl Pharmacol 120:55–61

Krishnan V, Narasimhan TR, Safe S (1992) Development of gel staining techniques for detecting the secretion of procathepsin D (52-kDa protein) in MCF-7 human breast cancer cells. Anal Biochem 204:137–142

Krishnan V et al (1995) Molecular mechanism of inhibition of estrogen-induced cathepsin D gene expression by 2,3,7,8-tetrachlorodibenzo-*p*-dioxin (TCDD) in MCF-7 cells. Mol Cell Biol 15:6710–6719

Kumar MB, Tarpey RW, Perdew GH (1999) Differential recruitment of coactivator RIP140 by *Ah* and estrogen receptors: absence of a role for LXXLL motifs. J Biol Chem 274:22155–22164

Lee DH et al (2007) Relationship between serum concentrations of persistent organic pollutants and the prevalence of metabolic syndrome among non-diabetic adults: results from the National Health and Nutrition Examination Survey 1999–2002. Diabetologia 50:1841–1851

Lew BJ et al (2009) Activation of the aryl hydrocarbon receptor during different critical windows in pregnancy alters mammary epithelial cell proliferation and differentiation. Toxicol Sci 111:151–162

Lewis BC et al (2001) In utero and lactational treatment with 2,3,7,8-tetrachlorodibenzo-p-dioxin impairs mammary gland differentiation but does not block the response to exogenous estrogen in the postpubertal female rat. Toxicol Sci 62:46–53

Liu H et al (1992) Inhibition of insulin-like growth factor-I responses in MCF-7 cells by 2,3,7,8-tetrachlorodibenzo-*p*-dioxin and related compounds. Mol Cell Endocrinol 87:19–28

Lu Y-F et al (1996) Inhibition of prolactin receptor gene expression by 2,3,7,8-tetrachlorodibenzo-*p*-dioxin in MCF-7 human breast cancer cells. Arch Biochem Biophys 332:35–40

Mazina O et al (2004) Studies on the mechanism of rapid activation of protein tyrosine phosphorylation activities, particularly c-Src kinase, by TCDD in MCF10A. J Biochem Mol Toxicol 18:313–321

McDougal A (2000) Aromatic hydrocarbon receptor-based antiestrogens as treatments for breast cancer. PhD dissertation, Texas A&M University

McDougal A, Wilson C, Safe S (1997) Inhibition of 7,12-dimethylbenz[*a*]anthracene-induced rat mammary tumor growth by aryl hydrocarbon receptor agonists. Cancer Lett 120:53–63

McDougal A et al (2000) Inhibition of carcinogen-induced rat mammary tumor growth and other estrogen-dependent responses by symmetrical dihalo-substituted analogs of diindolylmethane. Cancer Lett 151:169–179

McDougal A et al (2001) Tamoxifen-induced antitumorigenic/antiestrogenic action synergized by a selective Ah receptor modulator. Cancer Res 61:3901–3907
Moore M et al (1994) Benzo[a]pyrene-resistant MCF-7 human breast cancer cells. A unique aryl hydrocarbon-nonresponsive clone. J Biol Chem 269:11751–11759
Moore M et al (1996) Isolation and characterization of variant benzo[a]pyrene-resistant T47D human breast-cancer cells. Int J Cancer 66:117–123
Muto T et al (2002) Mammary gland differentiation in female rats after prenatal exposure to 3,3′,4,4′,5-pentachlorobiphenyl. Toxicology 177:197–205
Narasimhan TR et al (1991) Effects of 2,3,7,8-tetrachlorodibenzo-*p*-dioxin on 17β-estradiol-induced glucose metabolism in MCF-7 human breast cancer cells: ^{13}C-nuclear magnetic resonance studies. Mol Pharmacol 40:1029–1035
Nishiumi S, Yoshida K, Ashida H (2007) Curcumin suppresses the transformation of an aryl hydrocarbon receptor through its phosphorylation. Arch Biochem Biophys 466:267–273
Nodland KI, Wormke M, Safe S (1997) Inhibition of estrogen-induced activity by 2,3,7,8-tetrachlorodibenzo-*p*-dioxin (TCDD) in the MCF-7 human breast cancer and other cell lines transfected with vitellogenin A2 gene promoter constructs. Arch Biochem Biophys 338:67–72
Ohtake F et al (2007) Dioxin receptor is a ligand-dependent E3 ubiquitin ligase. Nature 446:562–566
Palermo CM et al (2003) Identification of potential aryl hydrocarbon receptor antagonists in green tea. Chem Res Toxicol 16:865–872
Park S et al (2004) TCDD causes suppression of growth and differentiation of MCF10A, human mammary epithelial cells by interfering with their insulin receptor signaling through c-Src kinase and ERK activation. J Biochem Mol Toxicol 18:322–331
Patterson DG Jr et al (2009) Levels in the U.S. population of those persistent organic pollutants (2003–2004) included in the Stockholm convention or in other long range transboundary air pollution agreements. Environ Sci Technol 43:1211–1218
Pesatori AC et al (2009) Cancer incidence in the population exposed to dioxin after the "Seveso accident": twenty years of follow-up. Environ Health 8:39
Phelan D et al (1998) Activation of the Ah receptor signal transduction pathway by bilirubin and biliverdin. Arch Biochem Biophys 357:155–163
Poland A, Knutson JC (1982) 2,3,7,8-Tetrachlorodibenzo-*p*-dioxin and related halogenated aromatic hydrocarbons. Examinations of the mechanism of toxicity. Annu Rev Pharmacol Toxicol 22:517–554
Poland A, Glover E, Kende AS (1976) Stereospecific, high affinity binding of 2,3,7,8-tetrachlorodibenzo-*p*-dioxin by hepatic cytosol: evidence that the binding species is receptor for induction of aryl hydrocarbon hydroxylase. J Biol Chem 251:4936–4946
Porter W et al (2001) Transcriptional activation of heat shock protein 27 gene expression by 17β-estradiol and modulation by antiestrogens and aryl hydrocarbon receptor agonists: estrogenic activity of ICI 164,384. J Mol Endocrinol 26:31–42
Ramamoorthy K et al (1999) 3,3′,4,4′-Tetrachlorobiphenyl exhibits antiestrogenic and antitumorigenic activity in the rodent uterus and mammary and in human breast cancer cells. Carcinogenesis 20:115–123
Rogers JM, Denison MS (2002) Analysis of the antiestrogenic activity of 2,3,7,8-tetrachlorodibenzo-p-dioxin in human ovarian carcinoma BG-1 cells. Mol Pharmacol 61:1393–1403
Romkes M, Safe S (1988) Comparative activities of 2,3,7,8-tetrachlorodibenzo-*p*-dioxin and progesterone on antiestrogens in the female rat uterus. Toxicol Appl Pharmacol 92:368–380
Romkes M, Piskorska-Pliszczynska J, Safe S (1987) Effects of 2,3,7,8-tetrachlorodibenzo-*p*-dioxin on hepatic and uterine estrogen receptor levels in rats. Toxicol Appl Pharmacol 87:306–314
Safe S (1986) Comparative toxicology and mechanism of action of polychlorinated dibenzo-*p*-dioxins and dibenzofurans. Annu Rev Pharmacol Toxicol 26:371–399
Safe S (1992) Toxicology, structure-function relationships, human and environmental health impacts of polychlorinated biphenyls (PCBs): progress and problems. Environ Health Perspect 100:259–268
Safe S (2005) 2,3,7,8-Tetrachlorodibenzo-*p*-dioxin (TCDD) and related environmental antiestrogens: characterization and mechanism of action. In: Naz RK (ed) Endocrine disruptors. CRC Press, Boca Raton, pp 249–287

Safe S, Kim K (2004) Nuclear receptor-mediated transactivation through interaction with Sp proteins. Prog Nucleic Acid Res Mol Biol 77:1–36

Safe S, McDougal A (2002) Mechanism of action and development of selective aryl hydrocarbon receptor modulators for treatment of hormone-dependent cancers. Int J Oncol 20:1123–1228

Safe S, Wormke M (2003) Inhibitory aryl hydrocarbon-estrogen receptor α cross-talk and mechanisms of action. Chem Res Toxicol 16:807–816

Safe S, Wormke M, Samudio I (2000) Mechanisms of inhibitory aryl hydrocarbon receptor - estrogen receptor crosstalk in human breast cancer cells. J Mammary Gland Biol Neoplasia 5:295–306

Safe S et al (2001) Selective Ah receptor modulators (SAhRMs): progress towards development of a new class of inhibitors of breast cancer growth. J Women's Cancer 3:37–45

Schecter A et al (2010) Perfluorinated compounds, polychlorinated biphenyls, and organochlorine pesticide contamination in composite food samples from Dallas, Texas, USA. Environ Health Perspect 118:796–802

Seidel SD et al (2001) Activation of the Ah receptor signaling pathway by prostaglandins. J Biochem Mol Toxicol 15:187–196

Spink DC et al (1990) 2,3,7,8-Tetrachlorodibenzo-*p*-dioxin causes an extensive alteration of 17β-estradiol metabolism in human breast cancer cells. Proc Natl Acad Sci USA 87:6917–6921

Spink DC et al (1992) 17β-Estradiol hydroxylation catalyzed by human cytochrome P4501A1: a comparison of the activities induced by 2,3,7,8- tetrachlorodibenzo-*p*-dioxin in MCF-7 cells with those from heterologous expression of the cDNA. Arch Biochem Biophys 293:342–348

Spink DC et al (1994) Stimulation of 17β-estradiol metabolism in MCF-7 cells by bromochloro- and chloromethyl-substituted dibenzo-*p*-dioxins and dibenzofurans: correlations with antiestrogenic activity. J Toxicol Environ Health 41:451–466

Sun G, Safe S (1997) Antiestrogenic activities of alternate substituted polychlorinated dibenzofurans in MCF-7 human breast cancer cells. Cancer Chemother Pharmacol 40:239–244

Tannheimer SL et al (1998) Benzo[a]pyrene- and TCDD-induced alterations in tyrosine phosphorylation and insulin-like growth factor signaling pathways in the MCF-10A human mammary epithelial cell line. Carcinogenesis 19:1291–1297

Taylor RT et al (2009) Roles of coactivator proteins in dioxin induction of CYP1A1 and CYP1B1 in human breast cancer cells. Toxicol Sci 107:1–8

Tritscher AM et al (1995) Persistence of TCDD-induced hepatic cell proliferation and growth of enzyme altered foci after chronic exposure followed by cessation of treatment in DEN initiated female rats. Carcinogenesis 16:2807–2811

Umbreit TH et al (1989) Alteration of the acute toxicity of 2,3,7,8-tetrachlorodibenzo-*p*-dioxin (TCDD) by estradiol and tamoxifen. Toxicology 59:163–169

Van den Berg M et al (1998) Toxic equivalency factors (TEFs) for PCBs, PCDDs, PCDFs for humans and wildlife. Environ Health Perspect 106:775–792

Van den Berg M et al (2006) The 2005 World Health Organization reevaluation of human and mammalian toxic equivalency factors for dioxins and dioxin-like compounds. Toxicol Sci 93:223–241

Van der Heiden E et al (2009) Food flavonoid aryl hydrocarbon receptor-mediated agonistic/antagonistic/synergic activities in human and rat reporter gene assays. Anal Chim Acta 637:337–345

Vorderstrasse BA et al (2004) A novel effect of dioxin: exposure during pregnancy severely impairs mammary gland differentiation. Toxicol Sci 78:248–257

Wakui S et al (2005) CYP1 and AhR expression in 7,12-dimethylbenz[a]anthracene-induced mammary carcinoma of rats prenatally exposed to 3,3′,4,4′,5-pentachlorobiphenyl. Toxicology 211:231–241

Wakui S et al (2006) Prenatal 3,3′,4,4′,5-pentachlorobiphenyl exposure modulates induction of rat hepatic CYP 1A1, 1B1, and AhR by 7,12-dimethylbenz[a]anthracene. Toxicol Appl Pharmacol 210:200–211

Walker KB (2004) Inhibitory actions of Ah receptor agonists and indole-containing compounds in breast cancer cell lines and mouse models. Ph.D. Thesis, Texas A&M University

Wang X et al (1993) Mechanism of 2,3,7,8-tetrachlorodibenzo-*p*-dioxin (TCDD)-mediated decrease of the nuclear estrogen receptor in MCF-7 human breast cancer cells. Mol Cell Endocrinol 96:159–166

Wang W et al (1997a) Mechanism of inhibition of MDA-MB-468 breast cancer cell growth by 2,3,7,8-tetrachlorodibenzo-*p*-dioxin. Carcinogenesis 18:925–933
Wang W et al (1997b) 17β-Estradiol-mediated growth inhibition of MDA-MB-468 cells stably transfected with the estrogen receptor: cell cycle effects. Mol Cell Endocrinol 133:49–62
Wang W, Smith R, Safe S (1998) Aryl hydrocarbon receptor-mediated antiestrogenicity in MCF-7 cells: modulation of hormone-induced cell cycle enzymes. Arch Biochem Biophys 356:239–248
Wang SL et al (2008) Increased risk of diabetes and polychlorinated biphenyls and dioxins: a 24-year follow-up study of the Yucheng cohort. Diabetes Care 31:1574–1579
Watanabe H et al (2004) Comparative uterine gene expression analysis after dioxin and estradiol administration. J Mol Endocrinol 33:763–771
Whitlock JP et al (1996) Induction of cytochrome P4501A1: a model for analyzing mammalian gene transcription. FASEB J 10:809–818
Wilson CL, Safe S (1998) Mechanisms of ligand-induced aryl hydrocarbon receptor-mediated biochemical and toxic responses. Toxicol Pathol 26:657–671
Wormke M et al (2000) Crosstalk between estrogen receptor α and the aryl hydrocarbon receptor in breast cancer cells involves unidirectional activation of proteosomes. FEBS Lett 478:109–112
Wormke M et al (2003) The aryl hydrocarbon receptor mediates degradation of the estrogen receptor α through activation of proteasomes. Mol Cell Biol 23:1843–1855
Wu X et al (2003) Gene expression profiling of the effects of castration and estrogen treatment in the rat uterus. Biol Reprod 69:1308–1317
Zacharewski TR et al (1994) Antiestrogenic effects of 2,3,7,8-tetrachlorodibenzo-*p*-dioxin on 17β-estradiol-induced pS2 expression. Cancer Res 54:2707–2713
Zhang S, Qin C, Safe SH (2003) Flavonoids as aryl hydrocarbon receptor agonists/antagonists: effects of structure and cell context. Environ Health Perspect 111:1877–1882
Zhang S et al (2009) The aryl hydrocarbon receptor as a target for estrogen receptor-negative breast cancer chemotherapy. Endocr Relat Cancer 16:835–844

Chapter 8
Mammary Gland as a Sensitive Tissue to Developmental Exposures of Perfluorooctanoic Acid (PFOA) in the Mouse

Sally S. White, Suzanne E. Fenton, Chengfeng Yang, and Sandra Z. Haslam

Abstract The persistence in the environment, combined with the ubiquity of perfluorinated products in the marketplace, has caused what is now recognized as the widespread contamination of human and wildlife tissues with perfluorooctanoic acid (PFOA). The global presence of PFOA has raised concern about adverse health effects that may result from unavoidable human exposures. In this review, we cover the sources of PFOA, its prevalence, and current knowledge about human PFOA exposures and associated health consequences. Examined in detail are PFOA-induced effects on mammary gland in animals. Studies of other environmental agents indicate that late fetal and early postnatal mammary gland development is particularly sensitive to environmental insult. Early life exposures that alter mammary gland development are thought to have a potential impact on the development of mammary cancers later in life in animal models. This is also thought to be the case in humans. Recent research in the mouse examining the effects of in utero, lactational and peripubertal exposures, impact of genetic background, and putative mechanisms of action has made substantial discoveries regarding the effects of PFOA exposure on the mammary gland with high relevancy to human health.

Keywords PFOA • Exposure • Health effects • Mice • Mammary gland • In utero • Lactation • Peripuberty • Endocrine disruptor

S.Z. Haslam (✉)
Department of Biomedical and Integrative Physiology, Michigan State University, East Lansing, MI 48824, USA

Breast Cancer and the Environment Research Center, Michigan State University, East Lansing, MI 48824, USA
e-mail: shaslam@msu.edu

J. Russo (ed.), *Environment and Breast Cancer*, DOI 10.1007/978-1-4419-9896-5_8,

8.1 Introduction

8.1.1 Perfluorooctanoic Acid (PFOA): Sources, Prevalence, and Half-Life

Perfluorooctanoic acid (PFOA) is a man-made environmental pollutant sometimes also referred to as C8, or its salt, ammonium perfluorooctanoate (APFO). As a fully-fluorinated eight-carbon chain – either linear or branched – with a single carboxylic acid functional group, PFOA exhibits structural homology with naturally occurring fatty acids. PFOA has been in industrial use since the late 1940s and early 1950s prior to the establishment of the Toxic Substances Control Act (TSCA) (EPA 1976). PFOA is most often employed for its surfactant properties, and it remains a vital ingredient in the production of many consumer products including nonstick cookware coatings, all-weather clothing, and paper coatings on food packaging to repel grease, as well as industrial applications such as fire-fighting foams, electrical insulation, and insecticides.

PFOA is a waste product in the production of many perfluorinated chemicals (PFCs) and may be released in the effluent from production facilities (Hansen et al. 2002), and is also a final environmental degradation product of many PFCs, which may occur via aerobic, microbial metabolism (Dinglasan et al. 2004), or by photolysis in the lower atmosphere (Ellis et al. 2004). PFOA, however, represents a final product of the processes, and resists further degradation in the ambient environment by biotic or physical processes (Liou et al. 2010). These facts may explain the global distribution of PFOA.

This persistence in the environment, combined with the ubiquity of perfluorinated products in the marketplace, has caused what is now recognized as the widespread contamination of human and wildlife tissues with PFOA. Many studies have demonstrated the presence of PFOA in both abiotic and biotic media, including isolated bodies of water and mammalian populations, as well as the ubiquity of PFOA in organisms across taxonomic classes, particularly when in greater proximity to industrialized areas of the world (Hansen et al. 2002; Moody et al. 2003; Moriwaki et al. 2003; Boulanger et al. 2004; Saito et al. 2004; So et al. 2004; Loewen et al. 2005). In larger organisms, PFOA bioaccumulation is well documented. However, PFOA does not bioaccumulate in fat, but rather is stored in the liver and is bound to circulating blood proteins such as B-lipoproteins, albumin, and fatty acid binding proteins, resulting in extended half-lives in most mammals. Because of this tendency, even low-level exposures in humans can lead to elevated body burdens over time.

A comparison of common perfluoroalkyl acids (PFAA) half-lives is summarized in Table 8.1 (Ohmori et al. 2003; Butenhoff et al. 2004a; Chang et al. 2008; Olsen et al. 2009; USEPA 2009). Reported half-life estimates illustrate patterns of human > monkey > mouse ≥ rat. Across the PFAAs there is a significant species difference in elimination, and clearance is greatly reduced in humans. Importantly, there is a gender difference in the elimination of PFOA and other carboxylated

Table 8.1 Comparative PFAA elimination half-lives[a]

Serum half-life	PFBS (C4) (days)	PFBA (C4)	PFHxS (C6)	PFOS (C8)	PFOA (C8)	PFNA (C9) (days)	PFDA (C10) (days)
Rat	**4.0**	**6.4–9.2 h**		7 days	**2–4 h**	**2**	**59**
	4.5	*1.0–1.8 h*			*6–7 days*	*31*	*40*
Mouse		**5–13 h**			**16 days**	**41**	
		2.8–3.1 h			*22 days*	*64*	
Monkey	**3.5**	**1.7 days**	**87 days**	**110 days**	**33 days**		
	4.0	*1.7 days*	*141 days*	*132 days*	*21 days*		
Human	25.8	**3.0 days**	8.5 years	5.4 years	2.3–3.8 years		
		3.6 days					

PFBS perfluorobutane sulfonate; *PFBA* perfluorobutanoic acid; *PFHxS* perfluorohexane sulfonate; *PFOS* perfluorooctane sulfonate; *PFNA* perfluorononanoic acid; *PFDA* perfluorodecanoic acid
[a]Bold – females; italics – males

PFAAs in rats; with respect to PFOA, this gender difference is developmentally regulated, with the adult pattern becoming apparent by sexual maturation. The differences are hormonally dependent, and are likely regulated by the actions of organic anion transporters, and their total expression in the kidney, where they expedite PFOA elimination. A gender difference has not been detected in humans, but uncertainty exists due to the small sample size evaluated. It is critical to note that the half-lives of these compounds are measured in hours to days to months in rats, mice, and monkeys, but years in humans, with the exception of the C4 PFAAs (Table 8.1).

8.1.2 Human PFOA Exposures and Associated Health Consequences

The global presence of PFOA has raised concern about adverse health effects that may result from unavoidable human exposures (USEPA 2006). Potential sources of human exposure may include contact between food and PFC-treated packaging, ingestion of contaminated drinking water or household dust (believed due to prevalence of PFOA in consumer products), and possibly dietary sources including fresh-water fish consumption, among other unknown pathways (Begley et al. 2005; Gulkowska et al. 2006). Interestingly, the potential for transference of PFOA from surrounding soils into plant tissues has recently been demonstrated, and may explain an additional source of human exposure (Stahl et al. 2009). Whatever the means of exposure, it is now recognized and accepted that PFOA is widely distributed in the natural environment (Kannan et al. 2002, 2004; So et al. 2004; Yamashita et al. 2005) and may represent a significant health issue. An increasing number of occupational and epidemiological studies have evaluated the potential latent health consequences of these exposures.

In studies of occupationally exposed populations among definitively PFOA-exposed employees slight increases were observed for cancers of the pancreas, prostate, and large intestine, as well as cerebrovascular disease mortality (Alexander 2001). In a multi-year study of 69,000 West Virginia and Ohio residents exposed environmentally through drinking water contaminated by a fluorochemical manufacturing plant (West Virginia University School of Medicine 2008; Frisbee et al. 2009; Steenland et al. 2009), mean serum PFOA concentrations ranged from about 300 to 400 ng/mL (ppb) (Emmett et al. 2006a); lower serum PFOA concentrations were found in residents who drank noncontaminated, bottled water (mean concentration of <80 ng/mL). This study examined adult individuals with PFOA exposure in recent years, for various health parameters with respect to serum PFOA concentration. No association between current PFOA levels was found for what they considered to be markers for adverse health conditions, measured by clinical blood chemistry. Increased total cholesterol with increasing serum PFOA concentration was observed, suggesting that PPARα-activation (resulting in hypolipidemia) is not occurring (Steenland et al. 2010b).

A study of the general population at various locations throughout the U.S. between 1990 and 2002, found that PFOA was present in every human serum sample and ranged from 2.8 to 23.7 μg/L (Calafat et al. 2006). The U.S. National Health and Nutrition Examination Survey (NHANES), conducted by the Centers for Disease Control and Prevention, has measured PFOA in human tissue samples collected from across the country since 1999. The mean concentration of PFOA in the blood of nonoccupationally exposed Americans is 3.9 ng/mL (Calafat et al. 2007), but little information is available on mean serum concentrations of infants, children, or adolescents.

Multiple other epidemiological studies have investigated the potential relationship between blood serum PFOA concentration and potential adverse human health effects. Elevated cholesterol and other lipids in people exposed to PFOA occupationally or via drinking water have been found (Sakr et al. 2007a, b; Costa et al. 2009; Steenland et al. 2009, 2010b; Nelson et al. 2010), suggesting a possible link between perfluorinated compound levels, cholesterol levels, and increased risk of cardiovascular disease. Additionally, these studies have reported positive relationships of PFOA with other lipids (i.e., LDL cholesterol and triglycerides), with the exception of HDL cholesterol. Decreased concentrations of estradiol in women and in girls (West Virginia University School of Medicine 2008), clinically elevated uric acid (Steenland et al. 2010a), and immune system changes have also been alluded to (West Virginia University School of Medicine 2008). A number of epidemiological studies have examined fertility and developmental endpoints. Maternal PFOA was known to reach the fetus, because PFOA was present in umbilical cord blood, when also present in maternal blood (Apelberg et al. 2007; Monroy et al. 2008). However, no association was found between maternal PFOA and various developmental indices in a Danish National Cohort study (Fei et al. 2007). The most recent study found associations of elevated PFOA concentrations with lower sperm quality in reportedly healthy men (Joensen et al. 2009).

Associations with serum PFOA levels in the general population (<20 μg/L) have been reported for increased incidence of thyroid disease (Melzer et al. 2010), and decreased fertility as measured by time to pregnancy (Fei et al. 2009). While these epidemiologic studies have identified associations between PFOA exposure and adverse health outcomes, they do not demonstrate either cause and effect or potential modes of action.

8.1.2.1 PFOA-Induced Developmental Effects in Animals and Putative Mechanisms of Action (PPARα vs. Other)

Controlled laboratory studies have addressed the possible health effects of human relevance, examining PFOA exposure in multiple model organisms. PFOA does not appear to have significant mutagenic activity (Lawlor 1995, 1996). In nonhuman primates, chronic exposure studies have revealed a capacity for systemic toxicity and even death. Detrimental dose-dependent effects on body weight, bone marrow, spleen, heart brain and pituitary and hepatocellular hyperthrophy were observed (Butenhoff et al. 2004b). The liver weight changes were reversible. No hormonal or metabolic end point changes were observed, though triiodothyronine levels were decreased in the highest exposure group during the dosing period.

In rats, PFOA may be absorbed via dermal, inhalational, or oral exposure (Hinderliter et al. 2006). PFOA is eliminated intact, and not metabolized (Kudo and Kawashima 2003). PFOA is distributed primarily to the liver and serum in males, but also substantially to the kidney in females (Vanden Heuvel et al. 1991). Female rats do not exhibit the pronounced hepatomegaly and peroxisomal beta-oxidation observed in male rats (Kawashima et al. 1989). Rather, PFOA urinary excretion occurs rapidly in the female rat and in an estrogen-dependent manner (Ylinen et al. 1989). The gender-specific difference in PFOA elimination results from higher renal expression of organic anion transport 2 (Oat2) in the female rat. In mice, PFOA is partitioned primarily to the liver and serum, irrespective of gender, and no gender differences in urinary PFOA excretion nor renal Oat2 expression are observed in either mice or humans (Kudo et al. 2002). A pharmacokinetic analysis in pregnant Sprague–Dawley rats measured PFOA levels in amniotic fluid, placenta, embryos, milk and fetal, neonatal, and maternal blood (Butenhoff et al. 2004a) and provided the first evidence of transmission of PFOA from the dam to the offspring both during and subsequent to pregnancy. Interestingly, milk PFOA concentrations were about one tenth that of maternal serum, and were comparable to pup serum levels at mid-lactation.

Due to greater similarities in urinary excretion patterns in humans and mice, the mouse has been adopted as the more appropriate model of human health, when considering the reproductive and developmental toxicity of carboxylated PFAAs.

In mice, prenatal PFOA exposure induced reductions in percentage of live offspring born and birth weight, decreased postnatal survival, growth deficits, and delayed eye opening among offspring. Also, liver enlargement was observed in dams exposed throughout gestation (Lau et al. 2006; Wolf et al. 2007).

A long-term study of a range of PFOA doses and exposure in utero, exposure in utero followed by ovariectomy (OVX) or adult exposure was carried out in CD-1 mice (Hines et al. 2009). The main observed effects were on body weight. In utero exposures caused reduced early age body weight, with the lowest exposures causing increased body weight, and serum leptin and insulin levels between 20 and 40 weeks of age. There was no exposure effect on body weight in OVX animals or in animals exposed as adults. At 18 months of age, there was no effect of PFOA on body weight and internal PFOA concentrations were at control level. Liver weight was unaffected in late life by these exposure paradigms.

A thorough disposition study of PFOA levels in serum, urine, amniotic fluid, milk, mammary tissue, and whole pups at varying time points was performed in CD-1 mice given a single oral bolus of a range of PFOA doses on gestation day 17 (Fenton et al. 2009). Pups exhibited significantly higher serum PFOA concentrations than their respective dams, and their body burden increased for 8 days after birth, regardless of dose, indicative of PFOA transmission through milk.

In general toxicity studies of PFOA in rodents, the most prominent and reproducible observation is hepatomegaly and hepatic necrosis. These liver changes are believed to occur through activation of the peroxisome proliferator-activated receptor alpha (PPARα). The PFOA-induced histopathologic changes in liver are consistent with exposure to PPAR agonists (Kennedy et al. 2004). PPARα, a nuclear receptor of the steroid hormone receptor superfamily, binds and can be activated by both endogenous and exogenous ligands, such as dietary fatty acids. PPARα activation results in a number of metabolic changes including increased fatty acid beta-oxidation, and inhibition of hepatic secretion of very low-density lipoproteins and cholesterol (Kennedy et al. 2004). Agonism of PPARα by PFOA is thought to also explain the thymic and splenic atrophy often observed in exposed rodents (Yang et al. 2001).

Long-term chronic PFOA exposure has also been associated with a common tumor triad in exposed rats, including hepatocellular adenomas, pancreatic acinar-cell tumors, and Leydig cell tumors (Sibinski 1987). The PPARα action believed to be responsible for hepatocellular tumors, is generally not thought to be relevant to human health, given the tenfold lower expression of PPARα mRNA in the human liver, as compared to the rodent (Kennedy et al. 2004). For this reason, there is some question whether hepatotoxicity, when the observed hepatotoxic endpoints are demonstrated to be PPARα-mediated, should be considered relevant to human health. The human relevance of nonhepatic end points has not yet been determined.

Studies of other environmental agents indicate that late fetal and early neonatal mammary gland development is particularly sensitive to environmental insult (reviewed in Fenton 2006). Early life exposures that alter mammary gland development are thought to have a potential impact on the development of mammary cancers later in life in animal models. This is also thought to be the case in humans (Hiatt et al. 2009). Recent research in the mouse has made substantial discoveries regarding the effects of PFOA exposure on the mammary gland with high relevancy to human health. PFOA effects on the mammary gland are the remaining focus of this review.

8.1.3 *Studies of PFOA Effects on Mammary Gland*

8.1.3.1 Mammary Gland Effects of PFOA from In Utero/Lactational Exposures

In studies of overall dose response for maternal and developmental toxicity to PFOA, prenatal (GD 1–17) exposure reduced postnatal weight gain and survival among offspring beginning at 5 mg/kg. It was unclear if those effects were mediated by interference with dam lactation or if they were the result of general developmental impairment (Lau et al. 2006). Neonatal body weight gain is highly dependent upon the quantity and quality of milk received from the dam. Thus, the early postnatal effects could have been due either to nutritional deficits associated with mammary gland alterations in lactating dams or in utero toxicity, or some combination of the two. The specific effects of PFOA on the lactating mouse mammary gland and potential for consequences on neonatal mammary gland development in female offspring were examined. CD-1 mice were treated via oral gavage of the dam during known gestational windows of sensitivity for mammary gland development (dam mammary gland differentiation, GD 8–17; offspring mammary bud formation; GD 12–17) (Borellini and Oka 1989), or over the entirety of gestation. A 5-mg PFOA/kg body weight/day exposure delivered throughout gestation or during the second half of gestation significantly altered normal lactational mammary gland development in the dam (White et al. 2007). Mammary gland and milk protein gene expression was altered; epidermal growth factor, a gene associated with mammary proliferation was elevated at PND 10 (the normal peak of lactation in the mouse) and lactoferrin, a milk protein found at elevated levels at the beginning and end of lactation was elevated at mid-lactation and significantly downregulated at weaning compared to controls. These exposures also significantly retard neonatal growth and halt proliferation of the female pup mammary epithelium, even for as short an exposure as the final 6 days of gestation (GD 12–17; see Figs. 8.1 and 8.2).

These studies identified severe PFOA-induced delays in the mammary gland development of female offspring (White et al. 2007) independent of body growth retardation. The effects were apparent following a GD 12–17 oral exposure, indicating that for mammary gland responses, an entire gestational exposure is not necessary.

Further experiments were carried out in order to examine the timing, route of exposure, and persistence of the mammary gland effects in PFOA-exposed offspring. In a cross-foster study (White et al. 2009), pregnant CD-1 mice received either vehicle or 5 mg PFOA/kg body weight by oral gavage on GD 8–17. At parturition, litters were cross-fostered to yield the following four exposure groups: (1) control litters nursed by control dams; (2) control litters nursed by dams dosed with PFOA during gestation (lactational exposure); (3) litters exposed in utero nursed by control dams (intrauterine exposure); (4) litters exposed in utero to PFOA nursed by dams dosed with PFOA during gestation (intrauterine and lactational exposure). The litters and their dams were necropsied on PND 1, 3, 5, and 10. A similar cross-foster study examined effects later in life. This study was performed as described

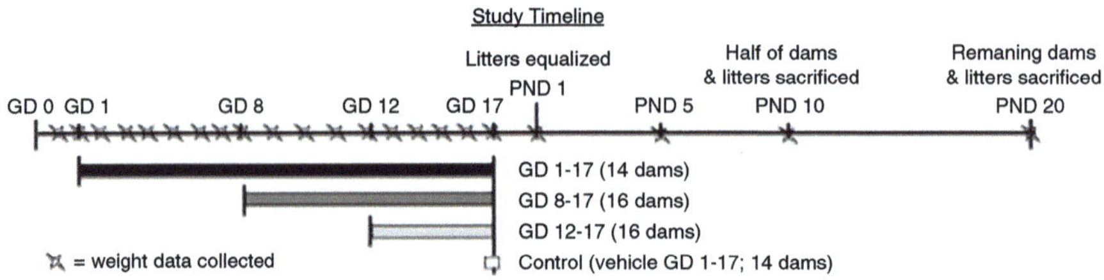

Fig. 8.1 Study design. Time-pregnant CD-1 mice received 5 mg PFOA/kg BW/day for different periods of gestation, depicted by bar lengths, ending on GD 17. *Stars* represent BW data collection (for both dams and offspring after PND 1). Other data collection time points are also shown. From White et al. (2007) by permission of Oxford University Press

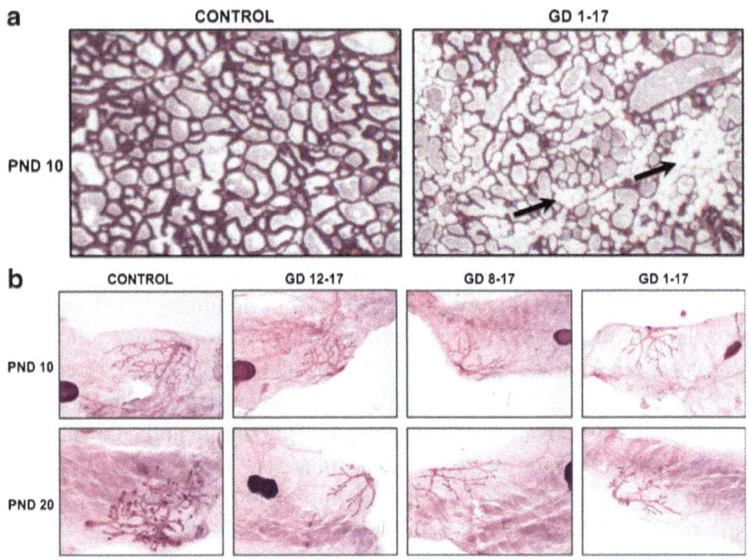

Fig. 8.2 Dam and offspring mammary gland morphology following PFOA exposure. (**a**) Maternal mouse mammary gland development on PND 10 following GD 1–17 PFOA exposure. (**a**) H & E – stained sections of mammary glands at 70× showing significantly ($p<0.001$) delayed development stemming from PFOA exposure. *Arrows* indicate adipose tissue. (**b**) Female pup mammary gland development after exposure during three segments of gestation. Whole mount preparations of mammary tissue from female offspring at PND 10 and 20 at 20×. From White et al. (2007) by permission of Oxford University Press

above, but included the additional dose of 3 mg PFOA/kg body weight, with exposure at GD 1–17. Another study addressed only the critical period of exposure, and pregnant dams received vehicle or 5 mg PFOA/kg on GD 1–17, GD 7–17, GD 10–17, GD 13–17, or GD 15–17. Female offspring were necropsied on PND 22, 29, 32, 42, and 62, as well as at 18 months postnatally.

Together these latter studies demonstrated the capacity for both short duration (3 days) prenatal and exclusively lactational PFOA exposure (5 mg/kg dam body weight) to delay mammary gland development in offspring. Delayed mammary gland development was observed as early as PND 1 and as late as 9 weeks postnatally, when body weight deficits caused by treatment were overcome. In the 9-week-old sexually mature mice, mammary gland deficits were still apparent, despite the fact that PFOA serum concentrations were relatively low (<350 ng/mL), and of the same order of magnitude as concentrations reported in humans exposed occupationally or residentially (highly contaminated areas) (Emmett et al. 2006b). Furthermore, the deficit in mammary gland development was evident even when the internal PFOA dose dropped to near background levels, suggesting a permanent effect. Sparse epithelial filling of the mammary gland fat pad observed in 18-month-old PFOA-exposed offspring, combined with increased stromal density and inflammation provided further evidence that early-life PFOA exposures result in permanent, long-term effects in the mammary gland.

The early-life effects cross-foster study also showed that in all four groups of PFOA-exposed female offspring the delay in mammary gland development started as early as PND 1, a time when the mammary epithelium normally undergoes allometric growth and development. Interestingly, only hours of lactational exposure from dams receiving 5 mg/kg BW led to significant delays in development that persisted through PND 10. Taken together these results suggest that deficits in mammary gland development resulting from intrauterine, lactational, or combined PFOA exposures occur early, and persist into sexual maturation. Branching morphogenesis and ductal outgrowth are highly sensitive to PFOA exposure. Interestingly, among the 3 mg/kg lactationally exposed group deficits in mammary gland development were evident at PND 42 and 63 in the absence of any body growth retardation over life. Thus, the threshold for effects on mammary gland development may be lower compared to that for body growth deficits, and that the mechanisms responsible for those effects differ.

The findings from these studies are consistent with previous work (White et al. 2007) that reported delays in mammary gland development resulting from developmental PFOA exposure, independent of body weight deficits. These findings are also in agreement with studies of other environmental agents that indicate that late fetal and early neonatal mammary gland development is particularly sensitive to environmental insult (reviewed in Fenton 2006). Furthermore, they showed for the first time that PFOA exposure transmitted through milk produces effects that persist into adulthood and late-life. Importantly the dosimetry data showed that offspring with intrauterine PFOA exposure exhibited higher serum PFOA concentrations on PND 1 than did the treated dams they nursed on, a novel observation vital to the understanding of the pharmacokinetics of PFOA in the fetus and neonate.

Further dosimetry studies (single bolus exposure on GD 17) (Fenton et al. 2009) described several novel findings: (1) The amount of PFOA in amniotic fluid is about half that concentration found in the dam serum. (2) Dam PFOA concentrations in serum, urine, and milk peak just after birth (PND 1–2). (3) Concentrations of PFOA in dam serum, urine, mammary tissue, and milk do not decline in a linear fashion over time, but follow a U-shaped curve with highest measured concentrations early and late in lactation. (4) The body burden of the offspring increases until the peak of lactation, and precipitously declines once nursing slows. The body burden (total measurable PFOA in the entire animal) and the serum concentrations (per mL serum) of the offspring do not follow a similar pattern, and this is due to exponential growth and increased blood volume in the growing neonate. Also, this study was the first to report milk to serum ratios for mice, ranging from 0.2 to 0.6 early and late in lactation (low milk volumes) to 0.1–0.2 between PND 8 and 11 (peak milk volumes).

8.1.4 *Effects of PFOA Peripubertal Exposure on Mammary Gland Development*

In addition to in utero and lactational exposure, the peripubertal period of breast development is considered to be an important window of susceptibility of the developing breast to environmental exposures that may predispose humans to increased breast cancer risk later in life (Selevan et al. 2000; Fenton 2006). Since PFOA is persistent in the environment, and there is wide-spread human exposure to PFOA, its effect on the mammary gland during this sensitive period of mammary gland development was examined. It is also increasingly recognized that genetic background could be another important susceptibility factor that determines human responses to environmental pollutants (Kleeberger 2003). To address these issues, the effect of peripubertal exposure to PFOA on mammary gland development was examined in two mouse strains: C57BL/6 and BALB/C.

To determine the effect of peripubertal PFOA exposure on mouse mammary gland development, BALB/C and C57BL/6 mice were treated with a wide dose range of PFOA by oral gavage, once daily, 5 days/week for 4 weeks starting at 21 days of age (Yang et al. 2009; Zhao et al. 2010). Both mouse strains displayed normal behavior, looked healthy and showed similar BW gains at all PFOA doses with the exception of a significant decrease in BW at the 10 mg/kg dose.

However, analysis of mammary gland whole mounts revealed that 2.5, 5, 7.5, and 10 mg/kg doses of PFOA treatment caused significant inhibition on mammary gland growth in the BALB/C strain, as evidenced by reduced ductal length, as well as decreased numbers of terminal end buds (TEBs) (Fig. 8.3a). No morphological changes were observed with treatment at lower doses.

In striking contrast, PFOA treatment in the C57BL/6 strain resulted in significantly increased numbers of TEBs and enlarged terminal ducts (TDs) at the 5 mg/kg doses (Fig. 8.3b). Ductal length was not different among the control, 1 and 5 mg/kg doses. A significant inhibitory effect on all measures of mammary gland development (ductal length, numbers of TEBs and enlarged TDs) was seen at the 7.5 and 10 mg/kg doses.

The effect of PFOA treatment on mammary gland epithelial cell proliferation was determined by BrdU incorporation assay (Fig. 8.3c). The mammary glands of BALB/C mice treated with 5 mg/kg PFOA had significantly fewer proliferating cells in TEBs/TDs and ducts. The same dose of PFOA slightly increased the number of proliferating cells in C57BL/6 mammary glands. However, given the fact that

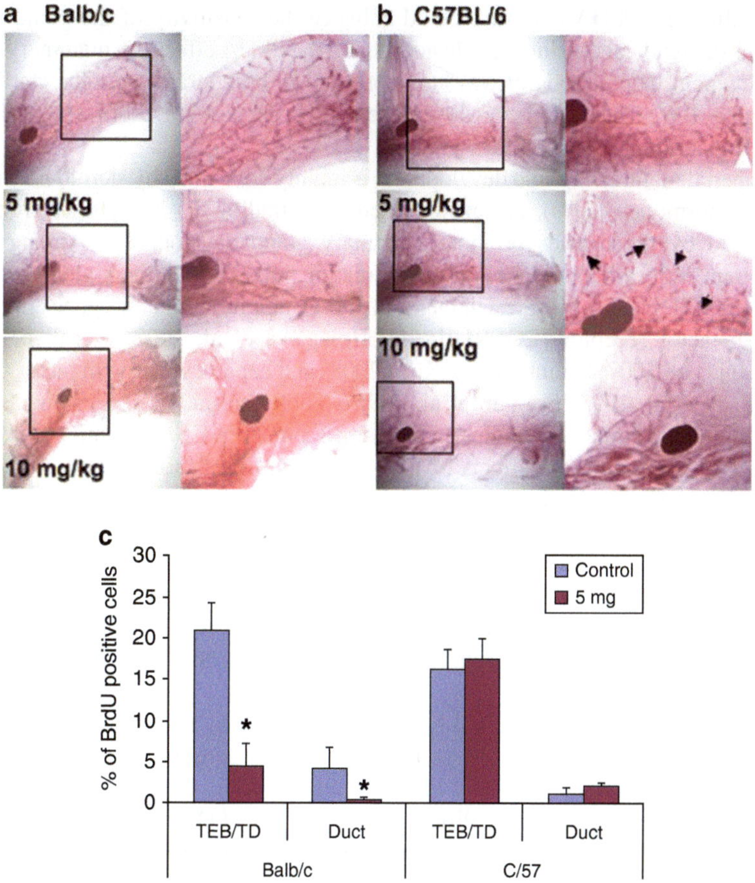

Fig. 8.3 Effect of peripubertal PFOA treatment on mammary gland development and mammary epithelial cell proliferation. BALB/C and C57BL/6 female mice were treated with vehicle control or 5 mg/kg BW PFOA by oral gavage daily from 3 to 7 weeks of age. Twenty-four hours after the last vehicle control or PFOA treatment, mice were killed and mammary gland whole mounts were prepared. Representative mammary gland whole mount photomicrographs from control- or PFOA-treated (**a**) Balb/c or (**b**) C57BL/6 mice. *Black arrows* indicate stimulated terminal ducts (TD) and *white arrows* indicate terminal end buds (TEBs) (Mag. 2.5×; Mag. of insets 4.5×). Mouse mammary epithelial cell proliferation was determined by BrdU incorporation assay and quantitated in TEBs, stimulated TDs, and ducts (**c**). Data are presented as Mean ± S.E.M. ($n=5$). $^*p<0.05$ compared to the control group. From Yang et al. (2009)

PFOA treatment significantly increased the numbers of TEBs/TDs, more overall cell proliferation occurred in PFOA-treated C57BL/6 mammary glands (Fig. 8.3).

Accumulating evidence has shown that TEB structures are sensitive to chemical carcinogen treatment and their presence at the time of carcinogen exposure is positively associated with mammary tumor multiplicity in rodent models (Fenton 2006). The increased numbers of TEBs in the PFOA-treated developing glands raise the possibility that PFOA exposure could enhance the sensitivity of the gland to the actions of chemical carcinogens. In addition to the PFOA effects on mammary gland development, hepatotoxicity was also observed in both strains of mice starting at 1 mg/kg BW. The inhibitory dose-dependent effects were more severe in the C56BL/6 strain.

Pubertal mammary gland development is mainly controlled by steroid hormones, growth hormones (GHs) and growth factors. Estradiol (E) and progesterone (P) produced by the ovaries promote mammary gland development. Among other important factors that are involved in stimulating pubertal mammary gland development are GH, insulin-like growth factor I (IGF-I), amphiregulin (Areg, an epidermal growth factor receptor [EGFR] ligand) (Imagawa et al. 2002; Sternlicht 2006; Ciarloni et al. 2007; Kleinberg and Ruan 2008) and hepatocyte growth factor (HGF) (Niranjan et al. 1995; Soriano et al. 1998). Thus, the underlying mechanism by which PFOA stimulates mammary gland development in C57BL/6 mice was investigated by examining the effects of PFOA exposure on factors known to regulate pubertal mammary gland development.

PFOA by itself (5 mg/kg BW) does not stimulate mammary gland development in OVX pubertal C57BL/6 mice. There was no outgrowth of ducts or presence of TEBs compared to control-treated mice and in sharp contrast to the stimulatory effect of PFOA observed in the ovary intact mice. These results indicate that PFOA does not have an independent direct stimulatory effect on C57BL/6 mouse mammary gland development.

E and P are two major steroid hormones produced by the ovaries that promote pubertal mammary gland development. We found that serum total E levels between ovary intact vehicle control- and PFOA-treated mice in proestrus or estrus cycle stages were not significantly different. However, PFOA treatment significantly increased serum P levels (~3-fold) at both proestrus and estrus stages. The effect of PFOA treatment on mammary gland response to exogenous hormones was also examined (Zhao et al. 2010). Ovary intact C57BL/6 mice were dosed with vehicle control or PFOA 5 mg/kg BW for 4 weeks starting at 21 days of age, OVX 24 h after the last dose of PFOA and 1 week later the mice were injected s.c. daily for 5 days with vehicle control, E, P, or E+P. There were more stimulated TDs in the mammary glands of mice treated with PFOA and E or P, compared with control mice treated with E or P. The mammary glands of mice treated with PFOA and P or E+P also had more side branches, a hallmark of P action. These results indicate that in addition to increasing serum P levels, PFOA treatment also increases mammary gland responses to E and P.

The effects of PFOA treatment on the expression levels of Areg, IGF-I and HGF, growth factors critically involved in mammary gland development, were also investigated. Western blot analysis showed that PFOA treatment significantly increased the protein levels of Areg, IGF-I and HGF by 3.5 ± 2.1, 4.1 ± 1.7, and 1.4 ± 0.3 fold, respectively. Areg expression induced by E is an essential mediator of estrogen receptor α (ERα) function in mammary gland development (Ciarloni et al. 2007) and Areg may mediate EGFR activation. We found that PFOA treatment also caused two- to threefold increases of ERα and EGFR proteins in mammary glands.

As PFOA is an agonist of PPARα, and studies have shown that PPARα mediates various toxicities of PFOA in rodents (Abbott et al. 2007), the dependence of PFOA-induced mouse mammary gland development on the expression of PPARα was investigated. To this end, PPARα knockout mice in C57BL/6 background were given the same PFOA treatment as described above for wildtype mice (PFOA 5 mg/kg BW for 4 weeks starting at 21 days of age). The same stimulatory effect of PFOA on mammary gland development was observed in knockout and wildtype mice, indicating that the stimulatory effect of peripubertal PFOA treatment on mammary gland development in C57BL/6 mice is independent of the expression of PPARα. Protein levels of Areg, IGF-I, HGF, ERα, and EGFR in PPARα knockout mammary glands were increased by PFOA to a level similar to that observed in wildtype mice.

Additionally to examine the effect of PFOA on mammary gland cell proliferation, mammary gland protein levels of cyclin D1 and proliferating cell nuclear antigen (PCNA), two of the most commonly used markers reflecting active cell proliferation, were also analyzed. Consistent with increased levels of P, growth factors, EGFR and ERα, PFOA induced similar and significant increases of cyclin D1 and PCNA protein levels in both wildtype and PPARα knockout mammary glands. Taken together, these results indicate that PFOA-induced increases in serum P, growth factors, and receptors contribute to pubertal mammary epithelial cell proliferation and that these PFOA effects are PPARα-independent. These results demonstrate for the first time PPARα-independent endocrine disrupting activity of PFOA. In contrast, the hepatotoxic effects of PFOA on the liver were not observed in the PPARα knockout mice indicating that the liver effects were PPARα-dependent.

8.1.5 Discussion and Integration

The widespread presence of PFOA in wildlife and humans and its accumulative and persistent properties have raised considerable health concerns over recent years. Effects of PFOA exposure on human health have not yet been fully elucidated. Most epidemiological studies have examined for health effects resulting from adult exposures. Because PFOA can potentially be transferred transplacentally and through nursing (Apelberg et al. 2007; Monroy et al. 2008; Fenton et al. 2009), potential effects on fetal and postnatal developmental are of concern in humans. In this regard, animal studies in mice have revealed effects of PFOA exposure on mammary gland development in offspring resulting from in utero, and lactational exposure, as well postnatal exposure during the peripubertal period. This is of particular concern because studies have shown that many environmental pollutants can affect mammary gland development in experimental animals, and the effect can be especially significant if chemical exposure occurs during critical stages of mammary gland development such as the gestational, neonatal, and peripubertal periods, as well as during pregnancy (Fenton 2006).

One critical stage of mammary gland development in the rodent and humans is formation and outgrowth of the mammary epithelial bud, which occurs around GD

13 in the mouse. The developmental exposures defined above (White et al. 2007, 2009) encompass this critical period, and identified the period of GD 15–17 as sufficient to cause long-lasting delays in epithelial branching and outgrowth. The effect of in utero and lactational PFOA exposure (3–5 mg/kg BW) in outbred CD1 mice results in delayed or inhibited mammary gland development (reduced ductal length and branching) in the exposed offspring, even at doses 10–100-fold lower than doses already reported (Macon et al. 2011). These exposures affect the mammary gland during critical times of development: embryonic development in utero and through lactation during postnatal allometric growth of gland prior to onset of ovarian cycles. PFOA exposure during pregnancy also reduced postpartum lactational function in the exposed dams. In CD1 mice, the inhibitory effect on mammary gland development in offspring persists in sexually mature adult and aged mice. These changes persist even after the PFOA body burden has returned to control levels pointing to the permanence of the effects of early PFOA exposure. The severity of late-life effects are not fully understood, but on-going studies will address these issues. It is also not currently known what effect adult PFOA exposure might have in the adult mammary gland. However, the detrimental effects on lactational function in mice exposed during pregnancy indicate that this is an additional stage of mammary gland development that is sensitive to PFOA effects. The peripubertal period is considered to be an important window of susceptibility of the developing breast to environmental exposures that may predispose humans to increased breast cancer risk later in life (Selevan et al. 2000; Fenton 2006). Peripubertal PFOA exposure over a range of doses in inbred BALB/C strain mice resulted in inhibition of mammary gland development (2.5–10 mg/kg BW) with no observable gross effect at lower doses (0.1, 1 mg/kg/BW). In striking contrast, peripubertal PFOA exposure (5 mg/kg BW) in inbred C57BL/6 strain mice results in a stimulation of mammary gland development and proliferation. No gross observable effects were seen at lower doses, yet higher doses (7.5 mg/kg BW) inhibited mammary gland development similar to the BALB/C strain. The stimulatory effect in C57BL/6 mice was evident in the increased number of proliferating TEBs, raising the possibility that peripubertal exposure could enhance the sensitivity of the gland to the actions of chemical carcinogens.

Further studies of peripubertal PFOA exposure in C57BL/6 mice show that PFOA is not directly stimulatory, but requires the presence of the ovaries (Zhao et al. 2010). CD1 mice exposed throughout gestation to 0.01–1.0 mg/kg BW PFOA also required the presence of functional ovaries for chemical-induced increases in serum leptin and insulin, and excessive weight gain in young adult mice (Hines et al. 2009). PFOA exposure significantly increased serum levels of progesterone in C57BL/6 mice and their mammary glands exhibited elevated levels of Areg, IGF-I and HGF, ERα and EGF-R, all factors that promote pubertal mammary gland development. Furthermore, PFOA exposure to the pregnant mammary gland caused altered milk protein production in CD1 mice (White et al. 2007). Thus, PFOA exhibits many of the characteristics of an endocrine disruptor.

Although it is clear that PFOA adversely affects the mammary glands of developing mice, the different effects of PFOA exposures and doses in different strains of mice (CD1, BALB/C, and C57BL/6) point to the importance of genetic background. These observations suggest that in human populations with heterogeneous genetic backgrounds, individuals may respond differentially to the same exposure. Thus, genetic diversity may have a role in determining the effects of PFOA on normal mammary development. This also points to the importance of considering strain differences in future studies to elucidate the mechanisms responsible for inhibitory vs. stimulatory effects on the mammary gland.

Studies have shown that PPARα plays critical roles in various toxicities of PFOA. For example, it was found by using PPARα knockout 129S1/SvlmJ mice that impaired postnatal body weight gain, delayed eye opening among pups, and postnatal mortality were dependent upon PPARα expression (Abbott et al. 2009), whereas, early prenatal loss was PPARα independent. Dam lactation and mammary gland morphology of female offspring were not examined, but PPARα knockout mice reproduce normally and exhibit normal mammary gland development. It is noteworthy that MG effects have been observed to occur in the absence of growth deficits that have been identified as PPARα-dependent effects.

Whether the effects of PFOA treatment on mouse mammary gland development depend upon the expression of PPARα is an important area of investigation. Knockout and transgenic mice have provided some clues as to possible modes of action for PFOA in the mammary gland. In C57BL/6 PPARα knockout mice, the effect of PFOA to stimulate peripubertal mammary gland development is PPARα independent (Zhao et al. 2010). The increased levels of Areg, IGF-I and HGF, ERα, and EGF-R in the mammary gland induced by PFOA exposure are observed in both C57BL/6 PPARα knock out and wildtype mice. On the other hand, in the same study, PFOA-induced hepatotoxicity was PPARα-dependent. PPARα action believed to be responsible for liver effects are generally not believed to be relevant to human health, given the tenfold lower expression of PPARα mRNA in the human liver, as compared to the rodent (Kennedy et al. 2004). In this context, it is particularly noteworthy that the observed peri-pubertal stimulatory effects of PFOA on the mammary gland are independent of associated hepatoxicity and PPARα-independent.

PPARα transgenic FVB/N mouse dams exhibiting constitutively activated PPARα, experience profound impairment of lobuloalveolar differentiation and impaired lactation with no offspring surviving until weaning (Yang et al. 2006). Altered PPAR-signaling has the potential to greatly interfere with proper functional differentiation of the lactating gland. However, as stated above, mammary gland effects of PFOA appear to be mouse strain-dependent and highly dependent on genetic background. Thus, the results obtained in PPARα knockout and transgenic mice need to be interpreted in this context.

PFOA has been slated for removal from emissions and products by 2015, under a voluntary agreement between the U.S. Environmental Protection Agency and eight major manufacturers (USEPA 2006, 2009). Because of the absence of federal regulatory standards for PFOA in drinking water, state environmental health departments have initiated the process of developing (North Carolina) or have already set their own standards (New Jersey, Minnesota, West Virginia) for this common water contaminant.

An important unresolved issue is the PFOA body burden in mice vs. humans, in relation to adverse health effects such as the observed effects on mammary development. There are significant differences in PFOA elimination half-lives in mice (days) vs. humans (years). Thus the potential exists that even low level exposures in humans can lead to elevated body burdens over time. Further studies that examine dose–response relationships, routes and timing of exposure, and the underlying mechanisms of PFOA-induced effects in animals in the context of different genetic backgrounds are needed. This is particularly true for critical periods of mammary gland development, as well as a careful analysis of long-term effects. It is anticipated that such studies can provide information relevant to identifying previously unrecognized potential human health hazards.

Acknowledgments This work was supported by the Breast Cancer and the Environment Research Centers Grant U01 ES/CA 012800 from the National Institute of Environment Health Science (NIEHS) and the National Cancer Institute (NCI), National Institutes of Health, Department of Health and Human Services (to S.Z.H.).

Disclaimer The views expressed in this chapter are those of the author(s) and do not necessarily reflect the views or policies of the NIEHS, NCI or the NIH.

References

Abbott BD, Wolf CJ, Schmid JE et al (2007) Perfluorooctanoic acid induced developmental toxicity in the mouse is dependent on expression of peroxisome proliferator activated receptor-alpha. Toxicol Sci 98(2):571–581

Abbott BD, Wolf CJ, Das KP et al (2009) Developmental toxicity of perfluorooctane sulfonate (PFOS) is not dependent on expression of peroxisome proliferator activated receptor-alpha (PPAR alpha) in the mouse. Reprod Toxicol 27(3–4):258–265

Alexander B (2001) Mortality of workers employed at the 3M Cottage Grove facility. Minneapolis (MN):University of Minnesota. U.S. EPA docket AR-226-1030a018 and 226-1030a019

Apelberg BJ, Witter FR, Herbstman JB et al (2007) Cord serum concentrations of perfluorooctane sulfonate (PFOS) and perfluorooctanoate (PFOA) in relation to weight and size at birth. Environ Health Perspect 115(11):1670–1676

Begley TH, White K, Honigfort P et al (2005) Perfluorochemicals: potential sources of and migration from food packaging. Food Addit Contam 22(10):1023–1031

Borellini F, Oka T (1989) Growth control and differentiation in mammary epithelial cells. Environ Health Perspect 80:85–99

Boulanger B, Vargo J, Schnoor JL et al (2004) Detection of perfluorooctane surfactants in Great Lakes water. Environ Sci Technol 38(15):4064–4070

Butenhoff JL, Kennedy GL Jr, Frame SR et al (2004a) The reproductive toxicology of ammonium perfluorooctanoate (APFO) in the rat. Toxicology 196(1–2):95–116

Butenhoff JL, Kennedy GL Jr, Hinderliter PM et al (2004b) Pharmacokinetics of perfluorooctanoate in cynomolgus monkeys. Toxicol Sci 82(2):394–406

Calafat AM, Needham LL, Kuklenyik Z et al (2006) Perfluorinated chemicals in selected residents of the American continent. Chemosphere 63(3):490–496

Calafat AM, Wong LY, Kuklenyik Z et al (2007) Polyfluoroalkyl chemicals in the U.S. population: data from the National Health and Nutrition Examination Survey (NHANES) 2003–2004 and comparisons with NHANES 1999–2000. Environ Health Perspect 115(11):1596–1602

Chang SC, Thibodeaux JR, Eastvold ML et al (2008) Thyroid hormone status and pituitary function in adult rats given oral doses of perfluorooctanesulfonate (PFOS). Toxicology 243(3):330–339

Ciarloni L, Mallepell S, Brisken C (2007) Amphiregulin is an essential mediator of estrogen receptor alpha function in mammary gland development. Proc Natl Acad Sci USA 104(13):5455–5460

Costa G, Sartori S, Consonni D (2009) Thirty years of medical surveillance in perfluooctanoic acid production workers. J Occup Environ Med 51(3):364–372

Dinglasan MJ, Ye Y, Edwards EA et al (2004) Fluorotelomer alcohol biodegradation yields poly- and perfluorinated acids. Environ Sci Technol 38(10):2857–2864

Ellis DA, Martin JW, De Silva AO et al (2004) Degradation of fluorotelomer alcohols: a likely atmospheric source of perfluorinated carboxylic acids. Environ Sci Technol 38(12): 3316–3321

Emmett EA, Shofer FS, Zhang H et al (2006a) Community exposure to perfluorooctanoate: relationships between serum concentrations and exposure sources. J Occup Environ Med 48(8):759–770

Emmett EA, Zhang H, Shofer FS et al (2006b) Community exposure to perfluorooctanoate: relationships between serum levels and certain health parameters. J Occup Environ Med 48(8):771–779

EPA US (1976) Toxic Substances Control Act

Fei C, McLaughlin JK, Tarone RE et al (2007) Perfluorinated chemicals and fetal growth: a study within the Danish National Birth Cohort. Environ Health Perspect 115(11):1677–1682

Fei C, McLaughlin JK, Lipworth L et al (2009) Maternal levels of perfluorinated chemicals and subfecundity. Hum Reprod 24(5):1200–1205

Fenton SE (2006) Endocrine-disrupting compounds and mammary gland development: early exposure and later life consequences. Endocrinology 147(6 Suppl):S18–S24

Fenton SE, Reiner JL, Nakayama SF et al (2009) Analysis of PFOA in dosed CD-1 mice. Part 2. Disposition of PFOA in tissues and fluids from pregnant and lactating mice and their pups. Reprod Toxicol 27(3–4):365–372

Frisbee SJ, Brooks AP Jr, Maher A et al (2009) The C8 health project: design, methods, and participants. Environ Health Perspect 117(12):1873–1882

Gulkowska A, Jiang Q, So MK et al (2006) Persistent perfluorinated acids in seafood collected from two cities of China. Environ Sci Technol 40(12):3736–3741

Hansen KJ, Johnson HO, Eldridge JS et al (2002) Quantitative characterization of trace levels of PFOS and PFOA in the Tennessee River. Environ Sci Technol 36(8):1681–1685

Hiatt RA, Haslam SZ, Osuch J (2009) The breast cancer and the environment research centers: transdisciplinary research on the role of the environment in breast cancer etiology. Environ Health Perspect 117(12):1814–1822

Hinderliter PM, DeLorme MP, Kennedy GL (2006) Perfluorooctanoic acid: relationship between repeated inhalation exposures and plasma PFOA concentration in the rat. Toxicology 222(1–2):80–85

Hines EP, White SS, Stanko JP et al (2009) Phenotypic dichotomy following developmental exposure to perfluorooctanoic acid (PFOA) in female CD-1 mice: low doses induce elevated serum leptin and insulin, and overweight in mid-life. Mol Cell Endocrinol 304(1–2): 97–105

Imagawa W, Pedchenko VK, Helber J et al (2002) Hormone/growth factor interactions mediating epithelial/stromal communication in mammary gland development and carcinogenesis. J Steroid Biochem Mol Biol 80(2):213–230

Joensen UN, Bossi R, Leffers H et al (2009) Do perfluoroalkyl compounds impair human semen quality? Environ Health Perspect 117(6):923–927

Kannan K, Corsolini S, Falandysz J et al (2002) Perfluorooctanesulfonate and related fluorinated hydrocarbons in marine mammals, fishes, and birds from coasts of the Baltic and the Mediterranean Seas. Environ Sci Technol 36(15):3210–3216

Kannan K, Corsolini S, Falandysz J et al (2004) Perfluorooctanesulfonate and related fluorochemicals in human blood from several countries. Environ Sci Technol 38(17):4489–4495

Kawashima Y, Uy-Yu N, Kozuka H (1989) Sex-related difference in the inductions by perfluoro-octanoic acid of peroxisomal beta-oxidation, microsomal 1-acylglycerophosphocholine acyltransferase and cytosolic long-chain acyl-CoA hydrolase in rat liver. Biochem J 261(2):595–600

Kennedy GL Jr, Butenhoff JL, Olsen GW et al (2004) The toxicology of perfluorooctanoate. Crit Rev Toxicol 34(4):351–384

Kleeberger SR (2003) Genetic aspects of susceptibility to air pollution. Eur Respir J Suppl 40:52s–56s

Kleinberg DL, Ruan W (2008) IGF-I, GH, and sex steroid effects in normal mammary gland development. J Mammary Gland Biol Neoplasia 13(4):353–360

Kudo N, Kawashima Y (2003) Toxicity and toxicokinetics of perfluorooctanoic acid in humans and animals. J Toxicol Sci 28(2):49–57

Kudo N, Katakura M, Sato Y et al (2002) Sex hormone-regulated renal transport of perfluorooctanoic acid. Chem Biol Interact 139(3):301–316

Lau C, Thibodeaux JR, Hanson RG et al (2006) Effects of perfluorooctanoic acid exposure during pregnancy in the mouse. Toxicol Sci 90(2):510–518

Lawlor T (1995) Mutagenicity test with T-6342 in the Salmonella-*Escherichia coli*/mammalian-microsome reverse mutation assay. Laboratory Number: 17073-0-409. Corning Hazleton Inc., Vienna

Lawlor T (1996) Mutagenicity test with T-6564 in the Salmonella-*Escherichia coli*/mammalian-microsome reverse mutation assay. Final report. CHV Study No.17750-0-409R. Corning Hazleton Inc., Vienna, 13 Sept 1996

Liou JS, Szostek B, DeRito CM et al (2010) Investigating the biodegradability of perfluorooctanoic acid. Chemosphere 80(2):176–183

Loewen M, Halldorson T, Wang F et al (2005) Fluorotelomer carboxylic acids and PFOS in rainwater from an urban center in Canada. Environ Sci Technol 39(9):2944–2951

Macon MB, Villanueva LR, Tatum-Gibbs K et al Prenatal perfluorooctanoic acid exposure in CD-1 mice: low dose developmental effects and internal dosimetry. Toxicol Sci, Accepted March 22, 2011; doi:10.1093/toxsci/kfr076

Melzer D, Rice N, Depledge MH et al (2010) Association between serum perfluorooctanoic acid (PFOA) and thyroid disease in the U.S. National Health and Nutrition Examination Survey. Environ Health Perspect 118(5):686–692

Monroy R, Morrison K, Teo K et al (2008) Serum levels of perfluoroalkyl compounds in human maternal and umbilical cord blood samples. Environ Res 108(1):56–62

Moody CA, Hebert GN, Strauss SH et al (2003) Occurrence and persistence of perfluorooctanesulfonate and other perfluorinated surfactants in groundwater at a fire-training area at Wurtsmith Air Force Base, Michigan, USA. J Environ Monit 5(2):341–345

Moriwaki H, Takatah Y, Arakawa R (2003) Concentrations of perfluorooctane sulfonate (PFOS) and perfluorooctanoic acid (PFOA) in vacuum cleaner dust collected in Japanese homes. J Environ Monit 5(5):753–757

Nelson JW, Hatch EE, Webster TF (2010) Exposure to polyfluoroalkyl chemicals and cholesterol, body weight, and insulin resistance in the general US population. Environ Health Perspect 118(2):197–202

Niranjan B, Buluwela L, Yant J et al (1995) HGF/SF: a potent cytokine for mammary growth, morphogenesis and development. Development 121(9):2897–2908

Ohmori K, Kudo N, Katayama K et al (2003) Comparison of the toxicokinetics between perfluorocarboxylic acids with different carbon chain length. Toxicology 184(2–3):135–140

Olsen GW, Chang SC, Noker PE et al (2009) A comparison of the pharmacokinetics of perfluorobutanesulfonate (PFBS) in rats, monkeys, and humans. Toxicology 256(1–2):65–74

Saito N, Harada K, Inoue K et al (2004) Perfluorooctanoate and perfluorooctane sulfonate concentrations in surface water in Japan. J Occup Health 46(1):49–59

Sakr CJ, Kreckmann KH, Green JW et al (2007a) Cross-sectional study of lipids and liver enzymes related to a serum biomarker of exposure (ammonium perfluorooctanoate or APFO) as part of a general health survey in a cohort of occupationally exposed workers. J Occup Environ Med 49(10):1086–1096

Sakr CJ, Leonard RC, Kreckmann KH et al (2007b) Longitudinal study of serum lipids and liver enzymes in workers with occupational exposure to ammonium perfluorooctanoate. J Occup Environ Med 49(8):872–879

Selevan SG, Kimmel CA, Mendola P (2000) Identifying critical windows of exposure for children's health. Environ Health Perspect 108(Suppl 3):451–455

Sibinski LJ (1987) Two-Year oral (diet) toxicity/carcinogenicity study of fluorochemical FC-143 (perfluorooctane ammonium carboxylate) in rats. Reviewed in US EPA "Revised Draft PFOA Hazard Assessment-Robust Study Annex" AR226-1137 (pp 260–267; PDF pp 157–164)

So MK, Taniyasu S, Yamashita N et al (2004) Perfluorinated compounds in coastal waters of Hong Kong, South China, and Korea. Environ Sci Technol 38(15):4056–4063

Soriano JV, Pepper MS, Orci L et al (1998) Roles of hepatocyte growth factor/scatter factor and transforming growth factor-beta1 in mammary gland ductal morphogenesis. J Mammary Gland Biol Neoplasia 3(2):133–150

Stahl T, Heyn J, Thiele H et al (2009) Carryover of perfluorooctanoic acid (PFOA) and perfluorooctane sulfonate (PFOS) from soil to plants. Arch Environ Contam Toxicol 57(2):289–298

Steenland K, Tinker S, Frisbee S et al (2009) Association of perfluorooctanoic acid and perfluorooctane sulfonate with serum lipids among adults living near a chemical plant. Am J Epidemiol 170(10):1268–1278

Steenland K, Fletcher T, Savitz DA (2010a) Epidemiologic evidence on the health effects of perfluorooctanoic acid (PFOA). Environ Health Perspect 118(8):1100–8

Steenland K, Tinker S, Shankar A et al (2010b) Association of perfluorooctanoic acid (PFOA) and perfluorooctane sulfonate (PFOS) with uric acid among adults with elevated community exposure to PFOA. Environ Health Perspect 118(2):229–233

Sternlicht MD (2006) Key stages in mammary gland development: the cues that regulate ductal branching morphogenesis. Breast Cancer Res 8(1):201

USEPA (2006) SAB review of EPA's draft risk assessment of the potential human health effects associated with exposure to perfluroоctanoic acid and its salts (EPA-SAB-06-006). Office of Pollution Prevention and Toxics RAD. http://www.epa.gov/opptintr/pfoa/pubs/pfoarisk.pdf. Accessed 29 June 2010

USEPA (2009) Provisional health advisories for perfluorooctanoic acid (PFOA) and perfluorooctane sulfonate (PFOS). http://water.epa.gov/action/advisories/drinking/upload/2009_01_15_criteria_drinking_pha-PFOA_PFOS.pdf. Accessed 29 June 2010

Vanden Heuvel JP, Kuslikis BI, Van Rafelghem MJ et al (1991) Tissue distribution, metabolism, and elimination of perfluorooctanoic acid in male and female rats. J Biochem Toxicol 6(2):83–92

West Virginia University School of Medicine (2008) The C8 health project: WVU Data Housing Website. http://www.hsc.wvu.edu/som/cmed/c8/. Accessed 29 June 2010

White SS, Calafat AM, Kuklenyik Z et al (2007) Gestational PFOA exposure of mice is associated with altered mammary gland development in dams and female offspring. Toxicol Sci 96(1):133–144

White SS, Kato K, Jia LT et al (2009) Effects of perfluorooctanoic acid on mouse mammary gland development and differentiation resulting from cross-foster and restricted gestational exposures. Reprod Toxicol 27(3–4):289–298

Wolf CJ, Fenton SE, Schmid JE et al (2007) Developmental toxicity of perfluorooctanoic acid in the CD-1 mouse after cross-foster and restricted gestational exposures. Toxicol Sci 95(2):462–473

Yamashita N, Kannan K, Taniyasu S et al (2005) A global survey of perfluorinated acids in oceans. Mar Pollut Bull 51(8–12):658–668

Yang Q, Xie Y, Eriksson AM et al (2001) Further evidence for the involvement of inhibition of cell proliferation and development in thymic and splenic atrophy induced by the peroxisome proliferator perfluorooctanoic acid in mice. Biochem Pharmacol 62(8):1133–1140

Yang Q, Kurotani R, Yamada A et al (2006) Peroxisome proliferator-activated receptor alpha activation during pregnancy severely impairs mammary lobuloalveolar development in mice. Endocrinology 147(10):4772–4780

Yang C, Tan YS, Harkema JR et al (2009) Differential effects of peripubertal exposure to perfluorooctanoic acid on mammary gland development in C57Bl/6 and Balb/c mouse strains. Reprod Toxicol 27(3–4):299–306

Ylinen M, Hanhijarvi H, Jaakonaho J et al (1989) Stimulation by oestradiol of the urinary excretion of perfluorooctanoic acid in the male rat. Pharmacol Toxicol 65(4):274–277

Zhao Y, Tan YS, Haslam SZ et al (2010) Perfluorooctanoic acid effects on steroid hormone and growth factor levels mediate stimulation of peripubertal mammary gland development in C57BL/6 mice. Toxicol Sci 115(1):214–224

Chapter 9
Atrazine: An Environmental Endocrine Disruptor That Alters Mammary Gland Development and Tumor Susceptibility

Jennifer L. Rayner and Suzanne E. Fenton

Abstract Atrazine, a widely used chlorotriazine herbicide, has been regulated and reviewed because of its ability to alter endocrine signaling and cause mammary tumors in female Sprague–Dawley rats. The ability of atrazine to cause breast cancer in humans has been studied and the results are equivocal. Rodent studies showed that atrazine alters the developing mammary gland, makes it susceptible to tumorigenesis or hyperplasia, alters lactational ability, and decreases weight gain in second-generation litters. This chapter reviews the proposed mode of action for mammary tumorigenesis in rodents, results of human studies, and potential modes of action for atrazine effects on the developing mammary gland.

Keywords Atrazine • HPG axis • Endocrine disruptor • Herbicide • Mammary gland • Lactation • Tumor development

9.1 Atrazine Background

Atrazine (2-chloro-4-ethylamino-6-isopropylamino-*s*-triazine, ATR) is a widely used herbicide due to its persistence and versatile application time. ATR is used primarily on commercial corn, sorghum, sugar cane, and fruit crops but can also be used on cotton, Christmas trees, recreational turf (parks and golf courses), and on other crops to control broadleaf and some grassy weeds by prohibiting photosynthesis (Gianessi 1998; ATSDR 2003). Approximately 76 million pounds of active ingredient are applied annually on cropland in the United States (US EPA 2002; USGS 2009a).

S.E. Fenton (✉)
National Toxicology Program, National Institute of Environmental Health Sciences, Research Triangle Park, NC 27709, USA
e-mail: suzanne.fenton@nih.gov

J. Russo (ed.), *Environment and Breast Cancer*, DOI 10.1007/978-1-4419-9896-5_9,

Atrazine is a pesticide of concern because it and its metabolites are detected in ground and surface water including those that serve as water sources for human consumption (Baker 1998; US EPA 2006; USGS 2006, 2009b; Vecchia et al. 2009). Atrazine was originally registered with the U.S. Environmental Protection Agency (US EPA) in 1958 to be used as an herbicide. As concerns regarding carcinogenic risk from exposure to ATR-contaminated drinking water increased, the US EPA asked the manufacturer for data to support continued review and registration (US EPA 2004). In 1990, ATR-containing products were classified as restricted use pesticides. In 1991, the US EPA's Office of Water set a Maximum Contaminant Level (MCL) for ATR of 3 ppb in water, under the Safe Drinking Water Act, and required frequent monitoring of watersheds (US EPA 2004). At low concentrations, ATR dissolves in water and can be washed from soils into bodies of water including streams, rivers, and lakes (ATSDR 2003). In areas of heavy use such as the Midwest, ATR concentrations in drinking water sources may exceed the MCL and/or the level of concern (LOC; 37.5 ppb; US EPA 2003); as such, these sources have to be monitored. No community drinking water systems monitored within the US EPA's Office of Pesticide Programs have exceeded the LOC, but one Nebraska and two Missouri watershed monitoring sites have (US EPA 2010).

Four major ATR metabolites are formed by plants, microbes, and animals; 2-chloro-4,6-diamino-s-chlorotriazine (DACT), hydroxyatrazine (HA), 2-chloro-4-amino-6-(isopropylamino)-s-triazine (DEA), and 2-chloro-4-amino-6-(ethylamino)-s-triazine (DIA) (Wu et al. 1998). These metabolites are formed by other chlorotriazine herbicides including propazine and simazine, adding to the risk for cumulative exposure (Fig. 9.1). Atrazine metabolites are not regulated, but DIA, DEA, and DACT were included in the Triazine Cumulative Risk Assessment (US EPA 2006), which also included ATR and simazine. The document concluded that cumulative exposure through drinking water and/or lawn and golf courses to triazine residues was not of concern in high use regions including the Midwest, California, and Florida (US EPA 2006).

Similar to regulations in the US, the European Union (EU) Directive 91/414 (Deb 2006) requires a review of the safety of active ingredients in pesticides and authorization of the ingredients before the product can be marketed or used in the EU (Ansell 2008). Under EU Directive 91/414, active substances and their breakdown products cannot exceed a concentration of 0.1 μg/L in groundwater (Deb 2006).

The EU reviewed ATR in 2003, and the Scientific Committee for Plants was asked to review the data regarding possible groundwater contamination (EU 2004). The Committee recommended withdrawing authorizations for herbicides containing ATR as an active ingredient because of its potential to pollute groundwater above the regulatory limit. There was lack of data supporting the theory that continued use of ATR products in places where groundwater levels already exceeded 0.1 μg/L would allow satisfactory recovery of groundwater quality. Authorizations for plant protection products containing ATR as an active ingredient were hence withdrawn (EU 2004). Limited use of plant products containing ATR was allowed until 2007 in places where no alternatives products were available (EU 2004).

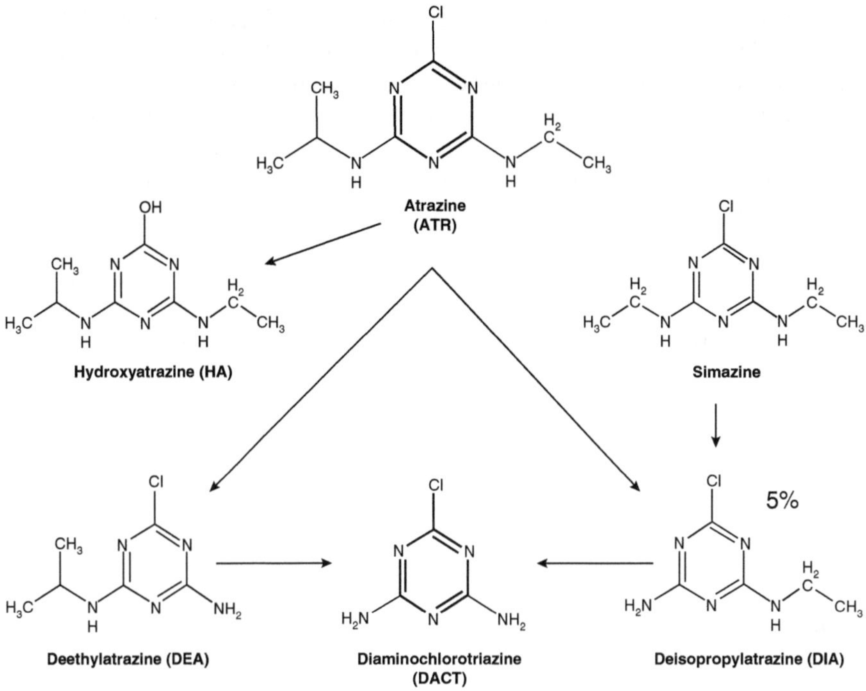

Fig. 9.1 Chemical structures of atrazine and its metabolites. Note that other parent compounds, such as simazine can produce the same set of metabolites

9.2 Atrazine is an Endocrine Disrupting Chemical

The Triazine Cumulative Risk Assessment grouped ATR and its chlorinated metabolites (DEA, DIA, and DACT) together based on a common mechanism of toxicity (US EPA 2006). The triazines alter luteinizing hormone (LH) in rats resulting in disruption of the hypothalamic-pituitary-gonadal (HPG) axis.

In the HPG axis, the hypothalamus secretes gonadotropin-releasing hormone (GnRH) which stimulates the pituitary gland to release follicle-stimulating hormone (FSH) and LH. FSH stimulates production of follicles and granulosa cells in the ovary, leading to increased estrogen secretion. LH causes ovulation, stimulates ovarian theca cell proliferation, and induces corpora lutea to form and secrete progesterone. As circulating concentrations of estradiol increase, they inhibit hypothalamic release of GnRH, creating a feedback loop. The cyclic release of these hormones in females regulates ovulation, and if fertilization does not occur, menstruation occurs in humans or estrus in rodents (Thomas and Thomas 2001).

In rodents, the estrous cycle occurs every 4–5 days from the time of sexual maturity (vaginal opening [VO]) until the end of the reproductive life span or pregnancy and is characterized by hormonal and vaginal cell changes. Several studies have examined the effects of ATR on the HPG axis using estrous cyclicity and hormone levels as outcomes. Early studies showed some strain differences in how ATR alters cyclicity. In Long-Evans (LE) rats, doses of ≥75 mg ATR/kg decreased the number of rats showing regular 4-day estrous cycles compared to doses of 300 mg ATR/kg in Sprague–Dawley (SD) rats (Cooper et al. 1996). Days spent in diestrus increased in both strains at ≥150 mg ATR/kg. At 300 mg ATR/kg, LE rats displaying persistent diestrus had minimal serum progesterone and estradiol levels and ovaries with undeveloped follicles and no recent corpora lutea indicating an anestrous state. In SD rats with persistent diestrus at the same dose, serum progesterone was elevated and the ovaries contained well-developed corpora lutea indicating a pseudopregnant state, suggesting increased sensitivity of the LE strain for these effects.

In a short-term (up to 45 days) gavage study, a significant increase in the number of SD rats having ≥4 days of diestrus at 40 or 200 mg ATR/kg was reported (Eldridge et al. 1999a). In a chronic (26 weeks) feeding study, the percentage of total days in estrus was significantly increased and the percentage of total days in diestrus was decreased at 400 ppm beginning at weeks 13–14 and continuing through the end of the study. These studies reveal that short-term exposure to ATR caused prolonged diestrus and continued exposure resulted in prolonged estrus in SD rats (Eldridge et al. 1999a).

Serum LH and PRL were significantly reduced in ovariectomized LE rats up to 6 h following a single dose of 300 mg ATR/kg and three daily doses of ≥50 mg ATR/kg. At 6 h after the last of three daily doses of ≥50 mg ATR/kg, pituitary PRL in LE rats was significantly increased. After a 21-day exposure, serum LH was significantly reduced and pituitary PRL was significantly increased at all doses, but serum PRL was only reduced at ≥150 mg ATR/kg. If the animals were given exogenous GnRH, no reductions in LH were observed. In ovariectomized SD rats, serum PRL was reduced at 300 mg ATR/kg after three daily doses. After 21 daily ATR doses, serum LH and PRL were significantly decreased at ≥150 mg ATR/kg, and pituitary PRL was significantly increased at ≥75 mg ATR/kg (Cooper et al. 2000), again demonstrating the LE rat as a more sensitive strain to the effects of ATR.

Taken together, these studies provide strong support for the effects of high-dose ATR on perturbed hypothalamic control of LH and PRL, leading to suppression of the preovulatory LH surge, altered PRL regulation, and disruption of the estrous cycle. For more details regarding the neuroendocrine/endocrine-related mechanism of action of ATR on the HPG axis, see Cooper et al. (2007).

Additional studies examined the impact of ATR on the HPG axis-regulated process of pubertal development in rats. Laws et al. (2000) dosed Wistar rats with ATR from postnatal day (PND)22–41 and observed them for VO, a marker for female puberty, which usually occurs in rats around PND32–34. Atrazine (≥50 mg/kg) significantly delayed VO by 2–6 days. No differences were observed in serum or pituitary PRL levels at PND41. In Wistar rats exposed PND21–46, 100 mg ATR/kg delayed VO, but in SD rats, VO was delayed at ≥30 mg ATR/kg (Ashby et al. 2002). In late gestationally exposed LE rats cross-fostered at birth, delayed VO was observed in the offspring who suckled from a 100-mg ATR/kg-exposed dam (Rayner et al. 2004). The studies show that ATR alteration of the HPG axis results in female pubertal developmental delays. The mechanism(s) by which this occurs is unknown and any relationship of VO to reproductive end points in young women is unclear.

9.3 Mammary Gland Development and Critical Periods for EDC Exposures

Mammary gland development, another important part of pubertal progression, occurs through cell differentiation and migration, and this process is also dependent upon several hormones and growth factors. Fenton (2006) noted three time periods of development during which the mammary gland has been reported to be most susceptible to environmental chemical exposures. The time periods include prenatal development of the epithelial sprout, peripubertal development, and pregnancy. Perturbation of cell signaling, hormone receptor number or activity, or direct action of chemicals on the proliferating cells by environmental chemicals may alter the growth, development, and function of the mammary gland.

In the rat, at approximately gestation day (GD) 10, a single-layered ectoderm enlarges creating the mammary streak, and extends from the anterior limb bud to the posterior limb bud on both sides of the animal (Sakakura 1987; Imagawa et al. 1994; Hovey et al. 2002). Cells migrate along the mammary streak and form six pairs of mammary buds in the rat (Imagawa et al. 1994) which increase in size due to continued cell migration through GD13–16 (Hovey et al. 2002; Fenton 2006). From GD16–21, the epithelial cells proliferate rapidly forming a sprout or cord (Sakakura 1987) that grows into the mesenchyme (Imagawa et al. 1990). The cord canalizes and branches, forming the mammary tree (Sakakura 1987; Imagawa et al. 1994).

Following birth (GD21), the mammary gland consists of 15–20 ducts branching off of a primary duct (Hovey et al. 2002). The branching ducts ends are shaped liked clubs (Imagawa et al. 1994; Hovey et al. 2002), and the ducts regress but reappear during the peri-pubertal time period (Imagawa et al. 1994; Hovey et al. 2002). Growth during this period of time (birth to PND22) is isometric meaning that the epithelium and the mesenchyme grow at the same rate as the body (Daniel and Silberstein 1987; Borellini and Oka 1989) and is hormone independent (Imagawa et al. 1994).

Following PND22, the approximate beginning of the peri-pubertal period, the mammary gland begins to grow allometrically, characterized by growth that occurs at a rate two to three times faster than body weight (Borellini and Oka 1989; Hovey et al. 2002). Ovarian estrogen stimulates ductal growth and stromal proliferation (Imagawa et al. 1990; Silberstein 2001; Hovey et al. 2002). The club-shaped end buds reappear at this time and these terminal end buds (TEBs) are clusters of epithelial cells, multiple layers thick (unlike other mammary gland epithelial structures) from which ductal elongation and branching occur (Masso-Welch et al. 2000). They are highly proliferative structures consisting of a basal surface and cuboidal epithelial cap cells (Daniel and Silberstein 1987). Cap cells are a type of stem cell stimulated by epidermal growth factor (EGF; Imagawa et al. 1994) to differentiate into luminal epithelial and myoepithelial cells (Masso-Welch et al. 2000), giving form to ductal structures (Imagawa et al. 1994). Ductal side branching, proliferation, and TEB formation are stimulated by progesterone, pituitary PRL, growth hormone, insulin-like growth factor I, and other hormone-regulated peptide growth factors (Imagawa et al. 1994; Atwood et al. 2000; Kleinberg et al. 2000; Silberstein 2001).

During the early stages of puberty, TEB cells undergo mitosis and cell migration to form ductules. Apoptosis of the innermost cells occurs to form the lumen of the ductules (Masso-Welch et al. 2000). This ductile elongation occurs until the ducts reach the end of the fat pad (Imagawa et al. 1990) and is regulated by transforming growth factor-β and interactions with the stromal portion of the gland (Silberstein 2001). As puberty ends, the TEBs bifurcate to form terminal ductules, which cluster together to form alveolar buds (Masso-Welch et al. 2000). Over time, the number of alveolar buds increases and the buds differentiate into lobuloalveolar structures until the animal reaches sexual maturity. Estrogen and progesterone are necessary for lobuloalveolar development (Topper and Freeman 1980; Silberstein 2001), and mammary-produced PRL regulates lobulalveoli cell proliferation (Naylor et al. 2003). Other growth factors are also involved in mammary gland growth regulation but their mechanisms of action are not fully understood.

After sexual maturity is reached, a cyclic remodeling takes place in the mammary gland that corresponds to the estrous cycle, but the gland is considered to be in a semi-resting state. At diestrus, terminal ends are present and during proestrus, the ends differentiate into alveolar buds. Estrus is marked by lobuloalveolar structures and rapid apoptosis of these structures. The terminal ends reappear at the beginning of the next cycle (Hovey et al. 2002). This remodeling continues until pregnancy occurs or a constant state of estrus is reached in the aged rat.

In the early stages of pregnancy, alveoli increase in number and size to fill the space between the ducts within the gland (Masso-Welch et al. 2000). During the late stages of pregnancy, alveolar cells fill with lipids and luminal cells fill with a basophilic substance. The number of blood vessels increases to provide nutrients to the cells of the rapidly growing gland (Imagawa et al. 1990; Masso-Welch et al. 2000), and many endogenous substances are transported to the mammary gland for milk production. At parturition, alveolar cells produce milk proteins and milk, which are expelled into the alveolar lumen. Processes of the myoepithelial cells contract and push the contents of the lumen (milk) into collecting ducts (Masso-Welch et al. 2000).

Mammary gland development is a very complex process and the current knowledge that we have of the interplay of hormones and other factors necessary for growth is growing. It is clear from the information that we have that there are many processes that endocrine disruptors could alter.

9.4 Perinatal ATR Delays Mammary Gland Development in Rats and Mice

In studies to examine the impact of ATR on hormonally-regulated processes, gestational exposures were used to evaluate the effect of ATR on mammary gland development. Several studies demonstrated that an oral dose of 100 mg ATR/kg/day to pregnant LE rats during GD15–19 resulted in delayed mammary gland development in the female offspring that persisted into adulthood (see Fig. 9.2; Rayner et al.

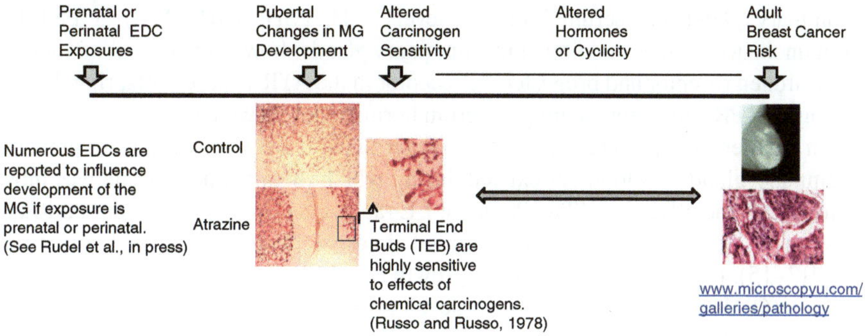

Fig. 9.2 Delayed differentiation of TEB can influence tumor development. Prenatal/perinatal exposure to a variety of EDCs is known to cause delayed mammary gland TEB differentiation, leaving the gland more susceptible to the effects of another "hit," such as a carcinogen. This influence, combined with altered hormonal regulation or perturbed cyclicity from the same early life exposures, may be the underpinnings for environmental breast cancer risk in adults

2004, 2005; Enoch et al. 2007; Moon et al. 2007). Importantly, body weight was not a significant variable influencing mammary gland developmental delays.

Rayner et al. (2004), cross-fostered prenatally exposed LE rat offspring at birth to determine if the mammary gland effects were the result of gestation and/or lactational exposures. Significantly delayed mammary gland development was observed as early as PND4 in prenatally and/or lactionally ATR-exposed offspring, as indicated by their smaller epithelial size and immature ductal structures. At PND22, the mammary glands in these animals were still smaller than the controls and exhibited sparse branching patterns with fewer TEBs. By PND33 and 40, only the female offspring exposed to ATR during gestation and throughout lactation had statistically significantly delayed mammary gland development. Numerous TEBs and inhibited longitudinal growth, indicated by a large amount of space between the fourth and fifth inguinal glands were observed in ATR animals at PND33. At this time, aromatase and EGF receptor expression were significantly reduced in prenatally and lactionally ATR-exposed offspring compared to control. At PND40, TEBs were abundant and the fat pad was not yet filled.

Immunohistochemical staining of the glands showed significantly increased BrdU incorporation in the gland on PND40 in offspring who nursed on an ATR-treated dam indicating that final differentiation of the gland had not occurred in those offspring. By PND58, very few differences between control and treated mammary glands were observed and no differences were observed in serum LH or PRL.

Similar delays in offspring mammary gland development were observed following low dose prenatal exposure to atrazine and metabolite mixtures (Enoch et al. 2007). The delays were observed as early as PND4 and as late as PND60 at which time TEBs were still present in the glands of treated animals. Moon et al. (2007) examined expression of hormone receptors (estrogen, PRL, progesterone) in the offspring mammary gland and serum hormone levels (LH, FSH, TSH, PRL) at PND41. Immunohistochemical staining of the mammary glands showed increased staining for the estrogen receptor and progesterone receptor in the ATR-exposed offspring, but no changes in PRL receptor staining or serum hormone levels were noted.

In another study, Rayner et al. (2005) determined if a critical window of prenatal mammary gland development existed during which the mammary tissue was most sensitive to the effects of ATR. Pregnant LE rats were dosed with 100 mg ATR/kg/day on GD13–19 or during the proposed times of rat mammary bud formation (GD13–15), bud size increase and outgrowth (GD15–17), and epithelial cell proliferation (GD17–19). Mammary gland development was delayed in all exposed offspring at PND4, 22, 25, 33, 46, and 67, but the most severe delays were observed in the offspring exposed GD17–19 and 13–19 indicating that GD17–19 may be a critical period of fetal mammary development for the effects of this endocrine disruptor. The offspring were bred starting on PND68 and produced litters (Rayner et al. 2005). F1 dams gestationally exposed to ATR GD17–19 and GD13–19 had smaller female pups whose mammary glands were underdeveloped as a result of lower body weights. The results suggested that ATR indirectly affects the body weight of the next generation.

Taken together, these studies showed that gestational ATR exposure altered prenatal mammary gland development and early postnatal development and resulted in developmental delays maintained throughout puberty and sexual maturity. The mechanism(s) through which this occurs has not been elucidated. Studies (Rayner et al. 2004; Moon et al. 2007) suggested that ATR-induced mammary gland delays may be the result of altered growth factor and steroid receptor expression, number, or activity, or more than likely a combination thereof.

Stoker and Cooper (2007) showed that ATR and/or its metabolites are transferred from the lactating dam to the offspring through the milk and reached the brains of the offspring. In the dams, the highest ATR concentrations were found in the mammary gland and liver. There are many pathways through which endogenous and exogenous substances enter milk including membrane or glucose transport, through mammary epithelial cell lipid secretion, or active transport mechanisms (McManaman and Neville 2003). Although ATR is nonlipophilic, it is possible that it acts in a manner similar to 1,1-dichloro-2,2-bis(*p*-chlorophenyl) ethylene, a compound stored in the dam's body and released with milk production (You et al. 1999) as ATR-induced delayed mammary gland development was observed in offspring exposed through lactational exposures (Rayner et al. 2004).

9.5 Chronic Adult Atrazine Exposure and Mammary Gland Tumors

ATR is not a direct carcinogen or mutagen, and has no reported estrogenic activity (Simpkins et al. 1998). However, in chronic ATR-dietary studies in adult SD rats (Gammon et al. 2005), an increased incidence of mammary adenocarcinomas was observed in the females consuming 2.28, 17.4, and 36.3 mg ATR/kg, but increased tumorigenesis was not evident in female F344 rats, male SD or F344 rats, or ovariectomized female SD rats in other studies (Eldridge et al. 1999b; Wetzel et al. 1994). The tumor incidence in control SD rats was 53%, while tumor incidence in high dose ATR rats was 89%. Mammary gland hyperplasia was also significantly increased in high dose males in the same study (Gammon et al. 2005).

It has been hypothesized that in SD rats, the ATR-induced suppression of the LH surge led to a state of persistent estrus (reproductive aging) in which ovarian estradiol was continually secreted (Eldridge et al. 1999b; US EPA 2006). This increase in estradiol was hypothesized to stimulate the mammary gland, causing the early formation of mammary tumors. Tumor formation is not expected to occur in humans via this mechanism because menopause (reproductive aging) is thought to proceed after ovarian follicles are depleted and estrogen levels decrease (Eldridge et al. 1999b; US EPA 2006). However, there is evidence by these same authors (Simpkins et al. 1998) that 4-week administration of ATR does not alter serum estradiol levels, and that "treatment-induced changes in estradiol metabolism are not a likely explanation for the ATR effects observed."

Two studies examined the impact of ATR in association with 7,12-dimethylbenz(a)-anthracene (DMBA)-induced tumors. Human c-HA-*ras* proto-oncogene transgenic rats (high susceptibility to tumorigenesis) were given a single dose of DMBA at 50 days of age and given a diet containing 0, 5, 50, or 500 ppm ATR (Fukamachi et al. 2004). The incidence of mammary adenomas and adenocarcinomas was significantly increased at 5 ppm and mammary adenocarcinoma incidence was increased at 50 ppm ATR in transgenic rats, but tumor incidence was not further increased at 500 ppm ATR. No tumors were observed in nontransgenic rats given the same ATR exposures.

Ueda et al. (2005) examined the modifying effects of ATR on tumors in ovariectomized SD rats. The rats received DMBA at 7 weeks of age and were ovariectomized at 19 weeks after DMBA administration. Rats with (DMBA+) and without (DMBA−) palpable tumors at ovariectomy were fed ATR diets for 34 weeks. In DMBA-rats, tumor incidence and volume were significantly increased at 500 ppm ATR (about 20 mg ATR/kg). A greater number of PCNA positive cells in adenocarcinomas were observed at 500 ppm ATR in DMBA+ rats and increased number of estrogen receptor-α positive tumors were observed at 50 ppm ATR in DMBA+ rats. Altered serum estrogen was not detected, and PRL, LH, and progesterone were not changed by ATR treatment. No tumors were observed in a subgroup of ATR-fed rats who had not received DMBA. These two studies suggest that ATR may have an enhancing effect on DMBA-induced mammary tumors at low dietary doses through an estrogen-independent mechanism.

9.6 Atrazine and Breast Cancer

An early occupational exposure study found a positive association between ATR and prostate cancer rates in workers at an ATR manufacturing plant, but additional epidemiological studies have shown no association between ATR and other cancers

(Rusiecki et al. 2004; US EPA 2010). Based on animal data and small amounts of epidemiological data, the US EPA and their Science Advisory Panel concluded that ATR exposure was not likely to be carcinogenic in humans (US EPA 2003). However, a new evaluation of ATR with regard to cancer and noncancer effects began in 2010 (US EPA 2010).

Although the specific mechanism of action for ATR-induced mammary gland tumors in female SD rats and hyperplasia in male SD rats is not fully known, it has been assumed irrelevant for humans. A concern remains for the development of breast cancer in humans from prolonged exposure to ATR, especially through contaminated drinking water. The studies by Fukamachi et al. (2004) and Ueda et al. (2005) highlight the possible proliferation effect of ATR on induced tumors. A few epidemiological studies have been conducted to look for associations between ATR and breast cancer risk and are summarized in Table 9.1.

Two ecologic studies of breast cancer incidence in rural populations of Kentucky have been conducted. In Kettles et al. (1997), county breast cancer incidence rates were calculated for the years 1991–1994 and the triazine exposure status of each county was categorized based on the water contamination (1991–1994), historical acres of corn planted in 1970, and pesticide use in 1970. Approximately 1.9 million women in the 120 counties were covered by the study. Detected triazines in surface water was positively associated with a significantly increased risk of breast cancer for low exposed counties (OR = 1.10) and high exposed counties (OR = 1.18) for the years 1991–1992. Low levels of groundwater contamination was associated with significantly increased breast cancer incidence (OR = 1.17). In 1993–1994, groundwater contamination – low (OR = 1.10), medium (OR = 1.15), and high (OR = 1.10) was associated with significantly increased breast cancer incidence, but no association was observed between surface water contamination and breast cancer incidence. It is unknown whether the women drank the water in which triazines were detected.

In Hopenhayn-Rich et al. (2002), the population of Kentucky was divided into 15 Area Development Districts (ADDs), as well as by county, and age-adjusted breast cancer incidence rates from the years 1993 to 1997 were obtained from the Kentucky Cancer Registry. Atrazine exposure indices were derived from public drinking water ATR levels, acreage of corn planted in 1970, and Kentucky ATR sales in 1997. In this study, no association was observed between ATR and breast cancer in the population of Kentucky.

Muir et al. (2004) used an ecologic study to explore the correlation between breast cancer in Lincolnshire and Leicestershire counties in the United Kingdom, and pesticide application. Population census and pesticide application data from 1991 were analyzed with breast cancer rates from Lincolnshire and Leicestershire from 1989 to 1991. Urban and rural electoral wards in each county were used as area units. No association between ATR application and breast cancer was observed for the urban wards in either county, however, a positive association was observed for ATR application and the rural wards of Leicestershire County. The slope coefficient was 0.17 (CI 0.03–0.31).

Table 9.1 Summary of epidemiological studies examining the relationship between atrazine exposure and human breast cancer rates

References	Study type	Estimated exposure	Breast cancer population	Association between exposure and breast cancer rate
Kettles et al. (1997)	Ecologic	Triazine by county Groundwater Surface water Acres of planted corn Pesticide use	County incidence rates for Kentucky 1991–1992, 1993–1994	1991–1992: Positive for groundwater-low levels, surface water-low, high counties 1993–1994: Positive for groundwater-low, medium, high levels, surface water-no association
Hopenhayn-Rich et al. (2002)	Ecologic	Atrazine Public drinking water 1992–1999 Acres of planted corn Atrazine sales	Area development district and county incidence rates for Kentucky 1993–1997	No associations
Muir et al. (2004)	Ecologic	Atrazine: Pesticide application in 1991	Incidence rates in Lincolnshire and Leicestershire Counties, UK, 1989–1991	Positive for rural areas in Leicestershire county
McElroy et al. (2007)	Case-control	Atrazine: Private well water 1994, 1996, 2001	Rural cases for Wisconsin 1988–2001 $n=3,275$ cases $n=3,669$ control	No associations

McElroy et al. (2007) studied the risk for breast cancer in women drinking ATR-contaminated well water in Wisconsin in a case-control study. The study population included 6,944 Wisconsin women, age 20–79 ($n=3{,}275$ cases, $n=3{,}699$ controls) who lived in rural areas of Wisconsin and received water from wells. Breast cancer cases (1988–2001) were obtained from the Wisconsin tumor registry. Atrazine concentrations were obtained from random well samples collected in 1994, 1996, and 2001, and natural neighbor interpolation was used to estimate yearly ATR exposure levels across the state. There was no association between breast cancer diagnosis and exposure to ATR contaminated well water in Wisconsin.

Overall, the results of the studies described were inconsistent and had many limitations. The studies examined triazine or ATR concentration in the water at the time of or after breast cancer diagnosis. As it takes years for breast cancer to develop and it is thought to be a "two hit" disease (Knudson 1996), ATR water concentrations were not a good proxy for what could have been early life exposure that led to breast cancer development. A causal relationship cannot be inferred from the ecologic studies because of ecologic and cross-level bias, temporal ambiguity, and lack of confounder control (Morgenstern 1995). Only one study (McElroy et al. 2007) looked at confounders, but the women may have been misclassified with regard to estimated ATR exposure. Better studies need to be conducted to clarify if a relationship exists between ATR and breast cancer.

9.7 Biological Activity of Atrazine Metabolites

As mentioned previously, ATR and its metabolites are persistent and have been detected in ground and surface waters (Fig. 9.1; Baker 1998; US EPA 2006; USGS 2006, 2009b; Vecchia et al. 2009). The mercapturate forms of ATR and its chlorinated metabolites have been detected in humans (Norrgran et al. 2006; Barr et al. 2007). Although not regulated, the chlorinated metabolites DIA, DEA, and DACT, have been grouped together with ATR as having the same mechanism of toxicity-disruption of the hypothalamic-pituitary-adrenal (HPA) axis through attenuation of LH (US EPA 2006). A few studies have investigated health effects of the metabolites in female offspring.

Treatment with DACT caused delayed VO, significantly increased ovary and uterus weights, and reduced pituitary weight in Wistar rats (Laws et al. 2003). Treatment with HA did not affect timing of puberty or organ weights. An increase in adrenocorticotropic hormone (ACTH), corticosterone, and progesterone were significantly increased following a 4-day exposure to ≥10 mg DIA/kg or ≥12.5 mg ATR/kg (Fraites et al. 2009). When given during the nadir of HPA axis activity, ACTH and corticosterone levels were significantly increased by DIA. Exposure to DACT had no effect on hormones of the HPA axis.

The metabolites also had an effect on mammary gland development and HPG hormone levels. In Enoch et al. (2007), LE rats were gavage dosed on GD15–19 with an ATR metabolite mixture (AMM) containing ATR (25%) and its metabolites DACT (35%), DIA (5%), DEA (15%), and HA (20%), based on reported concentrations detected in ATR-contaminated ground and surface water surveys. The doses 0.09, 0.87, and 8.73 mg AMM/kg corresponded to 2.5, 25, and 250 ppm, respectively, of an arbitrarily-set base concentration (combined maximum ATR and metabolite concentrations detected in water). The pituitary weight was significantly increased at all doses, but pituitary PRL was only increased at 0.87 mg ATR/kg. Significantly delayed mammary gland development was observed at all treatment doses on PND4, 25, 40, and 60. Mammary gland scores were low for the treated groups on PND33; however, scores for control mammary glands were unusually low at this time point and this prevented statistical significance at PND33. The results were observed at 0.09 and 0.87 mg/kg which are lower than the acute developmental NOAEL for ATR (6.25 mg ATR/kg; Stoker et al. 2002). Taken together these studies show that metabolites of ATR are biologically active individually and as an environmentally based mixture. As mentioned earlier, other parent compounds also make these metabolites. Whether the metabolites and parent compounds should be regulated together or separately has been the subject of debate and discussion (US EPA 2006).

9.8 Conclusions

Atrazine is a very popular herbicide that is a proven environmental endocrine disruptor. The detection of atrazine and its metabolites in ground and surface waters used for human consumption raises the concern for adverse health effects, including cancer. The action of ATR on the HPG axis may directly or indirectly result in alteration of hormones, delayed puberty, disrupted estrous cyclicity, and delayed mammary gland development in laboratory rodents. The delayed mammary gland development was persistent throughout the growth and development of the animals and was observed at lower doses than those that cause the other reproductive tissue effects (Enoch et al. 2007).

The TEBs were present for at least twice as long as normal in prenatally ATR-exposed mammary glands and the TEBs are known to be target sites for chemical carcinogens (Russo and Russo 1978). As shown in Fig. 9.2, the ATR-induced delays in mammary gland development are of concern because it is possible that increased sensitivity to chemical carcinogens and other environmental influences (another second hit) could affect breast tumor risk in adulthood (Fenton 2006). US girls are at an epidemic level of precocious puberty, typically detected as early breast bud development, then slowly progress through the stages of later pubertal development (Kaplowitz 2010). The undifferentiated breast epithelial ends (similar to TEBs in rats) are then also present for longer than normal periods of time in girls, potentially leaving them at increased risk for environmental influences to alter their breast cancer risk in later life.

In the case of adults, with fully developed mammary glands, ATR can alter the incidence of tumors that will occur in a species and dose-specific manner. The mode of action for ATR-induced tumors in adult females is proposed, but not fully elucidated. Furthermore, this mode of action would not explain hyperplasia in the mammary tissue of male SD rats. Data have shown that some metabolites of ATR found in ground and surface waters can cause the same effects as dietary and oral doses of ATR, and it is possible that the effects observed following ATR exposure are due to the metabolites and not the parent compound. More research is required to fully understand how ATR and its metabolites alter rodent mammary gland development, and what the possible mode of action might be for that sensitive tissue. The currently identified modes of action cannot explain the early mammary gland developmental changes that occur prior to hormone-dependent growth of the gland.

Epidemiological studies looking for an association between ATR exposure and breast cancer have had inconclusive results. The potential reasons for this are many of these studies did not evaluate early life exposure and completely missed all of the "critical periods" of breast development, nor did they actually measure the population's internal dose compared to the level in the water supplies. Studies such as the National Children's Study, Agricultural Health Study and the CHAMACOS study of California farm worker families have an opportunity to evaluate the breast health of the daughters of farm workers. Longitudinal follow-up would be invaluable for understanding the impact of environmental exposures on breast cancer risk.

References

Ansell C (2008) Pesticide regulation in the EU and California. Institute of Governmental Studies, UC Berkeley. http://escholarship.org/uc/item/7h47100p. Accessed 20 June 2010

Ashby J, Tinwell H, Stevens J, Pastoor T, Breckenridge CB (2002) The effects of atrazine on the sexual maturation of female rats. Reg Toxicol Pharmacol 35:468–473

ATSDR Agency for Toxic Substances and Disease Registry (2003) Toxicological profile for atrazine. U.S. Department of Health and Human Services, Public Health Service, Atlanta, Georgia

Atwood CS, Hovey RC, Glover JP, Chepko G, Ginsburg E, Robison WG, Vonderhaar BK (2000) Progesterone induces side-branching of the ductal epithelium in the mammary gland of peripubertal mice. J Endrocrinol 167:39–52

Baker DB (1998) Herbicides in drinking water: a challenge for risk communication. In: Ballantine LG, McFarland JE, Hackett DS (eds) Triazine herbicides risk assessment. American Chemical Society, Washington

Barr DB, Panuwet P, Nguyen JV, Udunka S, Needham LL (2007) Assessing exposure to atrazine and its metabolites using biomonitoring. Environ Health Perspect 115:1474–1478

Borellini F, Oka T (1989) Growth control and differentiation in mammary epithelial cells. Environ Health Perspect 80:85–89

Cooper RL, Stoker TE, Goldman JM, Parrish MB, Tyrey L (1996) Effect of atrazine on ovarian function in the rat. Reprod Toxicol 10:257–263

Cooper RL, Stoker TE, Tyrey L, Goldman JM, McElroy WK (2000) Atrazine disrupts the hypothalamic control of pituitary-ovarian function. Toxicol Sci 53:297–307

Cooper RL, Laws SC, Das PC, Narotsky MG, Goldman JM, Tyrey EL, Stoker TE (2007) Atrazine and reproductive function: mode and mechanism of action studies. Birth Defects Res B 80:98–112

Daniel CW, Silberstein GB (1987) Postnatal development of the rodent mammary gland. In: Neville M, Daniel C (eds) The mammary gland. Plenum Press, New York

Deb G (2006) Atrazine: a case study in the differences between regulations of endocrine disrupting chemicals in the EU and the US. Temple J Sci Tech Environ Law 25:173–190

Eldridge JC, Wetzel LT, Tyrey L (1999a) Estrous cycle patterns of Sprague-Dawley rats during acute and chronic atrazine administration. Reprod Toxicol 13:491–499

Eldridge JC, Wetzel LT, Stevens JT, Simpkins JW (1999b) The mammary tumor response in triazine-treated female rats: a threshold-mediated interaction with strain and species-specific reproductive senescence. Steroids 64:672–678

Enoch RR, Stanko JP, Greiner SN, Youngblood GL, Rayner JL, Fenton SE (2007) Mammary gland development as a sensitive end point after acute prenatal exposure to an atrazine metabolite mixture in female Long-Evans rats. Environ Health Perspect 115:541–547

EU European Union (2004) Commission decision of 10 March 2004 concerning the non-inclusion of atrazine in Annex I to Council Directive 91/414/EED and the withdrawal of authorizations for plant protection products containing this active substance (text with EEA relevance) (notified under document number C(2004)731). http://eur-lex.europa.eu/smartapi/cgi/sga_doc?smartapi!prod!CELEXnumdoc&lg=EN&numdoc=32004D0248&model=guichett. Accessed 27 June 2010

Fenton SE (2006) Endocrine-disrupting compounds and mammary gland development: early exposures and later life consequences. Endocrinology 147S:S18–S24

Fraites MJ, Cooper RL, Buckalew A, Jayaraman S, Mills L, Laws SC (2009) Characterization of the hypothalamic-pituitary-adrenal axis response to atrazine and metabolites in the female rat. Toxicol Sci 112:88–99

Fukamachi K, Han BS, Kim CK, Takasuka N, Matsuoka Y, Matsuda E, Yamasaki T, Tsuda H (2004) Possible enhancing effects of atrazine and nonylphenol on 7,12-dimethylbenz[a]-anthracene-induced mammary tumor development in human c-Ha-*ras* proto-oncogene transgenic rats. Cancer Sci 95:404–410

Gammon DW, Aldous CN, Carr WC Jr, Sanborn JR, Pfiefer KF (2005) A risk assessment of atrazine use in California: human health and ecological aspects. Pest Manag Sci 61:331–355

Gianessi LP (1998) Benefits of triazine herbicides. In: Ballantine LG, McFarland JE, Hackett DS (eds) Triazine herbicides risk assessment. American Chemical Society, Washington

Hopenhayn-Rich C, ML Stump, Browning SR (2002) Regional assessment of atrazine exposure and incidence of breast and ovarian cancers in Kentucky. Arch Environ Contam Toxicol 42:127–136

Hovey RC, Trott JF, Vonderhaar BK (2002) Establishing a framework for the functional mammary gland: from endocrinology to morphology. J Mammary Gland Biol Neoplasia 7:17–38

Imagawa W, Bandyopadhyay GK, Nandi S (1990) Regulation of mammary epithelial cell growth in mice and rats. Endocr Rev 11:494–523

Imagawa W, Yang J, Guzman R, Nandi S (1994) Control of mammary gland development. In: Knobin E, Neill JD (eds) The physiology of reproduction, 2nd edn. Raven Press, New York

Kaplowitz PB (2010) Precocious puberty. http://emedicine.medscape.com/article/924002-overview. eMedicine. 29 March 2010. Accessed 8 July 2010

Kettles MA, Browning SR, Prince TS, Horstman SW (1997) Triazine herbicide exposure and breast cancer incidence: an ecologic study of Kentucky counties. Environ Health Perspect 105:1222–1227

Kleinberg DL, Feldman M, Ruan W (2000) IGF-I: an essential factor in terminal end bud formation and ductal morphogenesis. J Mammary Gland Biol Neoplasia 5:7–17

Knudson AG (1996) Hereditary cancer: two hits revisited. J Cancer Res Clin Oncol 122:135–140

Laws SC, Ferrell JM, Stoker TE, Schmid J, Cooper RL (2000) The effects of atrazine on female Wistar rats: an evaluation of the protocol for assessing pubertal development and thyroid function. Toxicol Sci 58:366–376

Laws SC, Ferrell JM, Stoker TE, Cooper RL (2003) Pubertal development in female Wistar rats following exposure to propazine and atrazine biotransformation by-products, diamino-s-chlorotriazine and hydroxyatrazine. Toxicol Sci 76:190–200

Masso-Welch PA, Darcey KM, Stangle-Castor NC, Ip MM (2000) A developmental atlas of rat mammary gland histology. J Mammary Gland Biol Neoplasia 5:165–185

McElroy JA, Gangnon RE, Newcomb PA, Kanarek MS, Anderson HA, Brook JV, Trentham-Dietz A, Remington PL (2007) Risk of breast cancer for women living in rural areas from adult exposure to atrazine from well water in Wisconsin. J Expo Sci Environ Epidemiol 17:207–214

McManaman JL, Neville MC (2003) Mammary physiology and milk secretion. Adv Drug Deliv Rev 55:629–641

Moon HJ, Han SY, Shin J-H, Kang IH, Kim TS, Hong JH, Kim S-H, Fenton SE (2007) Gestational exposure to nonylphenol causes precious mammary gland development in female rat offspring. J Reprod Dev 53:333–344

Morgenstern H (1995) Ecologic studies in epidemiology: concepts, principles, and methods. Annu Rev Public Health 16:61–81

Muir K, Rattanamongkolgul S, Smallman-Raynor M, Thomas M, Downer S, Jenkinson C (2004) Breast cancer incidence and its possible spatial association with pesticide application in two counties of England. Public Health 118:512–520

Naylor MJ, Lockefeer JA, Horseman ND, Ormandy CJ (2003) Prolactin regulates mammary epithelial cell proliferation via autocrine/paracrine mechanism. Endocrine 20:111–114

Norrgran J, Bravo R, Bishop AM, Restrepo P, Whitehead RD, Needham LL, Barr DB (2006) Quantification of six herbicide metabolites in human urine. J Chromatogr B Analyt Technol Biomed Life Sci 18:185–195

Rayner JL, Wood C, Fenton SE (2004) Exposure parameters necessary for delayed puberty and mammary gland development in Long-Evans rats exposed in utero to atrazine. Toxicol Appl Pharmacol 195:23–34

Rayner JL, Enoch RR, Fenton SE (2005) Adverse effects of prenatal exposure to atrazine during a critical period of mammary gland growth. Toxicol Sci 81:255–266

Rusiecki JA, de Roos A, Lee WJ, Dosemeci M, Lubin JH, Hoppin JA, Blair A, Alavanja MCR (2004) Cancer incidence among pesticide applicators exposed to atrazine in the agricultural health study. J Natl Cancer Inst 96:1375–1382

Russo I, Russo J (1978) Developmental stage of the rat mammary gland as determinant of its susceptibility to 7,12-dimethylbenz[a]anthracene. J Natl Cancer Inst 61:1439–1449

Sakakura T (1987) Mammary embryogenesis. In: Neville M, Daniel C (eds) The mammary gland. Plenum Press, New York

Silberstein GB (2001) Postnatal mammary gland morphogenesis. Microsc Res Tech 52:155–162

Simpkins JW, Eldridge JC, Wetzel LT (1998) Role of strain-specific reproductive patterns in the appearance of mammary tumors in atrazine-treated rats. In: Ballantine LG, McFarland JE, Hackett DS (eds) Triazine herbicides risk assessment. American Chemical Society, Washington

Stoker TE, Cooper TL (2007) Distribution of 14C-atrazine following an acute lactational exposure in Wistar rats. Reprod Toxicol 23:607–610

Stoker TS, Guidici DL, Laws SC, Cooper RL (2002) The effects of atrazine metabolites on puberty and thyroid function in the male Wistar rat. Toxicol Sci 67:198–206

Thomas MG, Thomas JA (2001) Toxic responses of the reproductive system. In: Klaassen CJ (ed) Casarett and Doull's toxicology the basic science of poisons, 6th edn. McGraw-Hill, New York

Topper YJ, Freeman CS (1980) Multiple hormone interactions in the developmental biology of the mammary gland. Physiol Rev 60:1049–2000

Ueda M, Imai T, Takizawa T, Onodera H, Mitsumori K, Matsui T, Hirose M (2005) Possible enhancing effects of atrazine on growth of 7,12-dimethylbenz(a)anthracene-induced mammary tumors in ovariectomized Sprague-Dawley rats. Cancer Sci 96:19–25

US EPA United States Environmental Protection Agency (2002) Overview of atrazine risk assessment. 2 May 2002. Office of Prevention, Pesticides, and Toxic Substances. EPA Docket EPA-HQ-OPP-2007-0151

US EPA United States Environmental Protection Agency (2003) Revised atrazine interim reregistration eligibility decision. Oct 2003. Office of Prevention, Pesticides, and Toxic Substances. EPA Docket EPA-HQ-OPP-2007-0151

US EPA United States Environmental Protection Agency (2004) Memorandum errata/addendum sheet for changes to the atrazine interim reregistration eligibility decision. Jan 2003. Amended March 2004. Office of Prevention, Pesticides, and Toxic Substances. http://www.epa.gov/oppsrrd1/REDs/atrazine_ired.pdf. Accessed 15 June 2010

US EPA United States Environmental Protection Agency (2006) Triazine cumulative risk assessment. 28 March 2006. http://www.epa.gov/oppsrrd1/REDs/triazine_cumulative_risk.pdf. Accessed 15 June 2010

US EPA United States Environmental Protection Agency (2010) Atrazine updates. http://www.epa.gov/opp00001/reregistration/atrazine/atrazine_update.htm. Accessed 27 June 2010

USGS United States Geological Survey (2006) The quality of our nation's waters: pesticides in the nation's streams and groundwater, 1992–2001. Revised 15 Feb 2007. US Geological Circular 1291. Reston Virginia. http://pubs.usgs.gov/circ/2005/1291/pdf/circ1291.pdf. Accessed 15 June 2010

USGS United States Geological Survey (2009a) Watershed regressions for pesticides (WARP) atrazine model. http://infotrek.er.usgs.gov/warp. Accessed 15 June 2010

USGS United States Geological Survey (2009b) Trends in pesticide concentrations in Corn-Belt streams, 1996–2006. Scientific Investigations report 2009-5132. http://pubs.usgs.gov/sir/2009/5132/pdf/sir20095132.pdf. Accessed 15 June 2010

Vecchia AV, Gilliom RJ, Sullivan DJ, Lorenz DJ, Martin JD (2009) Trends in concentrations and use of agricultural herbicides for Corn Belt rivers, 1996–2006. Environ Sci Technol 43:9096–9102

Wetzel LT, Luempert LC III, Breckenridge CB, Tisdel MO, Stevens JT, Thakur AK, Extrom PJ, Eldridge JC (1994) Chronic effects of atrazine on estrus and mammary tumor formation in female Sprague–Dawley and Fischer 344 rats. J Toxicol Environ Health 43:182–196

Wu J, Robinson RA, Simoneaux B (1998) Metabolism of selected (s)-triazines in animals. In: Ballantine LG, McFarland JE, Hackett DS (eds) Triazine herbicides risk assessment. American Chemical Society, Washington

You L, Gazi E, Archibeque-Engle S, Casanova M, Conolly RB, Heck HA (1999) Transplacental and lactational transfer of p, p′-DDE in Sprague–Dawley rats. Toxicol Appl Pharmacol 157:134–144

Chapter 10
The Biological Impact of Radiation Exposure on Breast Cancer Development

David H. Nguyen, Irineu Illa Bochaca, and Mary Helen Barcellos-Hoff

Abstract Ionizing radiation is a well-established breast carcinogen in women and has been a widely studied cause of cancer in experimental models. Clinical data and experimental models are discussed to highlight radiation effects on the mammary gland and breast cancer as a system of heterotypic interactions among multiple cell types. Epidemiological data from different populations of women who were exposed to radiation during various stages of physiological development have offered insight into potential biological mechanisms that mediate radiation-induced breast cancer. This chapter discusses classic and current views of radiation's action within the mammary gland and how these effects interact biologically to inform a more comprehensive conceptualization of radiation as a carcinogen, including new emphasis on a defined adult stem cell population within the mammary gland.

Keywords Ionizing radiation • Stem cell • Mammary gland • Breast cancer

10.1 Epidemiological Evidence of Radiation as a Risk Factor of Breast Cancer

A fundamental challenge in radiation research related to human health is predicting the biological impact of exposure to low dose (<0.1 Gy) ionizing radiation (IR). Excess cancers have been observed in the Japanese atomic-bomb survivors at doses of 0.1–4 Gy, which are 40–1,600 times the average yearly background levels in the USA (Preston et al. 2007). However, predicting cancer risk in populations exposed to doses lower than ~0.1 Gy is limited by statistical considerations. Therefore, radiation

M.H. Barcellos-Hoff (✉)
Department of Radiation Oncology, New York University, Langone School of Medicine, 566 First Avenue, New York, NY 10016, USA
e-mail: mhbarcellos-hoff@nyumc.org

J. Russo (ed.), *Environment and Breast Cancer*, DOI 10.1007/978-1-4419-9896-5_10,

risk models extrapolate in the region below which epidemiological data are robust using an assumption of linearity. This linear-no-threshold (LNT) regulatory paradigm is based in large part on observations that cancer incidence increases with doses above 0.1 Gy, as well as pragmatic, regulatory, and societal considerations to protect the population. A recent review study of the National Academy of Sciences (BEIR VII) concluded that human health risks continue in a linear fashion at low doses without a threshold such that the smallest dose has the potential to increase risk in humans (NAS/NRC 2006).

IR is one of very few exogenous exposures consistently associated with greater breast cancer risk (reviewed in Ronckers et al. 2005). Diagnostic radiation in girls with scoliosis, usually beginning at the onset of the growth spurt through puberty and adolescence, and in TB patients who spanned a wide range of ages, increases the risk of developing breast cancer later in life (Boice et al. 1991; Morin Doody et al. 2000). The average dose to the breast was lower in the scoliosis cohort (0.11 Gy) compared to the fluoroscopy cohorts (0.79 and 0.89 Gy) but both were fractionated and appeared to have cumulative effects. Single exposures of Nagasaki–Hiroshima survivors who were peripubertal (approximately aged 10–14 years) also increased breast cancer risk. Notably, young girls were much more likely to develop breast cancer than older girls or adult women who were exposed to comparable radiation doses (Tokunaga et al. 1993). Furthermore, X-ray treatment of benign breast disease (BBD) and acute postpartum mastitis in women of childbearing ages reportedly increases breast cancer risk (Shore et al. 1986; Mattsson et al. 1993). Doses to the breast were considerably higher compared to the earlier mentioned studies. In the BBD cohort, exposed women were at 3.58-fold higher risk compared to a control group of women with BBD never treated with radiation (Mattsson et al. 1993). Women treated for postpartum mastitis who were exposed to more than 1.5 Gy were at 2–4-fold increased risk of breast cancer compared to a combined control group of siblings and unirradiated mastitis patients (Shore et al. 1986).

10.2 Risk of Secondary Cancer Associated with Medical Radiation Exposure

High dose radiation exposure to the breast from radiation therapy for Hodgkin's disease or other cancers during childhood greatly increases breast cancer risk (Hancock et al. 1993; Howe and McLaughlin 1996). Radiotherapy for breast cancer can result in several Gy of radiation exposure in the contralateral breast; radiation treatment for breast cancer was found to be related to the development of secondary breast cancers especially among women at ages younger than 45 years (Boice et al. 1992). Land et al. conducted a nested case–control study of 196 breast cancer patients and 566 matched controls among Japanese atomic-bomb survivors (Land et al. 1994a, b). Statistical modeling indicated that early first birth, multiple births and long cumulative lactation history protected not only against breast cancer per se but also against radiation-induced breast cancer in this population. The protective effect of age at first birth held for parous women at the time of exposure and for women who completed a first pregnancy only after radiation exposure. Studies in rats by Clifton et al. also showed that pregnancy following radiation-exposure reduced tumorigenesis (Clifton et al. 1975). They speculated that differentiation of a given mammary cell for milk secretion markedly reduces the proliferative potentiality of that cell; in other words, in the presence of hormones that stimulate end-differentiation of the mammary cells, irradiation-altered mammary cells are lost from the high proliferative potential population. Along these lines, Sivaraman et al. have proposed a cell-fate hypothesis to explain the protective effect of pregnancy on breast cancer risk in general (Sivaraman et al. 2001). Thus, while radiation exposure increases breast cancer risk, these events are unlikely to be sufficient as evidenced by the long latency (approximately 40 years) between exposure and disease, and the observation that subsequent tissue and reproductive processes can modify risk (Land et al. 1994a, b).

A major question arises from epidemiological analysis of one of the few known human carcinogens, IR in breast cancer, is: What is the biological basis for the window of susceptibility during adolescence? We have studied how radiation affects critical events and signals during puberty. IR is recognized as a breast carcinogen whose action is largely attributed to DNA damage that leads to mutations. However, there is increasing evidence that radiation also acts by altering signaling, which in turn can affect how cells behave and their microenvironment. We think that environmental carcinogens, like IR, can act indirectly via such signals (Barcellos-Hoff et al. 2005). One way that signals could affect cancer development is by deregulating mammary stem cells. Stem cells are "born" during puberty; more stem cells are thought to mean greater risk of developing cancer since they are the longest lived. Our preliminary evidence suggests that radiation could increase the number of stem cells in mammary glands. Consistent with this idea, we have also found that radiation can affect the frequency of a rare variant cell in human mammary epithelial cell cultures (Mukhopadhyay et al. 2010). These vHMEC appear to have a greater capacity to replicate, like stem cells, and therefore may increase the risk of developing cancer. Important signals from neighboring cells prevent these cells from growing rapidly, but radiation alters these stop signals so that the vHMEC can escape. Together our studies show that studying normal mammary biology and its response to radiation provides important new ideas about the radiation biology that promotes cancer.

10.3 Radiation Effects on Breast Cancer Type

Breast cancer is a heterogeneous disease, or rather a collection of neoplastic diseases. Since tumor characteristics are highly correlated with prognosis, there has been considerable investment in defining and standardizing characterization. Traditional pathology, marker analysis, imaging features, and molecular analysis contribute to classification. The presence of human epidermal growth factor receptor 2 (HER2) amplification distinguishes a specific breast cancer subtype as well as providing a distinct molecular target (Gusterson et al. 1992). Estrogen receptor (ER) status is important not only because ER-positive tumors are managed with antiestrogen treatments but because it also distinguishes cancers with two major clinical features. ER-positive tumors tend to occur in postmenopausal women and have a relatively slow progress, while ER-negative tumors are frequent in young women and have a worse prognosis (Rakha and Ellis 2007). Among ER-negative breast cancers there are also several diseases. ER-negative and progesterone receptor (PR)-negative cancers tend to be poorly differentiated and aggressive. Triple-negative (TN) invasive ductal carcinoma tumors lack all three markers, ER, PR, and HER2, and can be further subdivided by those that express basal markers, cytokeratin 5/6 (CK5/6) or alpha-smooth muscle actin, which are called basal-like, and those that do not (Rakha et al. 2009).

Given the growing evidence of distinct disease prognosis and response to therapy based on the markers expressed by the breast cancer at the time of diagnosis, it would be interesting to determine whether the dose, timing, or purpose of radiation exposure impacts the type of breast cancer in addition to the frequency. Women who were treated with radiation during childhood for diagnostic or therapeutic purposes represent cohorts in which to examine the delayed carcinogenic effects of IR on breast cancer development later in life (Boice et al. 1991; Tokunaga et al. 1993; Morin Doody et al. 2000), but the type of breast cancer was not assessed in most studies.

Notably, a recent study of survivors of childhood cancer who received radiation treatment shows that not only the frequency but also the type of breast cancer is affected (Castiglioni et al. 2007). Women who were irradiated during puberty (~10–14 years of age) were more likely to have breast cancer that contained HER2 amplifications. More interestingly, the breast cancers of women irradiated postpubertal (14–18 years of age) were much more likely to develop cancer at an earlier age (mean = 39 years) compared to spontaneous breast cancer (57 years) but were significantly more likely to have the so-called triple negative tumors, i.e., negative for ER, PR, and the overexpression of HER2, compared to age matched controls. This effect is highly intriguing in terms of both breast cancer biology and the mechanism by which radiation acts, but it is untested in populations who were exposed to lower doses. Interestingly, there is little evidence of disproportionate frequency of contralateral ER-negative breast cancer in women treated with radiation for breast cancer (M. Stoval, personal communication), suggesting a physiological basis for the shift identified in the Milan study.

10.4 Radiation Effects During Mammary Carcinogenesis

The tissue architecture of the mammary gland consists of the parenchyma (a ductal tree of epithelial cells) that is wrapped in a dense sheath of fibroblastic stroma, both of which are embedded in a larger stroma of adipocytes. The mammary ducts consist of a bilayer with columnar epithelial cells lining the inside of the duct, and a single layer of stratified myoepithelial cells that separate the ductal epithelial cells from the fibroblasts (Richert et al. 2000). The mouse mammary gland differs from the human breast in that human ducts are organized into lobules that are embedded in a much denser fibroblastic stroma than that found around mouse ducts, containing intra- and interlobular fibroblastic stromas. Mouse mammary ducts have only one dense sheath of fibroblastic stroma around them, but contain alveolar buds all along the length of the ducts, which are ductal cells arranged in grape-like clusters, and that are specialized for milk production; the equivalent of the milk-producing human ductal cells that are found only at the lobular ends of the human mammary ductal system (Howard and Gusterson 2000).

The processes of mammary gland development, differentiation, and neoplasia are regulated by the ovarian hormones, estrogen and progesterone (Shyamala 1997). Although the mouse mammary gland is organized differently than the human breast, these processes are ovarian hormone dependent in both human and rodent glands (Shyamala 1997). Estrogen provides the primary stimulus for ductal morphogenesis during puberty while concomitantly priming the gland for lobular–alveolar differentiation via its induction of PR. Progesterone is subsequently necessary for elaboration of the ductal tree via side-branching in the virgin animal and alveolar expansion during pregnancy (Lydon et al. 1995). While estrogen and progesterone are critical for proliferation, it is clear that mammary epithelial cells differ in their ability to respond to these signals. During both ductal and lobular–alveolar mammary growth, the distribution of proliferating cells is heterogeneous, suggesting the involvement of local factors in dictating the specific response to systemic hormones (Bresciani 1968; Daniel et al. 1987; Christov et al. 1993).

Ethier and Ullrich showed that dissociated cells from mouse mammary gland irradiated with 1 Gy, 24 h after exposure transplanted to unirradiated mice increased the frequency and persistence of dysplasia over that of intact tissues (Ethier and Cundiff 1987; Ethier et al. 1987). Clifton and colleagues showed that dissociated cells from irradiated rat mammary gland exhibited a very high frequency of initiation (i.e., 1/100) when transplanted into unirradiated tissue. These studies highlight the importance of radiation acting directly on the mammary epithelial cells to affect their morphology and behavior. However, IR also elicits effects in the mammary gland that are independent of its interaction with DNA. Radiation rapidly induces extracellular signaling via growth factors and cytokines that regulate stromal remodeling, vascular integrity, and inflammatory responses (reviewed in Hallahan et al. 1993; McBride 1995; Barcellos-Hoff 1998a, b; Dent et al. 2003). In particular, IR induces the activation of TGFβ1, a growth factor that is produced and widely distributed extracellularly as a latent complex (Barcellos-Hoff et al. 1994; Ehrhart et al. 1997). TGFβ1 mediates epithelial fate decisions by regulating proliferation and apoptosis (reviewed in Derynck et al. 2001). A 10 cGy dose of IR is enough to activate TGFβ1 in the extracellular matrix of the mammary gland, and this effect persists at least up to 2 weeks after exposure (Ehrhart et al. 1997). TGFβ1 acts as a sensor of oxidative damage caused by IR (Jobling et al. 2006) and once activated, signals to adjacent cells to alter the deposition of extracellular matrix components (Barcellos-Hoff 1993, 1998a, b).

10.5 Radiation Biology and Cancer Risk

The scientific rationale for linearly extrapolating radiation health effects is underpinned by biophysical theory of how energy interacts with DNA, which is thought to be the major biological target. This area of radiation biology has made significant progress in identifying the critical mechanisms, processes, and pathways by which DNA is damaged, repaired or misrepaired. The efficiency and frequency by which IR induces mutations and chromosomal aberrations is thought by most to be the best surrogate of its carcinogenic potential, in part because there is a clear mechanistic understanding of their induction from energy deposition, and in part because these events are strongly associated with cancer. A fundamental principle of target theory is that the effect (e.g., DNA damage, cell kill, mutation) is linear or linear/linear–quadratic as a function of dose due to biophysical considerations that energy deposition (i.e., dose) is proportional to damage. In terms of immediate damage, the so-called targeted radiation effects, this conclusion is very well supported for DNA damage that can be measured directly or indirectly over several logs of radiation exposure (1–100 Gy).

However, biological responses to radiation damage quickly evolve and amplify in a nonlinear manner, particularly at low doses, which has been broadly documented both in cell culture and in vivo (reviewed in Brooks 2005; Wright and Coates 2006). There are now myriad experimental reports that low dose radiation alters the response to subsequent challenge doses (i.e., adaptive responses, AR), affects daughter cell fates such as differentiation and senescence, induces long-range signals that affect nonirradiated cells, and generates a state of chronic genomic instability (GIN). Although there are several definitions of nontargeted effects, we define nontargeted effects as those that are inconsistent with either direct energy deposition, such as bystander phenomenon (Kaplan et al. 1956b; Hei et al. 1997; Barcellos-Hoff and Ravani 2000; Mothersill et al. 2001), or those that are exhibited in the daughters of irradiated cells, but not mediated by a mutational mechanism, such as radiation-induced GIN (Kadhim et al. 1992, 1994, 1995; Clutton et al. 1996; Limoli et al. 1997) and persistent phenotypic changes (Herskind and Rodemann 2000; Rave-Frank et al. 2001; Park et al. 2003; Tsai et al. 2005). Although the extent to which these phenomena reflect different molecular mechanisms is not clear, experimental results to date suggest that significant deviation from linearity at low doses may impact the ability to predict cancer risk in humans (Baverstock 2000; Wright 2000; Barcellos-Hoff and Brooks 2001; Huang et al. 2003; Little 2003).

Previous work from our group has shown that IR induces rapid remodeling of the mammary microenvironment (Barcellos-Hoff 1993, 1998a, b), which led us to hypothesize that the irradiated stroma modified tumorigenic potential in a nontargeted fashion. To test this hypothesis, we created a radiation chimera by transplanting unirradiated, preneoplastic mammary cells to the mammary glands of irradiated hosts (Barcellos-Hoff and Ravani 2000). The undeveloped mammary epithelium is surgically removed at puberty, the animal irradiated, and some time later nonirradiated mammary epithelial cells are transplanted into the irradiated host. These studies used COMMA-1D mammary epithelial cells, which are nontumorigenic if injected into the cleared fat pads of 3-week-old mice, or subcutaneously in immature, adult mice or into nude mice, and undergo mammary morphogenesis when transplanted into 3-week-old mammary gland. Although clonal in origin, COMMA-1D cells harbor two mutant *Trp53* alleles that may confer neoplastic potential (Jerry et al. 1994). When transplanted into mice irradiated 1–14 days earlier with 4 Gy, outgrowths rapidly developed tumors, ranging from a peak of 100% at day 3 and twice that of sham-irradiated mice at 14 days postirradiation. Furthermore, tumors from irradiated animals were nearly five times larger than the few tumors that arose in sham-irradiated hosts, indicating that tumor biology, as well as frequency, was affected. These data support the idea that high dose radiation promotes carcinogenesis by inducing a hospitable tissue environment. Furthermore, our recent data using the same radiation chimera approach, but transplanting mammary fragments of *Trp53* null mice into syngeneic hosts that were previously irradiated, show that even doses as low as 0.1 Gy are enough to promote rates of tumor development over those of transplants into unirradiated hosts, though these tumors occurred almost 1 year after irradiation event (Nguyen et al. 2011). This is the first report of a low dose in vivo nontargeted effect of IR promoting breast cancer.

To date, it is unclear how nontargeted effects can be incorporated in risk assessments, even though their existence is widely reported. The difficulty is inherent in the fact that risk assessment via the LNT model is based on the direct effects of radiation on DNA, and the subsequent carcinogenesis that ensues due to mutagenesis. Thus, if nontargeted effects are to be incorporated into current risk models, a proportionality relationship needs to be established between cancer rates (or other end-points) due to the effect of targeted events and those due to nontargeted events. If such a relationship shows that nontargeted effects can be additive or synergistic with the targeted effects of radiation, then this, in principle, allows the contribution of nontargeted effects to be incorporated as a weighting factor into current risk models that are based on targeted effects. A proof of principle may be feasible using in vivo mouse models that have clear carcinogenic read-outs in the form of tumor frequencies, latencies, etc., in which the effect of radiation directly on the carcinogenesis of the target tissue can be separated from the indirect effect of radiation on carcinogenesis through irradiating only the host environment. The advantage of such mouse models is that the measured read-outs of tumorigenesis are in vivo end-points similar to human cancers, as opposed to in vitro assays of GIN and clonogenic survival (though these assays are informative on their own merits). The ability to surgically remove and then transplant a target organ into a syngeneic host allows one to isolate the effect of radiation exposure to either tissue compartments alone, to both, or to neither. Conceptually, this allows for a comparison of radiation's effect in all four combinations of tissue-host exposures and an assessment of whether the nontargeted effects of host irradiation are additive or synergistic to targeted effects of tissue irradiation. There are at least two organs that have been amenable to such experimental investigations: the thymus (Kaplan et al. 1956a, b) and the mammary gland (DeOme et al. 1959; Barcellos-Hoff and Ravani 2000; Medina et al. 2002; Nguyen and Barcellos-Hoff, unpublished).

However, incorporating nontargeted effects into risks of cancer in mouse models is one thing, but doing so for human health is a separate challenge, since with humans we are unable to perform the same experiments due to ethical considerations. With human cancer, understanding the contribution of nontargeted effects to targeted effects will likely require a different approach in which one needs to be able to selectively perturb nontarget cells/tissues such as the angiogenic and inflammatory system, as opposed to the target epithelial cells that will later form a breast tumor, and then measure the reduced effect of radiation-induced cancer. Using this concept, one might be able to establish a proportionality relationship between targeted and nontargeted effects in human cancer, which would in principle allow for the incorporation of the contribution of nontargeted mechanisms as a weighting factor in risk calculations. However, radiation risk is assessed at the level of populations, and thus statistical considerations relative to reliable and repeatable measures of an end-point may require sample sizes that are unfeasible.

10.6 Experimental Determinants of Radiation Susceptibility of Breast Cancer

With regard to radiation-induced mammary cancer, studies by Ullrich and colleagues have shown that BALB/c mice are highly sensitive to radiation-induced benign and malignant mammary growth (Ethier and Ullrich 1982; Ullrich 1983, 1984; Ethier et al. 1984; Ullrich et al. 1996). Our early studies showed that irradiation of BALB/c host mice promotes tumorigenesis of unirradiated syngeneic mammary epithelial cells injected after hostirradiation (Barcellos-Hoff and Ravani 2000). The tumor-promoting effects of host irradiation have been repeated using transplants of unirradiated mammary fragments from *Trp53* null mice of the BALB/c strain into syngeneic hosts that had been previously irradiated with 10–100 cGy of ionizing irradiation (Nguyen et al. 2011). While the host radiation chimera experiments have not been conducted with other mouse strains, it is evident that both the mammary epithelia and the BALB/c host contribute to the susceptibility of this strain to radiation-induced carcinogenesis.

Compared to C57bl/6, mouse mammary epithelial cells from BALB/c also have higher levels of GIN after exposure to IR (Ponnaiya et al. 1997). The BALB/c mice have T lymphocytes that behave differently than those from C57bl/6 mice (Chen et al. 2005), and harbor a variant allele for *Cdkn2a* (p16/INK4a, p19/ARF) (Zhang et al. 1998), but little is known about the mechanisms that make mammary carcinogenesis in the BALB/c strain distinctly more sensitive to radiation than in the C57bl/6 background. Nonetheless, the difference in carcinogenic potential of the mammary gland as a function of mouse strain implicates the same unidentified genetic factors in understanding human breast cancer.

The susceptibility of mouse strains to certain types of cancer is enhanced by knockout of the *Trp53* tumor suppressor gene (Donehower et al. 1992; Jacks et al. 1994; Purdie et al. 1994; Kuperwasser et al. 2000). *Trp53* is a transcriptional regulator that controls DNA damage response, cell cycle progression, and apoptosis.

It is mutated in over 50% of all human cancers (Hollstein et al. 1991, 1994) and is associated with Li–Fraumeni syndrome (LFS) when inherited as a germline mutation in one allele (Malkin et al. 1990), in which LFS women exhibit early onset of cancers such as breast carcinomas, sarcomas, and lymphomas, of which breast cancer is most common. While sharing similarities in overall tumor occurrence and spectrum with LFS patients, the *Trp53* knockout mouse models also collectively reveal that different genetic backgrounds depending on strain significantly influence tumor outcomes. Donehower et al. (1992) initially generated the null allele in a C57Bl/6 × 129/Sv background and these mice had a median tumor-free survival of 4.5 months. However, they later crossed the allele into a pure 129/Sv background and found that not only did tumors occur sooner than in the mixed background, the pure 129/Sv background gave 50% testicular tumors, in accordance with the observation that 129/Sv mice have a natural susceptibility for testicular cancer (Donehower 1996). On the other hand, the pure C57bl/6 mouse strain has a predisposition for spontaneous lymphomas late in life (Stutman 1974), a feature that is dramatically accelerated in all *Trp53* knockout strains.

Interestingly, although LFS patients have a high incidence of breast cancer (Malkin et al. 1990), mammary tumors only very rarely develop in these mouse knockout models. Though most *Trp53* mutations in LFS are point mutations, a small fraction of the cases are frame-shift mutations resulting in a nonfunctional, truncated protein (Toguchida et al. 1992; Frebourg et al. 1995). This rarity of mammary carcinomas initially led investigators to conclude that *Trp53* null mice, the *Trp53*-deficient mice generated by Jacks and Donehower, do not develop mammary cancer because of the strain, since C57Bl/6 and/or 129Sv backgrounds have a predisposition for developing lymphomas and not mammary carcinomas, or that the null mice did not live long enough for mammary tumors to develop.

Hence, Medina and Jerry backcrossed the *Trp53* null allele from the Jacks model into the BALB/c background because BALB/c mice are a widely used model of mammary cancer due to their relatively high susceptibility (Jerry et al. 2000; Kuperwasser et al. 2000). Although the BALB/c *Trp53* nulls have a median tumor-free survival of less than 4 months and mammary tumors are rarely observed, more than half of the *Trp53* heterozygote BALB/c females develop mammary cancer, with a median tumor-free survival of 13.5 months. To test this, mammary glands from *Trp53* null mice were then transplanted into wild-type BALB/c female hosts that had normal life spans. As a result, 75% of the transplants developed mammary tumors with the earliest detected at 7 months. Thus, given the time to develop, mammary tumors would be a prominent outcome of loss of p53 as is the case in LFS patients (Kuperwasser et al. 2000).

10.7 Radiation Responses of Mammary Stem Cells

Based on the idea that stem cell transformation can lead to unlimited progeny, tissue-specific stem cells or early progenitors are thought to be the critical cellular target in carcinogenesis as has been discussed from many perspectives (Clifton et al. 1986;

Potten and Loeffler 1990; Sell and Pierce 1994; Zeps et al. 1996; Reya et al. 2001; Welm et al. 2002). The restricted window of carcinogen susceptibility that is evident during or around puberty in both rodents and humans has been postulated to simply contain the greatest density of target cells.

It is known that IR causes damage to DNA directly by induction of double-strand breaks or indirectly by generation of reactive oxygen species. The consequences of these lesions are mutations, translocations, deletions, and amplifications, which are also hallmarks of cancer cells. The mitotic index of stem cells makes them highly susceptible to mutagenesis. When a mutated stem cell divides, the damage can be "fixed" by passing it on to daughter cells that then expand further. Each round of replication represents an occasion to generate more mistakes increasing the probability of carcinogenesis. During puberty the ductal tree expands to fill the fat pad. That expansion implies expansion of the stem cell population through symmetrical division. This period of high stem cell proliferation is a perfect window frame to introduce alterations on the stem cell. As shown on several studies, treating rodents with carcinogens (Russo et al. 1982, 1983; Russo and Russo 1996) or radiation (Ullrich and Storer 1979) during ductal morphogenesis dramatically increases the onset of tumorigenesis.

Adult, tissue-specific stem cells (ASC) play a key role in tissue development and regeneration (Blanpain et al. 2004; Potten 2004). Two fundamental properties define these cells (Reya et al. 2001): the ability to self-renew, i.e., to maintain a constant pool of ASC in a certain tissue, and their multipotency, which confers the potential to generate all the differentiated cell types present in that tissue. Homeostasis is maintained through asymmetric division giving rise to differentiated progeny, while stem cell expansion, i.e., during ductal morphogenesis in puberty, is accomplished through symmetric division. It is now generally accepted that "stemness" is not a single property, but a number of properties that can be manifested under different conditions (Booth and Potten 2000). As stated by Potten, a stem cell must be undifferentiated (relative to other epithelial cell types, but not necessarily relative to embryonic cells) and capable of proliferation, self-maintenance, and regeneration of the tissue after injury (Potten and Loeffler 1990). It must be capable of producing many differentiated progeny and of retaining the ability to switch between these options when appropriate.

As mentioned previously, the mammary gland is relatively simple. The ductal tree consists of only three distinct cell types in both humans and rodents: a stem/progenitor cell capable of self-renewal, which gives rise to the more differentiated daughter cells, luminal and myoepithelial cells. At this point, there is no defined and unequivocal marker for the mammary stem cell. Researchers have used a combination of properties, function and marker exclusion to infer which populations are most consistent with the putative stem cell phenotype. A combination of cell surface marker analysis using isolated cells and functional repopulation assay was used by both Stingl et al. (2006) and Shackleton et al. (2006) to identify $CD24^{+}/CD49f^{hi}$ cell populations that enrich for mouse mammary repopulating cells.

Label retaining cells (LRC) are long-lived as defined by the capacity to retain a nuclear DNA synthesis label for long periods of time (over 13 weeks). LRC properties have been the basis for identifying ASC distribution in situ in many tissues (Potten et al. 2003; Tumbar et al. 2004; Shinin et al. 2006). LRC on the mammary gland have been shown to segregate their DNA strands (Smith 2005), a property attributed to ASC (Merok et al. 2002; Potten et al. 2002; Shinin et al. 2006). Several studies have attempted to locate the stem cell population in situ. In the mouse mammary gland, analysis of nuclear morphology of a luminal LRC population showed that suprabasal cells are enriched for both luminal and myoepithelial markers and are clustered in the ventral, larger ducts proximal to the embryonic origin of the gland (Fernandez-Gonzalez et al. 2009). In human specimens, colocalization of luminal and basal markers has been used to identify bipotent cells in the ducts (Villadsen et al. 2007) and aldehyde dehydrogenase-1 (Aldh1) marks undifferentiated cells in situ with the ability to generate mammospheres (Ginestier et al. 2007).

Stem cells have distinctive capabilities to respond and repair DNA damage. Wicha and colleagues described Aldh1, which is a detoxification enzyme, as a marker of normal and malignant human mammary stem cells (Ginestier et al. 2007). Cairns proposed that stem cells maintain a primordial strand to prevent "fixing" replication errors (Cairns 2002). According to Potten et al., stem cells in the skin, gut, and brain are most susceptible to cell killing by IR (Booth et al. 2000). Consistent with this, $CD24^{+}/CD29^{+}$ mammary cells, similar to those isolated as repopulating units by Shackleton et al. (2006), decreased after irradiation, although the "side-population" Sca^{+} cells increased (Woodward et al. 2007).

Basal-like breast cancers arising in women carrying mutations in the BRCA1 gene are thought to develop from a mammary stem/progenitor cell (Wright et al. 2008; Burga et al. 2009). Consistent with this, recent studies suggest that BRCA1 mutations can affect stem cell hierarchy. Knockdown of BRCA1 in primary breast epithelial cells leads to an increase in cells displaying ALDH1 and a decrease in cells expressing luminal epithelial markers and ER (Liu et al. 2008). In breast tissues, loss of heterozygosity for BRCA1 was seen in ALDH1-positive lobules but not in adjacent ALDH1-negative lobules, which suggests that the loss of BRCA1 function blocks epithelial lineage commitment of ER-positive cells. A recent study by Lindeman and colleagues identified a luminal progenitor cell using surface markers and provides evidence that suggests that these ER-negative cells are expanded in BRCA1 carriers (Lim et al. 2009). Thus, not only mutations like BRCA1 but also cell non-autonomous damage, such as inflammation, can affect stem cell hierarchy. A recent idea is that stem cell number could change as a function of life events that influence breast cancer risk since proliferation per se is not sufficient, because pregnancy, a period of rapid growth, is generally a protective factor in the long-term risk of developing breast cancer, but only if it occurs early (reviewed in Britt et al. 2007). Recent studies suggest that indeed an early pregnancy during ductal morphogenesis can reduce stem cell number (Siwko et al. 2008), while in another study in which pregnancy occurred after maturation showed no effect (Britt et al. 2009). If confirmed, these studies appear to suggest that changes in stem cell number could be associated with risk.

Relatively few studies have attempted to assess the radiation sensitivity of the mammary stem cell or progenitors. A comprehensive analysis of the radiosensitivity of rat mammary clonogens was conducted by Gould and colleagues (Kamiya et al. 1991a, b, 1998). In this model, monodispersed rat mammary epithelial cells are injected into the intrascarpal fat pad where they form clonogenic organoids that can be enumerated. When irradiated clonogenic mammary epithelial cells are transplanted and hormonally stimulated, they give rise to clonal glandular structures within which carcinomas may arise. The size of the clonogenic cell subpopulation increases during morphogenesis as the ductal tree is laid out and slows during differentiation of terminal mammary end buds and alveolar structures. The surviving fractions of clonogenic mammary cells of groups of virgin rats from 1 to 12 weeks after birth after single exposures to 137Cs rays were studied (Shimada et al. 1994). The radiosensitivity of clonogens from prepubertal rats was high and changed with the onset of puberty at between 4 and 6 weeks of age. Whether there is an association between the high sensitivity of the prepubertal and pubertal mammary clonogens to radiation killing and a high susceptibility to radiogenic initiation of cancer remains to be determined. However, recent studies suggest that the ability of immature tissue to process chemical carcinogen damage is also different than that of the mature tissue (Ariazi et al. 2005).

It has become increasingly evident that tissue structure, function, and dysfunction are highly intertwined with the microenvironment during cancer development (Bissell et al. 2002; Barcellos-Hoff and Medina 2005; Gonda et al. 2009) and that tissue biology and host physiology are subverted to drive malignant progression (Coussens and Werb 2001). A remarkable series of experiments by Smith and colleagues demonstrate that mammary epithelial cells can reprogram diverse cell types (Boulanger et al. 2007; Booth et al. 2008). Transplantation into the mammary fat pad of normal mammary epithelial cells mixed with marked cells isolated from mature testis induces conversion or reprogramming of the beta-galactosidase marked testis cells with mammary repopulating capacity. The idea that the niche can supersede established phenotype demonstrates phenotypic plasticity that could be the basis for the current debate on markers vs. function of stem cells (Smith and Medina 2008).

We speculate that aberrant heterotypic interactions can act even earlier, during tissue maturation, to set the stage for developing breast cancer. Radiation exposure not only causes DNA damage, but also alters the microenvironment and the response to signals (Barcellos-Hoff 1998a, b). At the multicellular level, IR induces persistent and nonmutagenic effects that may promote carcinogenesis (Barcellos-Hoff et al. 2005). Barcellos-Hoff and Ravani (2000) showed that IR alters the microenvironment; injecting a p53 mutant mammary cell line into an irradiated host increased the development of tumors. The effect of the irradiated microenvironment on neoplastic progression persisted for several weeks and was independent of systemic radiation effects, as shown by hemibody irradiation. These observations suggest the hypothesis that nonmutagenic effects of radiation contribute to radiation carcinogenesis in vivo. TGFβ has been identified as one of the major determinants for the mouse mammary gland response to IR (Barcellos-Hoff 1993; Barcellos-Hoff et al. 1994, 2005). Mammary proliferation is inhibited by TGFβ1 in response to ovarian hormones as estrogen and progesterone (Pierce et al. 1993; Ewan et al. 2002). In culture, if a human mammary epithelial cell population is irradiated shortly after plating in the presence of TGFβ, the expression of E-cadherin, an epithelial phenotype marker, decreased. These data suggest that radiation predisposes human mammary epithelial cells to undergo epithelial-to-mesenchymal transition (EMT) (Andarawewa et al. 2007). A recent study from Weinberg and colleagues observed that the EMT process is associated with the expression of stem cell features (Mani et al. 2008).

A pooled analysis of eight irradiated populations by Preston et al. showed that increased risk of breast cancer is inversely correlated with age at irradiation (Preston et al. 2002). We hypothesized that radiation exposure during puberty not only increases mutations, but that induced signaling could affect stem cell self-renewal and epithelial hierarchy, thus increasing the potential "targets" of neoplastic transformation. Preliminary data using cell surface markers and limiting dilution of repopulating cells support this hypothesis (Illa Bochaca and Barcellos-Hoff unpublished). These are the first data to our knowledge that a known human carcinogen may affect stem cell frequency. Taken together, these observations suggest that IR can operate at multiple levels deregulating the stem cell population.

10.8 Conclusion

Given the complex interactions of radiation with DNA, target cells, and nontarget cells in the causation of cancer, it is evident that no single perspective on the effects of radiation provides a complete understanding of the mechanism of carcinogenic action. Our overarching hypothesis is that cancer *emerges* as a result of a complex, but ultimately predictable, interplay between targeted and nontargeted effects in the context of host genetics and physiology (Barcellos-Hoff 2007). Just as DNA damage elicits a dramatic transition in signaling within a cell, each irradiated tissue has its own set of signals and cell types, distinct from those of unirradiated tissue and different from other irradiated tissues. The sum of these events, occurring in different organs and highly modulated by genotype, predicates the consequence to the organism. We propose that radiation exposure culminates in cancer as a result of oncogenic mutations from targeted DNA damage that occur in the context of the biology of irradiated tissues driven in large part by nontargeted radiation effects (Barcellos-Hoff 2005, 2007). Furthermore, the view of cancer as an emergent property is able to incorporate the role of stem cells in the development of radiogenic cancer, allowing the two seemingly separate paradigms to be merged. Regardless of whether a cell is a stem cell, somatic cell, cancer-initiating cell, or noncancer-initiating cell, heterotypic interactions with other cell types of the tumor environment determine its behavior, all of which are subject to the effects of radiation. Future studies will encompass both targeted and nontargeted mechanisms of radiation action and how they can be targeted for the prevention and treatment of breast cancer.

Acknowledgments This research was supported by a DOD-BCRP predoctoral fellowship to DHN and the Department of Energy, Office of Biological and Environment Research Low Dose program, the Breast Cancer and the Environment Research Centers grant number U01 ES/CA

012801 from the National Institute of Environmental Health Sciences and the National Cancer Institute of the National Institutes of Health to MHBH. Its contents are solely the responsibility of the authors and do not necessarily represent the official views of the funding agencies.

References

Andarawewa KL, Erickson AC, Chou WS et al (2007) Ionizing radiation predisposes nonmalignant human mammary epithelial cells to undergo transforming growth factor beta induced epithelial to mesenchymal transition. Cancer Res 67:8662–8670

Ariazi JL, Haag JD, Lindstrom MJ et al (2005) Mammary glands of sexually immature rats are more susceptible than those of mature rats to the carcinogenic, lethal, and mutagenic effects of *N*-nitroso-*N*-methylurea. Mol Carcinog 43(3):155–164

Barcellos-Hoff MH (1993) Radiation-induced transforming growth factor b and subsequent extracellular matrix reorganization in murine mammary gland. Cancer Res 53:3880–3886

Barcellos-Hoff MH (1998a) How do tissues respond to damage at the cellular level? The role of cytokines in irradiated tissues. Radiat Res 150(5):S109–S120

Barcellos-Hoff MH (1998b) The potential influence of radiation-induced microenvironments in neoplastic progression. J Mammary Gland Biol Neoplasia 3:165–175

Barcellos-Hoff MH (2005) Integrative radiation carcinogenesis: interactions between cell and tissue responses to DNA damage. Semin Cancer Biol 15(2):138–148

Barcellos-Hoff MH (2007) Cancer as an emergent phenomenon in systems radiation biology. Radiat Environ Biophys 47(1):33–38

Barcellos-Hoff MH, Brooks AL (2001) Extracellular signaling via the microenvironment: a hypothesis relating carcinogenesis, bystander effects and genomic instability. Radiat Res 156(5):618–627

Barcellos-Hoff MH, Medina D (2005) New highlights on stroma-epithelial interactions in breast cancer. Breast Cancer Res 7:33–36

Barcellos-Hoff MH, Ravani SA (2000) Irradiated mammary gland stroma promotes the expression of tumorigenic potential by unirradiated epithelial cells. Cancer Res 60:1254–1260

Barcellos-Hoff MH, Derynck R, Tsang ML-S et al (1994) Transforming growth factor-b activation in irradiated murine mammary gland. J Clin Invest 93:892–899

Barcellos-Hoff MH, Park C, Wright EG (2005) Radiation and the microenvironment – tumorigenesis and therapy. Nat Rev Cancer 5(11):867–875

Baverstock K (2000) Radiation-induced genomic instability: a paradigm-breaking phenomenon and its relevance to environmentally induced cancer. Mutat Res 454(1–2):89–109

Bissell MJ, Radisky D, Rizki A et al (2002) The organizing principle: microenvironmental influences in the normal and malignant breast. Differentiation 70:537–546

Blanpain C, Lowry WE, Geoghegan A et al (2004) Self-renewal, multipotency, and the existence of two cell populations within an epithelial stem cell niche. Cell 118(5):635–648

Boice JD, Preston D, Davis G et al (1991) Frequent chest x-ray fluoroscopy and breast cancer incidence among tuberculosis patients in Massachusetts. Radiat Res 125:214–222

Boice JD, Harvey EB, Blettner M et al (1992) Cancer in the contralateral breast after radiotherapy for breast cancer. N Engl J Med 326(12):781–785

Booth C, Potten CS (2000) Gut instincts: thoughts on intestinal epithelial stem cells. J Clin Invest 105(11):1493–1499

Booth D, Haley JD, Bruskin AM et al (2000) Transforming growth factor-B3 protects murine small intestinal crypt stem cells and animal survival after irradiation, possibly by reducing stem-cell cycling. Int J Cancer 86(1):53–59

Booth BW, Mack DL, Androutsellis-Theotokis A et al (2008) The mammary microenvironment alters the differentiation repertoire of neural stem cells. Proc Natl Acad Sci USA 105(39):14891–14896

Boulanger CA, Mack DL, Booth BW et al (2007) Interaction with the mammary microenvironment redirects spermatogenic cell fate in vivo. PNAS 104(10):3871–3876

Bresciani F (1968) Topography of DNA synthesis in the mammary gland of the C3H mouse and its control by ovarian hormones: an autoradiographic study. Cell Tissue Kinet 1(1):51–63

Britt K, Ashworth A, Smalley M (2007) Pregnancy and the risk of breast cancer. Endocr Relat Cancer 14(4):907–933

Britt K, Kendrick H, Regan J et al (2009) Pregnancy in the mature adult mouse does not alter the proportion of mammary epithelial stem/progenitor cells. Breast Cancer Res 11(2):R20

Brooks AL (2005) Paradigm shifts in radiation biology: their impact on intervention for radiation-induced disease. Radiat Res 164:454–461

Burga LN, Tung NM, Troyan SL et al (2009) Altered proliferation and differentiation properties of primary mammary epithelial cells from BRCA1 mutation carriers. Cancer Res 69(4): 1273–1278

Cairns J (2002) Somatic stem cells and the kinetics of mutagenesis and carcinogenesis. Proc Natl Acad Sci USA 99(16):10567–10570

Castiglioni F, Terenziani M, Carcangiu ML et al (2007) Radiation effects on development of HER2-positive breast carcinomas. Clin Cancer Res 13(1):46–51

Chen X, Oppenheim JJ, Howard OM (2005) BALB/c mice have more CD4+CD25+ T regulatory cells and show greater susceptibility to suppression of their CD4+CD25-responder T cells than C57BL/6 mice. J Leukoc Biol 78(1):114–121

Christov K, Swanson SM, Guzman RC et al (1993) Kinetics of mammary epithelial cell proliferation in pituitary isografted BALB/c mice. Carcinogenesis 14(10):2019–2025

Clifton KH, Sridharan BN, Douple EB (1975) Mammary carcinogenesis-enhancing effect of adrenalectomy in irradiated rats with pituitary tumor MtT-F4. J Natl Cancer Inst 55(2):485–487

Clifton KH, Tanner MA, Gould MN (1986) Assessment of radiogenic cancer initiation frequency per clonogenic rat mammary cell in vivo. Cancer Res 46:2390–2395

Clutton SM, Townsend KM, Goodhead DT et al (1996) Differentiation and delayed cell death in embryonal stem cells exposed to low doses of ionising radiation. Cell Death Differ 3(1):141–148

Coussens LM, Werb Z (2001) Inflammatory cells and cancer: think different! J Exp Med 193(6):23F–26F

Daniel CW, Silberstein GB, Strickland P (1987) Direct action of 17 beta-estradiol on mouse mammary ducts analyzed by sustained release implants and steroid autoradiography. Cancer Res 47(22):6052–6057

Dent P, Yacoub A, Contessa J et al (2003) Stress and radiation-induced activation of multiple intracellular signaling pathways. Radiat Res 159(3):283–300

DeOme KB, Faulkin LJ Jr, Bern HA et al (1959) Development of mammary tumors from hyperplastic alveolar nodules transplanted into gland-free mammary fat pads of female C3H mice. Cancer Res 19(5):515–520

Derynck R, Akhurst RJ, Balmain A (2001) TGF-b signaling in tumor suppression and cancer progression. Nat Genet 29:117–129

Donehower LA (1996) The p53-deficient mouse: a model for basic and applied cancer studies. Semin Cancer Biol 7(5):269–278

Donehower LA, Harvey M, Slagle BL et al (1992) Mice deficient for p53 are developmentally normal but susceptible to spontaneous tumours. Nature 356(6366):215–221

Ehrhart EJ, Carroll A, Segarini P et al (1997) Latent transforming growth factor-b activation in situ: quantitative and functional evidence following low dose irradiation. FASEB J 11:991–1002

Ethier SP, Cundiff KC (1987) Importance of extended growth potential and growth factor independence on in vivo neoplastic potential of primary rat mammary carcinoma cells. Cancer Res 47:5316–5322

Ethier SP, Ullrich RL (1982) Detection of ductal dysplasia in mammary outgrowths derived from carcinogen-treated virgin female BALB/c mice. Cancer Res 42:1753–1760

Ethier SP, Adams LM, Ullrich RL (1984) Morphological and histological characteristics of mammary dysplasias occurring in cell dissociation-derived murine mammary outgrowths. Cancer Res 44:4517–4522
Ethier SP, Kudla A, Cundiff KC (1987) Influence of hormone and growth factor interactions on the proliferative potential of normal rat mammary epithelial cells in vitro. J Cell Physiol 132:161–167
Ewan KB, Shyamala G, Ravani SA et al (2002) Latent TGF-b activation in mammary gland: regulation by ovarian hormones affects ductal and alveolar proliferation. Am J Pathol 160(6):2081–2093
Fernandez-Gonzalez R, Illa-Bochaca I, Welm BE et al (2009) Mapping mammary gland architecture using multi-scale in situ analysis. Integr Biol 1(1):80–89
Frebourg T, Barbier N, Yan YX et al (1995) Germ-line p53 mutations in 15 families with Li-Fraumeni syndrome. Am J Hum Genet 56(3):608–615
Ginestier C, Hur MH, Charafe-Jauffret E et al (2007) ALDH1 is a marker of normal and malignant human mammary stem cells and a predictor of poor clinical outcome. Cell Stem Cell 1(5):555–567
Gonda TA, Tu S, Wang TC (2009) Chronic inflammation, the tumor microenvironment and carcinogenesis. Cell Cycle 8(13):2005–2013
Gusterson BA, Gelber RD, Goldhirsch A et al (1992) Prognostic importance of c-erbB-2 expression in breast cancer. International (Ludwig) Breast Cancer Study Group [see comments]. J Clin Oncol 10(7):1049–1056
Hallahan DE, Haimovitz-Friedman A, Kufe DW et al (1993) The role of cytokines in radiation oncology. In: Devita VT, Hellman S, Rosenberg SA (eds) Important advances in oncology. J.B. Lippincott Company, Philadelphia, pp 71–90
Hancock SL, Tucker MA, Hoppe RT (1993) Breast cancer after treatment of Hodgkin's disease. J Natl Cancer Inst 85(1):25–31
Hei TK, Wu LJ, Liu SX et al (1997) Mutagenic effects of a single and an exact number of alpha particles in mammalian cells. Proc Natl Acad Sci USA 94(8):3765–3770
Herskind C, Rodemann HP (2000) Spontaneous and radiation-induced differentiation of fibroblasts. Exp Gerontol 35(6–7):747–755
Hollstein M, Sidransky D, Vogelstein B et al (1991) p53 mutations in human cancers. Science 253(5015):49–53
Hollstein M, Rice K, Greenblatt MS et al (1994) Database of p53 gene somatic mutations in human tumors and cell lines. Nucleic Acids Res 22(17):3551–3555
Howard BA, Gusterson BA (2000) Human breast development. J Mammary Gland Biol Neoplasia 5(2):119–137
Howe GR, McLaughlin J (1996) Breast cancer mortality between 1950 and 1987 after exposure to fractionated moderate-dose-rate ionizing radiation in the Canadian fluoroscopy cohort study and a comparison with breast cancer mortality in the atomic bomb survivor study. Radiat Res 145:694–707
Huang L, Snyder AR, Morgan WF (2003) Radiation-induced genomic instability and its implications for radiation carcinogenesis. Oncogene 22(37):5848–5854
Jacks T, Remington L, Williams BO et al (1994) Tumor spectrum analysis in p53-mutant mice. Curr Biol 4:1–7
Jerry DJ, Medina D, Butel JS (1994) p53 mutations in COMMA-D cells. In Vitro Cell Dev Biol 30A:87–89
Jerry DJ, Kittrell FS, Kuperwasser C et al (2000) A mammary-specific model demonstrates the role of the p53 tumor suppressor gene in tumor development. Oncogene 19(8):1052–1058
Jobling MF, Mott JD, Finnegan M et al (2006) Isoform specificity of redox-mediated TGF-b activation. Radiat Res 166(6):839–848
Kadhim MA, Macdonald DA, Goodhead DT et al (1992) Transmission of chromosomal instability after plutonium alpha-particle irradiation [see comments]. Nature 355(6362):738–740
Kadhim MA, Lorimore SA, Hepburn MD et al (1994) Alpha-particle-induced chromosomal instability in human bone marrow cells. Lancet 344(8928):987–988

Kadhim MA, Lorimore SA, Townsend KM et al (1995) Radiation-induced genomic instability: delayed cytogenetic aberrations and apoptosis in primary human bone marrow cells. Int J Radiat Biol 67(3):287–293

Kamiya K, Gould MN, Clifton KH (1991a) Differential control of alveolar and ductal development in grafts of monodispersed rat mammary epithelium. Proc Soc Exp Biol Med 196(3):284–292

Kamiya K, Kim ND, Gould MN et al (1991b) Repair of potentially lethal damage in rat mammary clonogens following irradiation in organoid culture. Int J Radiat Biol 59(5):1207–1216

Kamiya K, Gould MN, Clifton KH (1998) Quantitative studies of ductal versus alveolar differentiation from rat mammary clonogens. Proc Soc Exp Biol Med 219(3):217–225

Kaplan HS, Brown MB, Hirsch BB et al (1956a) Indirect induction of lymphomas in irradiated mice: II. Factor of irradiation of the host. Cancer Res 16(5):426–428

Kaplan HS, Carnes WH, Brown MB et al (1956b) Indirect induction of lymphomas in irradiated mice: I. Tumor incidence and morphology in mice bearing nonirradiated thymic grafts. Cancer Res 16(5):422–425

Kuperwasser C, Hurlbut GD, Kittrell FS et al (2000) Development of spontaneous mammary tumors in BALB/c p53 heterozygous mice. A model for Li-Fraumeni syndrome. Am J Pathol 157(6):2151–2159

Land CE, Hayakawa N, Machado SG et al (1994a) A case-control interview study of breast cancer among Japanese A-bomb survivors. I. Main effects. Cancer Causes Control 5(2):157–165

Land CE, Hayakawa N, Machado SG et al (1994b) A case-control interview study of breast cancer among Japanese A-bomb survivors. II. Interactions with radiation dose. Cancer Causes Control 5(2):167–176

Lim E, Vaillant F, Wu D et al (2009) Aberrant luminal progenitors as the candidate target population for basal tumor development in BRCA1 mutation carriers. Nat Med 15(8):907–913

Limoli CL, Kaplan MI, Corcoran J et al (1997) Chromosomal instability and its relationship to other end points of genomic instability. Cancer Res 57(24):5557–5563

Little JB (2003) Genomic instability and bystander effects: a historical perspective. Oncogene 22(45):6978–6987

Liu S, Ginestier C, Charafe-Jauffret E et al (2008) BRCA1 regulates human mammary stem/progenitor cell fate. Proc Natl Acad Sci USA 105(5):1680–1685

Lydon JP, DeMayo FJ, Funk CR et al (1995) Mice lacking progesterone receptor exhibit pleiotropic reproductive abnormalities. Genes Dev 9:2266–2278

Malkin D, Li FP, Strong LC et al (1990) Germ line p53 mutations in a familial syndrome of breast cancer, sarcomas, and other neoplasms. Science 250(4985):1233–1238

Mani SA, Guo W, Liao M-J et al (2008) The epithelial-mesenchymal transition generates cells with properties of stem cells. Cell 133(4):704–715

Mattsson A, Ruden B-I, Wilking N et al (1993) Radiation-induced breast cancer: long-term follow-up of radiation therapy for benign breast disease. J Natl Cancer Inst 85:1679–1685

McBride WH (1995) Cytokine cascades in late normal tissue radiation responses. Int J Radiat Oncol Biol Phys 33(1):233–234

Medina D, Kittrell FS, Shepard A et al (2002) Biological and genetic properties of the p53 null preneoplastic mammary epithelium. FASEB J 16(8):881–883

Merok JR, Lansita JA, Tunstead JR et al (2002) Cosegregation of chromosomes containing immortal DNA strands in cells that cycle with asymmetric stem cell kinetics. Cancer Res 62(23):6791–6795

Morin Doody M, Lonstein JE, Stovall M et al (2000) Breast cancer mortality after diagnostic radiography: findings from the U.S. Scoliosis Cohort Study. Spine 25(16):2052–2063

Mothersill C, Rea D, Wright EG et al (2001) Individual variation in the production of a "bystander signal" following irradiation of primary cultures of normal human urothelium. Carcinogenesis 22(9):1465–1471

Mukhopadhyay R, Costes S, Bazarov A, Hines WC, Barcellos-Hoff MH, Yaswen P (2010) Promotion of variant human mammary epithelial cell outgrowth by ionizing radiation: an agent-based model supported by in vitro studies. Breast Cancer Res 12:R11

NAS/NRC (2006) Health risks from exposure to low levels of ionizing radiation: phase 2. Board on radiation effects research (BEIRVII). National Academy Press, Washington

Nguyen DH, Oketch-Rabah HA, Illa-Bochaca I et al (2011) Radiation acts on the microenvironment to affect breast carcinogenesis by distinct mechanisms that decrease cancer latency and affect tumor type. Cancer Cell 19:640–651

Park CC, Henshall-Powell RL, Erickson AC et al (2003) Ionizing radiation induces heritable disruption of epithelial cell interactions. Proc Natl Acad Sci USA 100(19):10728–10733

Pierce DFJ, Johnson MD, Matsui Y et al (1993) Inhibition of mammary duct development but not alveolar outgrowth during pregnancy in transgenic mice expressing active TGF-b 1. Genes Dev 7:2308–2317

Ponnaiya B, Cornforth MN, Ullrich RL (1997) Radiation-induced chromosomal instability in BALB/c and C57BL/6 mice: the difference is as clear as black and white. Radiat Res 147(2):121–125

Potten CS (2004) Radiation, the ideal cytotoxic agent for studying the cell biology of tissues such as the small intestine. Radiat Res 161(2):123–136

Potten CS, Loeffler M (1990) Stem cells: attributes, cycles, spirals, pitfalls and uncertainties. Lessons for and from the crypt. Development 110(4):1001–1020

Potten CS, Booth D, Cragg NJ et al (2002) Cell kinetic studies in murine ventral tongue epithelium: cell cycle progression studies using double labelling techniques. Cell Prolif 35:16–21

Potten CS, Booth C, Tudor GL et al (2003) Identification of a putative intestinal stem cell and early lineage marker; musashi-1. Differentiation 71(1):28–41

Preston DL, Mattsson A, Holmberg E et al (2002) Radiation effects on breast cancer risk: a pooled analysis of eight cohorts. Radiat Res 158(2):220–235

Preston DL, Ron E, Tokuoka S et al (2007) Solid cancer incidence in atomic bomb survivors: 1958–1998. Radiat Res 168(1):1–64

Purdie CA, Harrison DJ, Peter A et al (1994) Tumour incidence, spectrum and ploidy in mice with a large deletion in the p53 gene. Oncogene 9(2):603–609

Rakha EA, Ellis IO (2007) An overview of assessment of prognostic and predictive factors in breast cancer needle core biopsy specimens. J Clin Pathol 60(12):1300–1306

Rakha EA, Elsheikh SE, Aleskandarany MA et al (2009) Triple-negative breast cancer: distinguishing between basal and nonbasal subtypes. Clin Cancer Res 15(7):2302–2310

Rave-Frank M, Virsik-Kopp P, Pradier O et al (2001) In vitro response of human dermal fibroblasts to X-irradiation: relationship between radiation-induced clonogenic cell death, chromosome aberrations and markers of proliferative senescence or differentiation. Int J Radiat Biol 77:1163–1174

Reya T, Morrison SJ, Clarke MF et al (2001) Stem cells, cancer, and cancer stem cells. Nature 414:105–111

Richert MM, Schwertfeger KL, Ryder JW et al (2000) An atlas of mouse mammary gland development. J Mammary Gland Biol Neoplasia 5(2):227–241

Ronckers CM, Erdmann CA, Land CE (2005) Radiation and breast cancer: a review of current evidence. Breast Cancer Res 7:21–32

Russo J, Russo IH (1996) Experimentally induced mammary tumors in rats. Breast Cancer Res Treat 39(1):7–20

Russo J, Tay LK, Russo IH (1982) Differentiation of the mammary gland and susceptibility to carcinogenesis. Breast Cancer Res Treat 2(1):5–73

Russo J, Tait L, Russo IH (1983) Susceptibility of the mammary gland to carcinogenesis. III. The cell of origin of rat mammary carcinoma. Am J Pathol 113(1):50–66

Sell S, Pierce GB (1994) Maturation arrest of stem cell differentiation is a common pathway for the cellular origin of teratocarcinomas and epithelial cancers. Lab Invest 70(1):6–22

Shackleton M, Vaillant F, Simpson KJ et al (2006) Generation of a functional mammary gland from a single stem cell. Nature 439(7072):84–88

Shimada Y, Yasukawa-Barnes J, Kim RY et al (1994) Age and radiation sensitivity of rat mammary clonogenic cells. Radiat Res 137:118–123

Shinin V, Gayraud-Morel B, Gomes D et al (2006) Asymmetric division and cosegregation of template DNA strands in adult muscle satellite cells. Nat Cell Biol 8(7):677–682

Shore RE, Hildreth N, Woodard E et al (1986) Breast cancer among women given X-ray therapy for acute postpartum mastitis. J Natl Cancer Inst 77(3):689–696

Shyamala G (1997) Roles of estrogen and progesterone in normal mammary gland development: insights from progesterone null receptor mutant mice and in situ localization of receptor. Trends Endocrinol Metab 8(1):34–39

Sivaraman L, Conneely OM, Medina D et al (2001) p53 is a potential mediator of pregnancy and hormone-induced resistance to mammary carcinogenesis. Proc Natl Acad Sci USA 98(22):12379–12384

Siwko SK, Dong J, Lewis MT et al (2008) Evidence that an early pregnancy causes a persistent decrease in the number of functional mammary epithelial stem cells–implications for pregnancy-induced protection against breast cancer. Stem Cells 26(12):3205–3209

Smith GH (2005) Label-retaining epithelial cells in mouse mammary gland divide asymmetrically and retain their template DNA strands. Development 132(4):681–687

Smith G, Medina D (2008) Re-evaluation of mammary stem cell biology based on in vivo transplantation. Breast Cancer Res 10(1):203

Stingl J, Eirew P, Ricketson I et al (2006) Purification and unique properties of mammary epithelial stem cells. Nature 439(7079):993–997

Stutman O (1974) Cell-mediated immunity and aging. Fed Proc Am Soc Exp Biol 33(9): 2028–2032

Toguchida J, Yamaguchi T, Dayton SH et al (1992) Prevalence and spectrum of germline mutations of the p53 gene among patients with sarcoma. N Engl J Med 326(20):1301–1308

Tokunaga M, Land CE, Aoki Y et al (1993) Proliferative and nonproliferative breast disease in atomic bomb survivors. Results of a histopathologic review of autopsy breast tissue. Cancer 72(5):1657–1665

Tsai KK, Chuang EY, Little JB et al (2005) Cellular mechanisms for low-dose ionizing radiation-induced perturbation of the breast tissue microenvironment. Cancer Res 65(15): 6734–6744

Tumbar T, Guasch G, Greco V et al (2004) Defining the epithelial stem cell niche in skin. Science 303(5656):359–363

Ullrich RL (1983) Tumor induction in BALB/c female mice after fission neutron or gamma irradiation. Radiat Res 93(3):506–515

Ullrich RL (1984) Tumor induction in BALB/c mice after fractionated or protracted exposures to fission-spectrum neutrons. Radiat Res 97(3):587–597

Ullrich RL, Storer JB (1979) Influence of gamma-irradiation on the development of neoplastic disease in mice. II. Solid tumors. Radiat Res 80:317–324

Ullrich RL, Bowles ND, Satterfield LC et al (1996) Strain-dependent susceptibility to radiation-induced mammary cancer is a result of differences in epithelial cell sensitivity to transformation. Radiat Res 146(3):353–355

Villadsen R, Fridriksdottir AJ, Ronnov-Jessen L et al (2007) Evidence for a stem cell hierarchy in the adult human breast. J Cell Biol 177(1):87–101

Welm BE, Tepera SB, Venezia T et al (2002) Sca-1(pos) cells in the mouse mammary gland represent an enriched progenitor cell population. Dev Biol 245(1):42–56

Woodward WA, Chen MS, Behbod F et al (2007) WNT/beta-catenin mediates radiation resistance of mouse mammary progenitor cells. PNAS 104(2):618–623

Wright EG (2000) Inducible genomic instability: new insights into the biological effects of ionizing radiation. Med Confl Surviv 16:117–130

Wright EG, Coates PJ (2006) Untargeted effects of ionizing radiation: implications for radiation pathology. Mutat Res 597(1–2):119–132

Wright MH, Calcagno AM, Salcido CD et al (2008) Brca1 breast tumors contain distinct CD44+/CD24– and CD133+ cells with cancer stem cell characteristics. Breast Cancer Res 10(1):R10

Zeps N, Dawkins HJS, Papadimitriou JM et al (1996) Detection of a population of long-lived cells in mammary epithelium of the mouse. Cell Tissue Res 286(3):525–536

Zhang S, Ramsay ES, Mock BA (1998) Cdkn2a, the cyclin-dependent kinase inhibitor encoding p16INK4a and p19ARF, is a candidate for the plasmacytoma susceptibility locus, Pctr1. Proc Natl Acad Sci USA 95(5):2429–2434

Chapter 11
Brain Estrogens and Metabolism

Yong Xu and Deborah J. Clegg

Abstract Recent observations have demonstrated that the ovarian steroid estrogen, acting through one of its receptors, specifically estrogen receptor-α (ERα), in distinct regions in the central nervous system (CNS), is responsible for body weight regulation. The ventral medial hypothalamus (VMH) contains two key nuclei, the arcuate (ARC), which contains populations of neurons that regulate food intake and body weight, and the ventral medial nucleus (VMN). The VMN alone has not been found to have a prominent role in the regulation of food intake and body weight, but does influence energy expenditure. ERα is expressed in the CNS, and estrogenic activation of ERα in discrete brain nuclei is required for the coordinated control of food intake and energy expenditure. Further, we discuss data suggesting that the effects of estrogens on food intake and energy expenditure are mediated by estrogenic enhancement/augmentation of peripheral and neuronal signals in distinct hypothalamic neurons. In sum, estrogens are critical regulators of body weight homeostasis.

Keywords Food intake • Body weight • Energy homeostasis • Estrogens • Estrogen receptor alpha • Central nervous system

11.1 Introduction

Obesity and its associated health disorders and costs are increasing. There is a sexual dimorphism with respect to obesity-associated diseases, with men and postmenopausal women having greater risk of developing complications from obesity than younger women. These findings suggest that there may be a role for estrogens

---

D.J. Clegg (✉)
Department of Internal Medicine, University of Texas Southwestern Medical Center, Touchstone Diabetes Center, 5323 Harry Hines Blvd., K5.252, Dallas, TX 75390-8854, USA
e-mail: deborah.clegg@utsouthwestern.edu

J. Russo (ed.), *Environment and Breast Cancer*, DOI 10.1007/978-1-4419-9896-5_11,

in protecting against obesity and diseases associated with it. Within the brain, the hypothalamus is an important regulator of body weight in that it responds to hormones and other signals to control energy intake and expenditure. Estrogen receptors have been demonstrated to be located throughout the brain, and specifically within the hypothalamus. There are two estrogen receptors, estrogen receptor alpha (ERα) and estrogen receptor beta (ERβ). We and others have previously demonstrated that activation of ERα by estrogens reduces food intake and increases body weight. This review focuses on the relative contribution of activation of ERα by estrogens within the brain for the regulation of food intake and body weight. Understanding the mechanisms by which estrogens regulate body weight will assist in determining potential therapeutic agents for menopausal women to decrease the propensity of diseases associated with obesity.

11.2 Estrogens Regulate Metabolism

Studies from human and animal models have established important roles for estrogens in the regulation of metabolism. For example, when women enter menopause, estrogens decline and this is accompanied by a dramatic increase in the prevalence of obesity (Flegal et al. 2002; Freedman et al. 2002; Carr 2003), type II diabetes (Flegal et al. 2002; Freedman et al. 2002; Carr 2003), and cardiovascular disorders (Kaaja 2008). In animals, removal of ovaries, ovariectomy (OVX), leads to increased body weight and hyperadiposity (Drewett 1973; Blaustein and Wade 1976; Wallen et al. 2001), effects that are prevented by replacement of estrogens (Geary et al. 2001). Although OVX induces a transient increase in food intake, the hyperphagia does not solely appear to account for the changes in metabolism and the development of obesity (Wallen et al. 2001). Endogenous estrogens may regulate body weight homeostasis by modulating energy expenditure, as is suggested by a recent study demonstrating OVX decreases energy expenditure but has no effect on food intake in mice (Rogers et al. 2009). However, estradiol replacement has also been demonstrated to decrease food intake in rodents (Clegg et al. 2003a; Gao et al. 2007), indicating that exogenous estrogens may promote energy balance by influencing both energy intake and energy expenditure.

One additional mechanism by which estrogens control energy homeostasis is by regulating lipid metabolism. D'Eon and coworkers have used pair-fed OVX mice treated with estradiol-17β (OVX-E) or with control/vehicle (OVX-C) treatment. While these mice display similar body weight, the OVX-E mice demonstrated significantly decreased body fat due to decreased lipogenic gene expression, increased catecholamine-stimulated lipolysis in adipocytes, and increased lipid oxidative pathways in muscle (D'Eon et al. 2005). Additionally, estrogens are also thought to play a role in regulating fat distribution. For example, female humans and rodents distribute relatively more fat in the subcutaneous depot, while males have more fat stored in the visceral depot, which is more likely to cause insulin resistance, glucose intolerance, and diseases associated with the metabolic syndromes (Andersson et al. 1997; Bjorntorp 1997a, b). Estrogens appear to account for this sexual dimorphism, because the differences in the fat distribution between premenopausal females and age-matched men are abolished in postmenopausal females (Kotani et al. 1994). Collectively, these findings suggest, in addition to the role of estrogens in energy intake and expenditure, there appears to be a role for estrogens in modulating adiposity.

11.3 Central Nervous System (CNS) and Hypothalamic Control of Body Weight

In an effort to identify targets for therapeutic treatments to reduce food intake and body weight, obesity research has focused on central metabolic and hormonal pathways that control energy homeostasis (Obici 2009). The hypothalamus is one area within the central nervous system (CNS) that has received attention as a region in the brain that controls food intake, energy expenditure and body weight homeostasis. Since the 1930s, several thousand reports have been published investigating the potential role of various hypothalamic nuclei in the regulation of energy homeostasis (Bray and York 1972; York and Bray 1972; Bray et al. 1982; Bray 1984). Early interest in the hypothalamus stemmed from findings that dramatic changes in food intake, body weight, and energy homeostasis could be produced by lesioning specific hypothalamic nuclei, such as the ventral medial hypothalamus (VMH) (as reviewed in Louis-Sylvestre 1980; Smith 2000) or the lateral hypothalamic area (LHA) (Danguir and Nicolaidis 1980; Milam et al. 1980). More recently, areas in the hypothalamus such as the ventral medial nucleus (VMN) and arcuate (ARC) nucleus (among others) have been identified as targets for hormonal and neuropeptide signals that can produce marked changes in energy homeostasis.

11.4 Estrogens Interact with the Adiposity Signal, Leptin

First described in 1994 (Zhang et al. 1994), leptin has proven to be a key metabolic protein with actions throughout the body. Importantly, leptin provides a powerful catabolic signal to the brain, resulting in inhibition of food intake and increasing energy expenditure (Ahima et al. 1999; Elias et al. 1999; Elmquist et al. 1999; Schwartz et al. 2000; Woods et al. 2000; Morton et al. 2003; Seeley and Woods 2003; Balthasar et al. 2004; Schwartz and Porte 2005). Leptin is secreted from adipose tissue in direct proportion to fat content, and it crosses the blood–brain barrier to interact with leptin receptors in the hypothalamus and brainstem (Tartaglia et al. 1995; Ahima et al. 1996, 1999; Seeley et al. 1996; Elias et al. 1999; Morton et al. 2003; Schwartz and Porte 2005). Although there are several splice variants of the leptin receptor, the long form (termed leprb) is the critical variant for regulating energy balance (Chen et al. 1996). Leprb is localized in several brain areas including the VMN and the ARC, and leprb is colocalized with several neuropeptides believed to be involved in controlling food intake and reproduction (van Dijk et al. 1996; Elmquist et al. 1998a, b). Leptin has the ability to activate or inhibit hypothalamic neurons (Elmquist et al. 1998a–c). Thus, leptin is ideally situated to link metabolic status and brain function. It has been reported that leprb expression in the ARC is colocalized with ERα (Diano et al. 1998), and estrogens have been reported to regulate the expression of leprb mRNA in the ARC (Bennett et al. 1999), possibly via an ERE on the leptin receptor gene (Lindell et al. 2001). The extensive hypothalamic colocalization of these two receptors suggests a closely coupled interaction between these peripheral signals in the regulation of energy homeostasis.

Leptin levels are higher in females, even before puberty, compared with males, and these levels are independent of differences in body composition (Shimizu et al. 1997; Demerath et al. 1999; Wu-Peng et al. 1999). After puberty, estrogens and testosterone further modulate leptin synthesis and secretion via sex steroid receptor-dependent transcriptional mechanisms (Machinal et al. 1999). Estrogens may be modulators of leptin's catabolic action in the brain. Higher levels of estrogens have been associated with increased leptin sensitivity (Ainslie et al. 2001; Clegg et al. 2003b, 2006). Although circulating leptin levels do not change appreciably during the estrous cycle, ARC leprb expression is highest during estrus and metestrus and is inversely correlated with neuropeptide Y (NPY) mRNA expression (Bennett et al. 1999). OVX lowers sensitivity to central leptin when compared to intact females, and this can be restored by estradiol-17β replacement (Clegg et al. 2006). Analogously, exogenous estradiol-17β administration to male rats will increase sensitivity to central leptin (Clegg et al. 2006). The differences in leptin sensitivity caused by the presence or absence of estrogens may occur downstream of leprb transcription and translation. Additionally, females have greater c-Fos (a marker of neuronal activation) and pSTAT3 (a marker of leptin receptor activation) immunoreactivity in the ARC than males following intrathird ventricular leptin (unpublished data), which suggests enhanced leptin sensitivity. Therefore, there may be a threshold for estrogens required to enhance the central sensitivity to leptin.

Leptin resistance may also occur during pregnancy (Ladyman and Grattan 2005). Ladyman et al. demonstrated that pregnant rats treated with leptin had impaired activation of pSTAT3 and reduced leprb mRNA in the VMH when compared to nonpregnant females (Ladyman and Grattan 2005). However, there were no changes in leptin activation of pSTAT3 in the ARC of pregnant females, nor were there changes in leprb in pregnant vs. nonpregnant females. Pregnancy is a state of relative deficiency of estrogens, and these data may support the idea that low levels of estrogens are associated with reduced leptin sensitivity.

11.5 Estrogen Interacts with the Melanocortin System

As previously indicated, the ARC has been well investigated with regard to central leptin action (Woods et al. 2000; Williams et al. 2001). Leprb is expressed by two populations of ARC neurons, those expressing proopiomelanocortin (POMC) (Cheung et al. 1997; Thornton et al. 1997) and those expressing NPY and agouti-related peptide

(NPY/AgRP neurons) (Baskin et al. 1999). POMC neurons secrete the catabolic melanocortin neuropeptide, α-melanocyte stimulating hormone (αMSH), which acts in the PVN and lateral hypothalamus on melanocortin 3 and melanocortin 4 (MC3/MC4) receptors to produce a profound catabolic effect by reducing food intake and increasing energy expenditure (Elmquist et al. 1998c, 1999; Elias et al. 1999, 2000). If administered chronically, MC3/MC4 agonists reduce body weight and adiposity (Pierroz et al. 2002). Leptin stimulates POMC neurons to synthesize and release αMSH (Seeley and Schwartz 1997; Korner et al. 1999). AgRP is an antagonist at MC3/MC4 receptors, and its administration increases food intake. Hence, within the ARC, leptin elicits a powerful catabolic effect by activating αMSH and simultaneously inhibiting anabolic NPY/AgRP production and release. This produces reduced feeding and increased energy expenditure (Elmquist 1999 #1487).

POMC levels are also responsive to gonadal steroids. POMC mRNA levels fluctuate over the course of the estrous cycle, with the most dramatic changes on the day of proestrus (Wise et al. 1990; Bohler et al. 1991; Korner et al. 1999; Slamberova et al. 2004). POMC neurons express ERα (Miller et al. 1995), and OVX decreases POMC mRNA, which is reversed by estradiol-17β replacement (Pelletier et al. 2007). Lower POMC levels are also observed in ERα knockout mice (Hirosawa et al. 2008). Using electron microcopy, the Horvath group has reported that the number of excitatory synaptic inputs to ARC POMC neurons rises as mice enter proestrus when estrogen levels are high (Gao et al. 2007). Further, central estradiol-17β administration rapidly increases the excitatory synapses on POMC neurons, an effect that is also reflected by increased miniature excitatory postsynaptic current recorded from POMC–GFP neurons (Gao et al. 2007). These synaptological rearrangements in POMC neurons are tightly paralleled with the effects of estrogens on food intake, energy expenditure, and body weight (Gao et al. 2007). Estrogens activate POMC neurons partly via PI3K-mediated mechanisms (Qiu et al. 2003; Malyala et al. 2008). Collectively, these findings suggest that ERα in POMC neurons may contribute to energy homeostasis and the effects of estrogens. Similarly, the Ronnekleiv group reported that estradiol-17β administration in hypothalamic slices increases excitability of identified POMC neurons by rapidly uncoupling $GABA_B$ receptors from their G-protein-gated inwardly rectifying K^+ channels (Malyala et al. 2008). These studies demonstrated that estrogens directly act on POMC neurons and regulate their cellular activity. However, whether this regulation is mediated by ERα or other estrogen receptors and whether this estrogen–POMC interaction is physiologically relevant in the regulation of energy homeostasis remain to be elucidated.

11.6 Estrogens Interact with Serotonin

Estrogens decrease food intake by selectively influencing the neural controls of meal size, which likely require the serotonergic system (Lee et al. 1998). Estrogens heighten the anorexia induced by increased serotonergic neurotransmission (Rivera and Eckel 2005) and decreases the hyperphagia induced by decreased serotonergic neurotransmission (Uphouse et al. 1991; Salamanca and Uphouse 1992).

Estrogens were reported to increase the expression of the serotonin transporter (5-HTT) in the dorsal and median raphe nuclei, allowing estrogens to regulate the serotonin system (Rivera et al. 2009). Other labs reported that acute injection of estradiol-17β increased 5-HTT mRNA levels in the dorsal raphe nuclei (DRV) of OVX rats (McQueen et al. 1997; Sumner et al. 1999). The DRV has reciprocal connections with the hypothalamus and parabrachial nucleus (Petrov et al. 1992; Peyron et al. 1998) putting the DRV in a position to directly regulate part of the neural network controlling food intake (Peyron et al. 1998). The estrogens/serotonin interaction may also have clinical relevance, since human 5-HTT promoter polymorphisms are associated with anorexia nervosa, an eating disorder that primarily affects women (Heils et al. 1996; Fumeron et al. 2001).

11.7 Estrogens Interact with Cholecystokinin (CCK)

Cholecystokinin (CCK) is synthesized and released from cells of the upper intestine and acts on abdominal CCK-A receptors. It plays a variety of roles in the digestive process, including slowing gastric emptying and intestinal motility (see review Moran 2009). CCK exerts its satiety action primarily by activating subdiaphragmatic vagal afferent neurons (Degen et al. 2001). Administration of CCK antagonists increases food intake by increasing meal size (Moran et al. 1993). Several experiments have highlighted interactions between estrogens and CCK. CCK-A antagonists decreased food intake to a greater extent when intact females were in proesteus or estradiol-17β-treated OVX rats, and this effect was lessened in diestrous rats (Huang et al. 1993; Asarian and Geary 1999, 2007; Eckel and Geary 1999).

Because CCK satiation depends on vagal afferents (Moran et al. 1990, 1992; Reidelberger 1992), upregulation of CCK receptors in the terminals of vagal afferent fibers may account for the increased CCK sensitivity. To investigate this hypothesis, in vitro quantitative autoradiography was used to measure the effects of estradiol-17β treatment on the binding characteristics of CCK receptors in the nucleus of the solitary tract (NTS), a brain area that receives terminal projections of abdominal vagal afferent fibers (Moran et al. 1990), and in two interconnected areas, the area postrema (AP) and the VMN. Estradiol-17β treatment in OVX animals did not alter the number or affinity of CCK receptors (Geary et al. 1996), suggesting the upregulation of CCK receptors does not mediate the increased sensitivity to CCK following estradiol-17β treatment. Estrogens increase the potency of CCK by increasing the sensitivity of vagal CCK-A receptors, but do not increase CCK secretion or the number of CCK-A receptors (Linden et al. 1990; Butera et al. 1993; Geary et al. 1996; Asarian and Geary 1999).

CCK also influences meal size, and this has been characterized in male rats by examining the pattern of c-Fos expression after consumption (Fraser and Davison 1993; Emond and Weingarten 1995; DiNardo and Travers 1997; Park and Carr 1998; Rinaman et al. 1998; Eckel and Geary 2001) or injection of CCK (Olson et al. 1992; Chen et al. 1993; Rinaman et al. 1993, 1995; Li and Rowland 1994). Estradiol-17β treatment in OVX rats increased the number of feeding- and CCK-induced c-Fos-positive cells within the NTS, PVN, and the central nucleus of the amygdala (Eckel and Geary 2001; Eckel et al. 2002). These data suggest that exogenous estradiol-17β may decrease meal size by selectively increasing neuronal activity in multiple brain areas that control meal size. It is currently unknown whether a similar mechanism underlies the decrease in meal size or increase in CCK satiation, which occurs during estrus in cycling rats.

Although there is solid evidence estrogens increase the potency by which CCK exerts its direct, inhibitory control over meal size, such an interaction does not completely account for the decrease in food intake during estrus in gonadally intact rats or following estradiol-17β treatment in OVX rats. For example, blocking the release of CCK during a meal attenuated, but did not block, the phasic inhibitory decrease in meal size observed during estrus in gonadally intact rats (Eckel and Geary 1999). Additionally, endogenous CCK does not appear to play a role in the tonic inhibitory action of estradiol-17β (Asarian and Geary 1999; Eckel and Geary 1999). Thus, estrogens must modulate the potency of other stimuli that directly generate negative feedback during a meal.

11.8 Estrogens in the Central Nervous System Regulate Energy Homeostasis

In order to assess if estrogens directly influenced energy homeostasis in the CNS, intranuclear microinjections of estradiol benzoate were performed (Wade and Zucker 1970). However, due to the difficulty in precisely placing cannulae or producing lesions in small but complex hypothalamic regions, findings obtained from these studies are somewhat controversial. For example, earlier studies showed that estradiol-17β implanted in the PVN decreases food intake and body weight in OVX rats (Butera and Beikirch 1989) in the absence of any signs of peripheral estrogenic stimulation. Additionally, the anorexigenic effects of subcutaneous estradiol-17β were blunted in rats with PVN lesions (Butera et al. 1992). However, subsequent studies failed to reproduce these phenotypes in rats with PVN implants (Hrupka et al. 2002). Effects of estrogens in the medial preoptic area (MPOA) are also controversial, with only one report showing an anorexigenic response of estradiol-17β (Dagnault and Richard 1997), whereas several other groups showed that estradiol-17β implanted in this nucleus has no effect on feeding (Butera and Beikirch 1989). However, additional research on the direct effects of estrogens in the CNS is required.

11.9 Estrogen Receptors in the Central Nervous System

The effects of estrogens on energy balance are primarily mediated by ERα, one of the "classical" estrogen receptors. Women or female mice with mutations in the ERα gene are obese (Heine et al. 2000; Okura et al. 2003). Further, deletion of

ERα in mice blocks the antiobesity effects of replacement of estrogens (Geary et al. 2001). Although no hyperphagia is observed in ERαKO mice (Heine et al. 2000; Ohlsson et al. 2000; Geary et al. 2001), ERα is clearly required to mediate normal satiation processes, because estradiol-induced hypophagia and CCK-induced satiation in OVX wild-type mice are blocked in OVX ERαKO mice (Geary et al. 2001). Another estrogen receptor, ERβ, does not appear to mediate the antiobesity effects of estrogen, since deletion of ERβ does not lead to obesity (Ohlsson et al. 2000). This is consistent with pharmacological studies which showed that while a selective ERα agonist suppresses food intake, inhibition of ERβ does not influence feeding behavior (Santollo et al. 2007; Thammacharoen et al. 2008).

11.10 ERα in the Central Nervous System

ERα is abundantly expressed in the rodent brain, and it has been hypothesized that ERα in the brain may play important roles in regulating body weight, fat distribution, and glucose balance. Early studies showed that microinjections of estrogens into brain regions changed animals' feeding behavior and body weight (Palmer and Gray 1986; Butera and Beikirch 1989; Butera et al. 1992; Dagnault and Richard 1994; Hrupka et al. 2002). However, the physiological significance of estrogens/ERα signals in the brain in the context of body weight control was not directly addressed in these studies.

ERα is expressed in the ventrolateral portion of the VMN, the ARC, the MPOA, and the paraventricular nuclei (PVN) (Simerly et al. 1990; Simonian and Herbison 1997; Voisin et al. 1997; Osterlund et al. 1998; Wilkinson et al. 2002; Shima et al. 2003; Merchenthaler et al. 2004). ERβ is found in the same hypothalamic nuclei as ERα, but ERβ expression is significantly lower relative to ERα.

To determine if ERα in the CNS is required to maintain normal body weight balance in preliminary experiments, we crossed the mice carrying loxP-flanked ERα alleles (ERα$^{lox/lox}$) (Feng et al. 2007) to the Nestin-Cre transgenic mice (Bruning et al. 2000; Kleinridders et al. 2009) to produce mice lacking ERα only in the brain (ERα$^{lox/lox}$/Nestin-Cre mice) unpublished data. Compared to their ERα$^{lox/lox}$ littermates (controls), both male and female ERα$^{lox/lox}$/Nestin-Cre mice displayed significant increases in body weight (unpublished data). Further characterizations in female mice revealed that increases in body weight were mainly reflected by increased body fat (unpublished data). In addition, we found ERα$^{lox/lox}$/Nestin-Cre mice displayed hyperphagia (unpublished data) and decreased heat production (when compared to their ERα$^{lox/lox}$ littermates with matched body weight and lean mass) (unpublished data), which may both contribute to the development of obesity. In preliminary findings, the lower energy expenditure may be partly caused by decreased physical activity, as we found the ambulatory movements and rearing activities in ERα$^{lox/lox}$/Nestin-Cre mice were significantly lower than those in controls (unpublished data). Collectively, these preliminary findings suggest that ERα expressed in the CNS is required to facilitate estrogenic effects on food intake, energy expenditure and physical activity.

ERα is known to mediate the negative feedback regulation of estrogens on the hypothalamus–pituitary–gonad (HPG) axis (Couse et al. 1995). Notably, we have preliminary unpublished findings that circulating estradiol-17β is significantly elevated in $ER\alpha^{lox/lox}$/Nestin-Cre mice compared to the controls (unpublished preliminary findings), which suggests that ERα in the brain may at least partly mediate the negative feedback of estrogens. More importantly, our preliminary observations that mice lacking ERα only in the CNS developed robust obese phenotypes despite the higher estradiol-17β levels in the circulation further argue that compared to ERα expressed in peripheral tissues, brain ERα plays predominant roles in the regulation of energy balance.

11.11 ERα in the Ventromedial Hypothalamic Nucleus

As previously mentioned, ERα is found in the ARC and VMN (Osterlund et al. 1998; Merchenthaler et al. 2004; Schlenker and Hansen 2006), which are structures in very close proximity in the ventral hypothalamus. Earlier microinjection studies may have not differentiated the effects of injection in these two regions, and therefore failed to provide definitive results (Wade and Zucker 1970; Palmer and Gray 1986; Butera and Beikirch 1989). The VMN (also known as the VMH) has long been thought to be an important component of the neural circuits responsible for the homeostatic regulation of body weight and food intake. As previously mentioned, numerous studies showed that lesions of the VMN produce obesity due to both increased food intake and decreased energy expenditure (see King 2006). However, many of these results were questioned because the electrolytic insults and knife cuts used to lesion the VMN likely damaged the surrounding regions (such as the ARC) as well as neuronal fibers passing through the VMN (Gold 1973). Recent mouse genetic studies have begun to circumvent these issues by performing deletion of key genes specifically in VMH neurons. These studies were based on the finding that a transcription factor, steroidogenic factor-1 (SF1), is expressed exclusively in the VMN neurons within the brain (Ikeda et al. 1995). Deletion of SF1 in mice disrupts the VMN structure (Dellovade et al. 2000) and leads to obesity (Majdic et al. 2002). These findings supported the model that UMN neurons are physiological regulators of body weight homeostasis.

Multiple metabolic signals have been demonstrated to regulate energy homeostasis via actions in the VMN. For example, leptin directly activates SF1 neurons in the VMN and selective deletion of leptin receptors from SF1 neurons produces obesity. Likewise, knockdown of brain-derived neurotrophic factor (BDNF) in the VMH and dorsomedial hypothalamic nucleus produces hyperphagic obesity (Unger et al. 2007). Estrogens have been shown to directly alter the electrophysiological properties of VMN neurons (Minami et al. 1990). Further, a recent study has used the shRNA-mediated gene silencing approach to examine the role of estrogens and ERα in the VMN in the regulation of energy balance (Musatov et al. 2007). In this study, ERα in the VMN is silenced with an adeno-associated virus (AAV) carrying ERα-specific shRNA, while ERα expression in the ARC and other hypothalamic regions is shown to be unaffected (Musatov et al. 2007). Animals with impaired ERα signaling in the VMN are less sensitive to estradiol-induced weight loss and develop obesity characteristic of increased visceral fat (Musatov et al. 2007). The increased body weight is likely caused by decreased physical activity and impaired diet-induced thermogenesis, whereas food intake of these animals is not directly affected (Musatov et al. 2007). These findings support the hypothesis that ERα signaling in VMN neurons plays an important role in regulating physical activity, thermogenesis, and fat distribution.

11.12 ERα in the Brainstem

ERα is also present in the brainstem, including the NTS and DMV (Osterlund et al. 1998; Merchenthaler et al. 2004; Schlenker and Hansen 2006). Roles of these ERα populations have not yet been fully illustrated. Geary and coworkers showed that replacement of estrogens in wild-type mice suppresses food intake and potentiates CCK-induced satiation, which are accompanied by increased activity in NTS neurons (Geary 2001; Asarian and Geary 2007). Interestingly, these responses are all abolished in mice lacking ERα (Geary 2001). Further, it is shown that direct administration of estrogens in the NTS potentiates CCK-induced satiety signals (Thammacharoen et al. 2008). Collectively, these findings support the notion that ERα in the brainstem, such as in the NTS, may be another physiologically important site to mediate the anorexigenic effects of estrogens.

11.13 Estrogens Interact with NPY

NPY is an effective anabolic peptide. Central administration of NPY potently increases food intake and decreases energy expenditure and fat oxidation (Chavez et al. 1995; Levin 1999; Cone et al. 2001; Herzog 2003). ARC neurons coexpress NPY mRNA and leprb protein. Leptin administration decreases, while lack of leptin or leptin signaling increases, NPY (and AgRP) mRNA, demonstrating that leptin is a critical determinant of ARC NPY functioning (Baskin et al. 1999).

NPY neurons in the hypothalamus not only affect feeding, but they also influence reproduction. Therefore, estradiol can modulate both of these neuroendocrine systems by regulating NPY gene expression. NPY neurons are activated by signals indicating reduced energy availability, such as decreased levels of circulating glucose, leptin, or insulin, which increase NPY release in the PVN to stimulate feeding (Acosta-Martinez et al. 2007). This may be due to estradiol stimulating NPY and NPY Y1 receptor (Hill et al. 2004) expression and NPY release (Bonavera et al. 1994).

In an ex vivo hypothalamic neuronal cell line, N-38, estradiol affected the expression of NPY in a biphasic manner, which corresponded to changes in the ERα:ERβ ratio. When the ERα:ERβ ratio was high, NPY transcription was repressed; conversely, when the ratio was low, NPY transcription was stimulated. Additionally, a recent study has demonstrated that NPY/AgRP neurons are required to mediate the anorexigenic effects of estrogens. In this study, Xu and coworkers showed that hypothalamic expression of NPY and AgRP is tightly regulated across the estrous cycle, with the lowest levels during estrus which coincides with the plasma estrogen peak and feeding nadir in wild-type mice (Olofsson et al. 2009). They further showed that central estradiol administration suppresses fasting-induced c-Fos activation in NPY/AgRP neurons and blunts the refeeding response (Olofsson et al. 2009). Importantly, the cyclic changes in food intake and estradiol-induced anorexia are blunted in mice with degenerated NPY/AgRP neurons (Olofsson et al. 2009). This study indicates that neurons coexpressing NPY and AgRP are functionally required for the cyclic changes in feeding across estrous cycle and that NPY/AgRP neurons are essential mediators of estrogen's anorexigenic function. Surprisingly, these authors also found that ERα is completely excluded from NPY/AgRP neurons in the mouse hypothalamus (Olofsson et al. 2009), suggesting that estrogen may regulate these neurons indirectly via presynaptic neurons that express ERα. However, these ERα-expressing neurons that act on NPY/AgRP neurons remain to be identified.

11.14 Estrogens Interact with Ghrelin

Ghrelin is produced in the stomach and acts on growth hormone secretagogue receptors (GHSRs) to increase food intake. While mainly synthesized by the stomach, ghrelin is also found in the hypothalamus, pituitary gland, hippocampus, brain cortex, adrenal gland, intestine, and pancreas (Howard et al. 1996; Kojima et al. 1999; Kojima and Kangawa 2005). Exogenous ghrelin is less potent in intact female rats than in male rats or OVX females (Clegg et al. 2007). Central intrathird ventricular (i3vt) or peripheral ghrelin administration reliably increased feeding in intact male rats and OVX females (Tschöp et al. 2000; Horvath et al. 2001; Nakazato et al. 2001; Wren et al. 2001a, b; Davidson et al. 2005; Arnold et al. 2006); however, the threshold for a significant increase in feeding using either administration route was significantly reduced in intact females than in males or OVX females (Clegg et al. 2007). When OVX rats were treated with estradiol-17β, moderate intraperitoneal (i.p.) or i3vt doses of ghrelin no longer stimulated eating. Together, these data demonstrate that estradiol-17β reduces the orexigenic potency of ghrelin. Lastly, estradiol-17β replacement reduced the eating-stimulatory effect of i3vt ghrelin in male rats, indicating that the estrogenic effect exists in both sexes, which is a point of potential therapeutic relevance (Clegg et al. 2007). Careful attention to sex differences and gonadal hormone status should be included in the development of any ghrelin-based clinical control for eating behaviors.

The eating-stimulatory effect of ghrelin varies across different phases of the ovarian cycle in intact rats (Clegg et al. 2007). Administration of i3vt ghrelin had no reliable overall effect when cycle day was not taken into account. However, when the cycle day was considered, i3vt ghrelin increased eating during diestrus 1 and diestrus 2, but not during proestrus or estrus. In addition, in estradiol-17β replacement in OVX rats, ghrelin increased food intake on the days that modeled diestrus in intact rats, but not on the days that modeled proestrus or estrus. This indicates that there are cyclic variations in eating in rats and mice, and spontaneous food intake is maximal during diestrus and minimal during estrus. Therefore, the analogous periovulatory decreases in eating in women may be due to changes in estrogenic tone that affect ghrelin's eating-stimulatory action (Clegg et al. 2007). To assess the importance of ghrelin signaling in OVX-induced hyperphagia and obesity, $Ghsr^{-/-}$ mice lacking GHSR were OVX'd (Clegg et al. 2007). The OVX GHSR mice, which were similar to wild-type mice in body weight and food intake presurgery, showed no increase in food intake or body weight gain after surgery. This indicates that estrogens tonically inhibit endogenous ghrelin signaling in mice and that release from this inhibition is necessary for OVX mice to increase food intake and body weight. This mechanism may account for other sex differences in eating and weight regulation previously reported in $Ghsr^{-/-}$ mice. For example, female $Ghsr^{-/-}$ mice accumulated less body weight and adiposity when given a high-fat diet (Zigman et al. 2005). Also, the magnitude of the differences in adiposity observed between $Ghsr^{-/-}$ and wild-type mice was greater in females than in males (Clegg et al. 2007). Ghrelin signaling appears to be a necessary component of the estrogenic control of eating and weight regulation (Clegg et al. 2007).

The site of the GHSR-mediated effects on eating remains unclear (Kamegai et al. 2000, 2001; Shintani et al. 2001; Arnold et al. 2006), so estrogens may influence ghrelin and its receptors either centrally or peripherally (Clegg et al. 2007). In male brains, GHSRs have been implicated in ghrelin's eating-stimulatory effect in the ARC, PVN, ventral tegmental area, and dorsal vagal complex (Willesen et al. 1999; Horvath et al. 2001, 2003; Shintani et al. 2001; Cowley et al. 2003; Faulconbridge et al. 2003; Naleid et al. 2005). However, in one report, Currie et al. failed to observe any sex difference following direct ghrelin microinjections to the ARC or PVN (Currie et al. 2005). However, since ovarian cycling was not monitored, it is possible that the female rats were acyclic, which may have caused an artificial increase in ghrelin-induced eating. It is also possible that estrogenic actions on nucleus tractus solitaries (NTS) neurons contribute to the observed effects.

11.15 Estrogens Interact with Melanin-Concentrating Hormone (MCH)

Since its discovery in hypothalamic neurons (Vaughan et al. 1989; Bittencourt et al. 1992), melanin-concentrating hormone (MCH) has been recognized as an important regulator of energy homeostasis (Pissios et al. 2006). Central administration of MCH promotes feeding, while genetic ablation of the Mch gene produces a lean phenotype (Jeon et al. 2006). In addition, MCH is upregulated by fasting (Qu et al. 1996). MCH neurons in the LHA receive inputs from NPY/AgRP and POMC neurons in the ARC (Broberger et al. 1998; Elias et al. 1998, 1999; Schwartz et al. 2000; Flier 2004). Therefore, MCH neurons are in a position to integrate the feeding response because they have projections from the ARC and to brain structures like the nucleus accumbens (Georgescu et al. 2005).

Messina et al. investigated the effect of centrally injected MCH on feeding in estradiol-17β- and vehicle-treated OVX and male rats. MCH increased the meal size in all three groups. Additionally, intake increased more in rats in diestrus than rats in estrus, although MCH increased food intake in both groups. Overall, estradiol-17β decreased the orexigenic effect of MCH, leading the authors to hypothesize that the decrease in food intake during estrus was mediated by a decrease in MCH signaling (Messina et al. 2006). In a second study, Santollo et al. examined whether the behavioral effects of MCH were sexually dimorphic. They observed a greater increase in food intake, meal size, and water intake following MCH treatment in male rats than in estradiol-17β-treated OVX rats (Santollo and Eckel 2008). Additionally, they observed that higher MCH doses were necessary to increase food intake in estradiol-17β-treated OVX rats, suggesting that estradiol-17β reduced MCH sensitivity in female rats (Santollo and Eckel 2008). Given that circulating levels of estrogens are lower in males than in females, this sex difference may contribute to the increased sensitivity to MCH in male rats.

There are several ways that estradiol-17β could decrease MCH signaling. By acting on nuclear ERs in the lateral hypothalamus (LH) and zona incerta (ZI) (Shughrue et al. 1997), estrogens can alter gene transcription. ERs can modulate gene expression locally by decreasing MCH synthesis. In support of this hypothesis, physiological doses of estradiol-17β decreased prepro MCH mRNA expression in the ZI of OVX rats (Murray et al. 2000) and the LH of obese male rats. In addition, chronic estradiol-17β treatment in male rats blocked increases in LH MCH mRNA expression induced by fasting (Morton et al. 2004). In contrast, pharmacological doses of estradiol-17β in male mice increased MCH mRNA within hypothalamic tissue punches (Tritos et al. 2004). These discrepancies emphasize the need for additional research in intact, cycling rats to determine the role of endogenous estrogens in regulating MCH mRNA expression. It is also possible that estrogens, acting at nuclear ERs in brain regions that express MCH-1 receptors (Osterlund et al. 1998; Hervieu et al. 2000), can decrease MCH signaling by decreasing the number or binding affinity of MCH-1 receptors. A recent study demonstrated that LH neurons containing MCH-1 receptors and ERs are not coexpressed, but are in close proximity to one another (Muschamp and Hull 2007).

Several studies evaluated whether MCH affects meal size or number (Smith 2000; Messina et al. 2006; Santollo and Eckel 2008). The size of the first meal increased following MCH treatment in male and estradiol-17β- or vehicle-treated OVX rats. In male and vehicle-treated OVX rats, MCH increased the average meal size throughout the period of increased food intake. There was no change in meal size in the estradiol-17β-treated OVX rats, and there were no differences in meal number in any group, indicating that MCH increases food intake by increasing meal size in both males and females (Santollo and Eckel 2008).

11.16 Cellular Mechanisms of Estrogens

The cellular mechanisms for ERα functions can be broadly divided into two modes: (1) actions as a nuclear receptor (or genomic actions) and (2) rapid signaling (or nongenomic actions). For the nuclear receptor mode, inactive ERα exists in the cytoplasm. Upon binding of its ligand (e.g., estradiol-17β), activated ERα will undergo a conformational change, which will promote ERα homodimerization and subsequent nuclear translocation. In the nucleus, ERα acts as a ligand-dependent transcription factor, binding cognate palindromic estrogen response elements (EREs) in the promoters of target genes. This results in the recruitment of specific coregulators, resulting in an increase or decrease of transcription from the target gene (Vasudevan and Pfaff 2008). The rapid signaling initiated by ERα, on the other hand, takes place in a time frame of milliseconds to minutes. It can be initiated at the plasma membrane or in the cytoplasm by the natural ligand, estradiol-17β, resulting in the activation of signal transduction pathways, including PKA, MAPK, PI3K and calcium flux, within target cells (Vasudevan and Pfaff 2008).

Efforts have been made to dissociate the contribution of these two cellular mechanisms in the control of energy balance. For example, Pedram and coworkers generated a transgenic mouse model expressing only a functional E domain of ERα (MOER mice). The mutated ERα only exists at the cell membrane and retains capacity of initiating rapid signalings (at least in peripheral tissues). No ERα activity is present in the cytoplasm and the nucleus in MOER mice, and therefore ERα actions as a transcription factor are eliminated. Interestingly, MOER mice show similar obese phenotypes as ERα knockout mice (Pedram et al. 2009). These findings suggest that ERα on the membrane alone is not sufficient to maintain normal body weight, and that ERα in the cytoplasm and/or the nucleus is required. One limitation of this study is that the transgenic mutant ERα may not be faithfully expressed in all the sites. Importantly, the expression and the functions of this mutant ERα in the brain are not clear. In addition, as the mutant ERα is only present on the cytomembrane, the possible contribution of rapid signaling initiated by cytoplasmic ERα may be underestimated.

In contrast, a knock-in NERKI mouse model was made to introduce a mutation that selectively eliminates ERα signaling as a nuclear receptor. In this model, an

E207A/G208A mutation was made into the P box of the first zinc finger of the DNA-binding domain of ERα, and therefore abolishes ERE binding. However, the rapid signaling initiated by ERα (both in the cytomembrane and the cytoplasm) is preserved (Jakacka et al. 2002). Interestingly, these NERKI mice do not develop obesity (Syed et al. 2007). These findings indicate that the nuclear receptor properties of ERα are not required to maintain energy homeostasis. Instead, the rapid signaling initiated by ERα may be sufficient to mediate the estrogenic regulation of body weight.

11.17 Estrogens in Males

One fact that may have been underappreciated is that estrogens are also important for the regulation of metabolism in males. For example, boys experience a robust estradiol surge during the first 3 months of life (Bidlingmaier et al. 1987). Animal studies indicated that this neonatal estradiol exposure in males produces metabolic and cardiovascular benefits during adulthood, including decreased body weight and adiposity, lower blood pressure, and improved glucose tolerance (Cederroth and Nef 2009). These findings raise the possibility that estrogens are important for programming metabolic and cardiovascular profiles in males. In addition, estrogens may also directly affect energy balance in adult males. Like menopausal women, aged men have a higher incidence of obesity, type II diabetes, and cardiovascular diseases (Yeap 2009). Obesity in middle-aged and older men is associated with lower testosterone levels (Yeap 2009), suggesting that testosterone may provide antiobesity benefits in adult men. However, these effects cannot be attributed to the direct actions of testosterone on its receptor (the androgen receptor), as activation of the androgen receptor promotes eating (Callewaert et al. 2009). One hypothesis is that testosterone in males is converted by aromatase into estradiol, which in turn acts on ER to produce antiobesity benefits. Indeed, circulating estradiol levels in adult men is estimated to be 110 ± 54 pmol/L, which is comparable to that observed during the early follicular phase of the menstrual cycle in women and is significantly higher than in postmenopausal women (Longcope et al. 1990; de Ronde et al. 2003). Sixty percent of male estradiol is formed by aromatization of testosterone through aromatase (Baird et al. 1969). Estrogens and ERα may contribute to the regulation of energy balance in males.

Aromatase activity is present in the gonad, fat, bone, and brain (Murata et al. 2002; Roselli et al. 2002). Importantly, mutations in aromatase (Grumbach and Auchus 1999; Jones et al. 2000) cause obesity and metabolic dysfunctions in males. Within the brain, aromatase-expressing neurons are found in the bed nucleus of the stria terminalis (BNST), the medial amygdala (MeA), preoptic hypothalamus (POA), and lateral septum. These aromatase-expressing neurons have projections to the anterior hypothalamus and the VMH (Wu et al. 2009). As aromatase is not only present in the cell bodies, but also in the fibers and presynaptic terminals (Naftolin et al. 1996; Peterson et al. 2005), regions containing either aromatase-expressing cell bodies or fibers are exposed to enriched local estradiol microenvironment. Besides neurons, aromatase is also found in the glial cells (Martinez-Cerdeno et al. 2006). These findings support the possibility that brain aromatase activity may provide high levels of estrogens in male brains (as well as in female brains), which may act on ER (e.g., ERα) to regulate body weight homeostasis.

11.18 Conclusions

In this chapter, we have discussed the importance of estrogens in the regulation of energy homeostasis. We have provided evidence suggesting one of the critical sites of estrogen action is the CNS. Lastly, we discussed the potential role of ERα, both nuclear and membrane-associated, in the regulation of body weight.

When women enter menopause, they dramatically increase their risk for developing obesity, type II diabetes, and the metabolic syndrome. Hormone replacement therapy (HRT) in postmenopausal women has become very controversial. Due to the ubiquitous expression of ERs, especially in peripheral tissues, and to complex intracellular events coupled to ERs ("genomic" and "nongenomic" actions), the metabolic benefits provided by HRT are often associated with increased risk of heart disease and breast cancer. Obviously, one solution to this dilemma would be to target only the ERs involved in energy balance and to develop estrogen-like drugs that only initiate intracellular events that would produce metabolic benefits without unwanted side effects. Therefore, future research should focus on identifying the critical sites where ERs regulate body weight homeostasis and delineate the intracellular signaling pathways that are required for estrogens' actions. Additionally, understanding the functional role of ERs in the periphery may reveal new pharmacological targets for the beneficial actions of therapeutic estrogens without the deleterious side effects.

References

Acosta-Martinez M, Horton T et al (2007) Estrogen receptors in neuropeptide Y neurons: at the crossroads of feeding and reproduction. Trends Endocrinol Metab 18(2):48–50

Ahima RS, Prabakaran D et al (1996) Role of leptin in the neuroendocrine response to fasting. Nature 382:250–252

Ahima RS, Kelly J et al (1999) Distinct physiologic and neuronal responses to decreased leptin and mild hyperleptinemia. Endocrinology 140(11):4923–4931

Ainslie DA, Morris MJ et al (2001) Estrogen deficiency causes central leptin insensitivity and increased hypothalamic neuropeptide Y. Int J Obes Relat Metab Disord 25(11):1680–1688

Andersson B, Mattsson LA et al (1997) Estrogen replacement therapy decreases hyperandrogenicity and improves glucose homeostasis and plasma lipids in postmenopausal women with non-insulin-dependent diabetes mellitus. J Clin Endocrinol Metab 82(2):638–643

Arnold M, Mura A et al (2006) Gut vagal afferents are not necessary for the eating-stimulatory effect of intraperitoneally injected ghrelin in the rat. J Neurosci 26(43):11052–11060
Asarian L, Geary N (1999) Cyclic estradiol treatment phasically potentiates endogenous cholecystokinin's satiating action in ovariectomized rats. Peptides 20(4):445–450
Asarian L, Geary N (2007) Estradiol enhances cholecystokinin-dependent lipid-induced satiation and activates estrogen receptor-alpha-expressing cells in the nucleus tractus solitarius of ovariectomized rats. Endocrinology 148(12):5656–5666
Baird DT, Horton R et al (1969) Steroid dynamics under steady-state conditions. Recent Prog Horm Res 25:611–664
Balthasar N, Coppari R et al (2004) Leptin receptor signaling in POMC neurons is required for normal body weight homeostasis. Neuron 42(6):983–991
Baskin DG, Schwartz MW et al (1999) Leptin receptor long form splice variant protein expression in neuron cell bodies of the brain and colocalization with neuropeptide Y mRNA in the arcuate nucleus. J Histochem Cytochem 47:353–362
Bennett PA, Lindell K et al (1999) Cyclical variations in the abundance of leptin receptors, but not in circulating leptin, correlate with NPY expression during the oestrous cycle. Neuroendocrinology 69(6):417–423
Bidlingmaier F, Strom TM et al (1987) Estrone and estradiol concentrations in human ovaries, testes, and adrenals during the first two years of life. J Clin Endocrinol Metab 65(5):862–867
Bittencourt JC, Presse F et al (1992) The melanin-concentrating hormone system of the rat brain: an immuno- and hybridization histochemical characterization. J Comp Neurol 319(2):218–245
Bjorntorp P (1997a) Body fat distribution, insulin resistance, and metabolic diseases. Nutrition 13:795–803
Bjorntorp P (1997b) Hormonal control of regional fat distribution. Hum Reprod 12(Suppl 1):21–25
Blaustein JD, Wade GN (1976) Ovarian influences on the meal patterns of female rats. Physiol Behav 17(2):201–208
Bohler HC Jr, Tracer H et al (1991) Changes in proopiomelanocortin messenger ribonucleic acid levels in the rostral periarcuate region of the female rat during the estrous cycle. Endocrinology 128(3):1265–1269
Bonavera JJ, Dube MG et al (1994) Anorectic effects of estrogen may be mediated by decreased neuropeptide-Y release in the hypothalamic paraventricular nucleus. Endocrinology 134(6):2367–2370
Bray GA (1984) Hypothalamic and genetic obesity: an appraisal of the autonomic hypothesis and the endocrine hypothesis. Int J Obes 8(Suppl 1):119–137
Bray GA, York DA (1972) Studies on food intake of genetically obese rats. Am J Physiol 223(1):176–179
Bray GA, Sclafani A et al (1982) Obesity-inducing hypothalamic knife cuts: effects on lipolysis and blood insulin levels. Am J Physiol 243(3):R445–R449
Broberger C, De Lecea L et al (1998) Hypocretin/orexin- and melanin-concentrating hormone-expressing cells form distinct populations in the rodent lateral hypothalamus: relationship to the neuropeptide Y and agouti gene-related protein systems. J Comp Neurol 402:460–474
Bruning JC, Gautam D et al (2000) Role of brain insulin receptor in control of body weight and reproduction. Science 289(5487):2122–2125
Butera PC, Beikirch RJ (1989) Central implants of diluted estradiol: independent effects on ingestive and reproductive behaviors of ovariectomized rats. Brain Res 491(2):266–273
Butera PC, Willard DM et al (1992) Effects of PVN lesions on the responsiveness of female rats to estradiol. Brain Res 576(2):304–310
Butera PC, Bradway DM et al (1993) Modulation of the satiety effect of cholecystokinin by estradiol. Physiol Behav 53(6):1235–1238
Callewaert F, Venken K et al (2009) Differential regulation of bone and body composition in male mice with combined inactivation of androgen and estrogen receptor-alpha. FASEB J 23(1):232–240

Carr MC (2003) The emergence of the metabolic syndrome with menopause. J Clin Endocrinol Metab 88(6):2404–2411
Cederroth CR, Nef S (2009) Soy, phytoestrogens and metabolism: a review. Mol Cell Endocrinol 304(1–2):30–42
Chavez M, van Dijk G et al (1995) Third ventricular insulin infusion attenuates NPY-induced feeding at the level of the paraventricular nucleus. Obes Res 3:335s
Chen DY, Deutsch JA et al (1993) The induction and suppression of c-fos expression in the rat brain by cholecystokinin and its antagonist L364,718. Neurosci Lett 149(1):91–94
Chen G, Koyama K et al (1996) Disappearance of body fat in normal rats induced by adenovirus-mediated leptin gene therapy. Proc Natl Acad Sci USA 93:14795–14799
Cheung CC, Clifton DK et al (1997) Proopiomelanocortin neurons are direct targets for leptin in the hypothalamus. Endocrinology 138:4489–4492
Clegg DJ, Benoit SC et al (2003a) Estrogen mediates body fat distribution and brain sensitivity to adiposity signals. Diabetes 52(Suppl 1):A24
Clegg DJ, Riedy CA et al (2003b) Differential sensitivity to central leptin and insulin in male and female rats. Diabetes 52(3):682–687
Clegg DJ, Brown LM et al (2006) Gonadal hormones determine sensitivity to central leptin and insulin. Diabetes 55(4):978–987
Clegg DJ, Brown LM et al (2007) Estradiol-dependent decrease in the orexigenic potency of ghrelin in female rats. Diabetes 56(4):1051–1058
Cone RD, Cowley MA et al (2001) The arcuate nucleus as a conduit for diverse signals relevant to energy homeostasis. Int J Obes Relat Metab Disord 25(Suppl 5):S63–S67
Couse JF, Curtis SW et al (1995) Disruption of the mouse oestrogen receptor gene: resulting phenotypes and experimental findings. Biochem Soc Trans 23(4):929–935
Cowley MA, Smith RG et al (2003) The distribution and mechanism of action of ghrelin in the CNS demonstrates a novel hypothalamic circuit regulating energy homeostasis. Neuron 37(4):649–661
Currie PJ, Mirza A et al (2005) Ghrelin is an orexigenic and metabolic signaling peptide in the arcuate and paraventricular nuclei. Am J Physiol Regul Integr Comp Physiol 289(2):R353–R358
D'Eon TM, Souza SC et al (2005) Estrogen regulation of adiposity and fuel partitioning. Evidence of genomic and non-genomic regulation of lipogenic and oxidative pathways. J Biol Chem 280(43):35983–35991
Dagnault A, Richard D (1994) Lesions of hypothalamic paraventricular nuclei do not prevent the effect of estradiol on energy and fat balance. Am J Physiol 267(1 Pt 1):E32–E38
Dagnault A, Richard D (1997) Involvement of the medial preoptic area in the anorectic action of estrogens. Am J Physiol 272(1 Pt 2):R311–R317
Danguir J, Nicolaidis S (1980) Cortical activity and sleep in the rat lateral hypothalamic syndrome. Brain Res 185(2):305–321
Davidson TL, Kanoski SE et al (2005) The interoceptive cue properties of ghrelin generalize to cues produced by food deprivation. Peptides 26(9):1602–1610
de Ronde W, Pols HA et al (2003) The importance of oestrogens in males. Clin Endocrinol (Oxf) 58(5):529–542
Degen L, Matzinger D et al (2001) The effect of cholecystokinin in controlling appetite and food intake in humans. Peptides 22(8):1265–1269
Dellovade TL, Young M et al (2000) Disruption of the gene encoding SF-1 alters the distribution of hypothalamic neuronal phenotypes. J Comp Neurol 423(4):579–589
Demerath EW, Towne B et al (1999) Serum leptin concentration, body composition, and gonadal hormones during puberty. Int J Obes Relat Metab Disord 23(7):678–685
Diano S, Kalra SP et al (1998) Leptin receptors in estrogen receptor-containing neurons of the female rat hypothalamus. Brain Res 812(1–2):256–259
DiNardo LA, Travers JB (1997) Distribution of fos-like immunoreactivity in the medullary reticular formation of the rat after gustatory elicited ingestion and rejection behaviors. J Neurosci 17(10):3826–3839

Drewett RF (1973) Sexual behaviour and sexual motivation in the female rat. Nature 242(5398):476–477

Eckel LA, Geary N (1999) Endogenous cholecystokinin's satiating action increases during estrus in female rats. Peptides 20(4):451–456

Eckel LA, Geary N (2001) Estradiol treatment increases feeding-induced c-Fos expression in the brains of ovariectomized rats. Am J Physiol Regul Integr Comp Physiol 281(3):R738–R746

Eckel LA, Houpt TA et al (2002) Estradiol treatment increases CCK-induced c-Fos expression in the brains of ovariectomized rats. Am J Physiol Regul Integr Comp Physiol 283(6):R1378–R1385

Elias CF, Saper CB et al (1998) Chemically defined projections linking the mediobasal hypothalamus and the lateral hypothalamic area. J Comp Neurol 402(4):442–459

Elias CF, Aschkenasi C et al (1999) Leptin differentially regulates NPY and POMC neurons projecting to the lateral hypothalamic area. Neuron 23(4):775–786

Elias CF, Kelly JF et al (2000) Chemical characterization of leptin-activated neurons in the rat brain [in process citation]. J Comp Neurol 423(2):261–281

Elmquist JK, Ahima RS et al (1998a) Leptin activates distinct projections from the dorsomedial and ventromedial hypothalamic nuclei. Proc Natl Acad Sci USA 95:741–746

Elmquist JK, Bjorbaek C et al (1998b) Distributions of leptin receptor mRNA isoforms in the rat brain. J Comp Neurol 395(4):535–547

Elmquist JK, Maratos-Flier E et al (1998c) Unraveling the central nervous system pathways underlying responses to leptin. Nat Neurosci 1:445–450

Elmquist JK, Elias CF et al (1999) From lesions to leptin: hypothalamic control of food intake and body weight. Neuron 22:221–232

Emond MH, Weingarten HP (1995) Fos-like immunoreactivity in vagal and hypoglossal nuclei in different feeding states: a quantitative study. Physiol Behav 58(3):459–465

Faulconbridge LF, Cummings DE et al (2003) Hyperphagic effects of brainstem ghrelin administration. Diabetes 52(9):2260–2265

Feng Y, Manka D et al (2007) Estrogen receptor-alpha expression in the mammary epithelium is required for ductal and alveolar morphogenesis in mice. Proc Natl Acad Sci USA 104(37):14718–14723

Flegal KM, Carroll MD et al (2002) Prevalence and trends in obesity among US adults, 1999–2000. JAMA 288(14):1723–1727

Flier JS (2004) Obesity wars: molecular progress confronts an expanding epidemic. Cell 116:337–350

Fraser KA, Davison JS (1993) Meal-induced c-fos expression in brain stem is not dependent on cholecystokinin release. Am J Physiol 265(1 Pt 2):R235–R239

Freedman DS, Khan LK et al (2002) Trends and correlates of class 3 obesity in the United States from 1990 through 2000. JAMA 288(14):1758–1761

Fumeron F, Betoulle D et al (2001) Association of a functional 5-HT transporter gene polymorphism with anorexia nervosa and food intake. Mol Psychiatry 6(1):9–10

Gao Q, Mezei G et al (2007) Anorectic estrogen mimics leptin's effect on the rewiring of melanocortin cells and Stat3 signaling in obese animals. Nat Med 13(1):89–94

Geary N (2001) Estradiol, CCK and satiation. Peptides 22(8):1251–1263

Geary N, Smith GP et al (1996) The increased satiating potency of CCK-8 by estradiol is not mediated by upregulation of NTS CCK receptors. Brain Res 719(1–2):179–186

Geary N, Asarian L et al (2001) Deficits in E2-dependent control of feeding, weight gain, and cholecystokinin satiation in ER-alpha null mice. Endocrinology 142(11):4751–4757

Georgescu D, Sears RM et al (2005) The hypothalamic neuropeptide melanin-concentrating hormone acts in the nucleus accumbens to modulate feeding behavior and forced-swim performance. J Neurosci 25(11):2933–2940

Gold RM (1973) Hypothalamic obesity: the myth of the ventromedial nucleus. Science 182(4111):488–490

Grumbach MM, Auchus RJ (1999) Estrogen: consequences and implications of human mutations in synthesis and action. J Clin Endocrinol Metab 84(12):4677–4694

Heils A, Teufel A et al (1996) Allelic variation of human serotonin transporter gene expression. J Neurochem 66(6):2621–2624

Heine PA, Taylor JA et al (2000) Increased adipose tissue in male and female estrogen receptor-alpha knockout mice. Proc Natl Acad Sci USA 97(23):12729–12734
Hervieu GJ, Cluderay JE et al (2000) The distribution of the mRNA and protein products of the melanin- concentrating hormone (MCH) receptor gene, slc-1, in the central nervous system of the rat. Eur J Neurosci 12(4):1194–1216
Herzog H (2003) Neuropeptide Y and energy homeostasis: insights from Y receptor knockout models. Eur J Pharmacol 480(1–3):21–29
Hill JW, Urban JH et al (2004) Estrogen induces neuropeptide Y (NPY) Y1 receptor gene expression and responsiveness to NPY in gonadotrope-enriched pituitary cell cultures. Endocrinology 145(5):2283–2290
Hirosawa M, Minata M et al (2008) Ablation of estrogen receptor alpha (ERalpha) prevents upregulation of POMC by leptin and insulin. Biochem Biophys Res Commun 371(2):320–323
Horvath TL, Diano S et al (2001) Minireview: ghrelin and the regulation of energy balance – a hypothalamic perspective. Endocrinology 142(10):4163–4169
Horvath TL, Diano S et al (2003) Ghrelin in hypothalamic regulation of energy balance. Curr Top Med Chem 3(8):921–927
Howard AD, Feighner SD et al (1996) A receptor in pituitary and hypothalamus that functions in growth hormone release. Science 273(5277):974–977
Hrupka BJ, Smith GP et al (2002) Hypothalamic implants of dilute estradiol fail to reduce feeding in ovariectomized rats. Physiol Behav 77(2–3):233–241
Huang YS, Doi R et al (1993) Effect of cholecystokinin on food intake at different stages of the estrous cycle in female rats. J Assoc Acad Minor Phys 4(2):56–58
Ikeda Y, Luo X et al (1995) The nuclear receptor steroidogenic factor 1 is essential for the formation of the ventromedial hypothalamic nucleus. Mol Endocrinol 9(4):478–486
Jakacka M, Ito M et al (2002) An estrogen receptor (ER)alpha deoxyribonucleic acid-binding domain knock-in mutation provides evidence for nonclassical ER pathway signaling in vivo. Mol Endocrinol 16(10):2188–2201
Jeon JY, Bradley RL et al (2006) MCH–/– mice are resistant to aging-associated increases in body weight and insulin resistance. Diabetes 55(2):428–434
Jones ME, Thorburn AW et al (2000) Aromatase-deficient (ArKO) mice have a phenotype of increased adiposity. Proc Natl Acad Sci USA 97(23):12735–12740
Kaaja RJ (2008) Metabolic syndrome and the menopause. Menopause Int 14(1):21–25
Kamegai J, Tamura H et al (2000) Central effect of ghrelin, an endogenous growth hormone secretagogue, on hypothalamic peptide gene expression. Endocrinology 141(12):4797–4800
Kamegai J, Tamura H et al (2001) Chronic central infusion of ghrelin increases hypothalamic neuropeptide Y and Agouti-related protein mRNA levels and body weight in rats. Diabetes 50(11):2438–2443
King BM (2006) The rise, fall, and resurrection of the ventromedial hypothalamus in the regulation of feeding behavior and body weight. Physiol Behav 87(2):221–244
Kleinridders A, Konner AC et al (2009) CNS-targets in control of energy and glucose homeostasis. Curr Opin Pharmacol 9(6):794–804
Kojima M, Kangawa K (2005) Ghrelin: structure and function. Physiol Rev 85(2):495–522
Kojima M, Hosoda H et al (1999) Ghrelin is a growth-hormone-releasing acylated peptide from stomach. Nature 402(6762):656–660
Korner J, Chua SC Jr et al (1999) Regulation of hypothalamic proopiomelanocortin by leptin in lean and obese rats. Neuroendocrinology 70(6):377–383
Kotani K, Tokunaga K et al (1994) Sexual dimorphism of age-related changes in whole-body fat distribution in the obese. Int J Obes Relat Metab Disord 18(4):207–212
Ladyman SR, Grattan DR (2005) Suppression of leptin receptor messenger ribonucleic acid and leptin responsiveness in the ventromedial nucleus of the hypothalamus during pregnancy in the rat. Endocrinology 146(9):3868–3874
Lee MD, Aloyo VJ et al (1998) Infusion of the serotonin1B (5-HT1B) agonist CP-93,129 into the parabrachial nucleus potently and selectively reduces food intake in rats. Psychopharmacology (Berl) 136(3):304–307

Levin BE (1999) Arcuate NPY neurons and energy homeostasis in diet-induced obese and resistant rats. Am J Physiol 276(2 Pt 2):R382–R387

Li BH, Rowland NE (1994) Cholecystokinin- and dexfenfluramine-induced anorexia compared using devazepide and c-fos expression in the rat brain. Regul Pept 50:223–233

Lindell K, Bennett PA et al (2001) Leptin receptor 5′ untranslated regions in the rat: relative abundance, genomic organization and relation to putative response elements. Mol Cell Endocrinol 172(1–2):37–45

Linden A, Uvnas-Moberg K et al (1990) Involvement of cholecystokinin in food intake: III. Oestradiol potentiates the inhibitory effect of cholecystokinin octapeptide on food intake in ovariectomized rats. J Neuroendocrinol 2(6):797–801

Longcope C, Goldfield SR et al (1990) Androgens, estrogens, and sex hormone-binding globulin in middle-aged men. J Clin Endocrinol Metab 71(6):1442–1446

Louis-Sylvestre J (1980) Neuroendocrinology of hyperphagias and obesities. Reprod Nutr Dev 20(5B):1545–1562

Machinal F, Dieudonne MN et al (1999) In vivo and in vitro ob gene expression and leptin secretion in rat adipocytes: evidence for a regional specific regulation by sex steroid hormones. Endocrinology 140(4):1567–1574

Majdic G, Young M et al (2002) Knockout mice lacking steroidogenic factor 1 are a novel genetic model of hypothalamic obesity. Endocrinology 143(2):607–614

Malyala A, Zhang C et al (2008) PI3K signaling effects in hypothalamic neurons mediated by estrogen. J Comp Neurol 506(6):895–911

Martinez-Cerdeno V, Noctor SC et al (2006) Estradiol stimulates progenitor cell division in the ventricular and subventricular zones of the embryonic neocortex. Eur J Neurosci 24(12):3475–3488

McQueen JK, Wilson H et al (1997) Estradiol-17 beta increases serotonin transporter (SERT) mRNA levels and the density of SERT-binding sites in female rat brain. Brain Res Mol Brain Res 45(1):13–23

Merchenthaler I, Lane MV et al (2004) Distribution of estrogen receptor alpha and beta in the mouse central nervous system: in vivo autoradiographic and immunocytochemical analyses. J Comp Neurol 473(2):270–291

Messina MM, Boersma G et al (2006) Estradiol decreases the orexigenic effect of melanin-concentrating hormone in ovariectomized rats. Physiol Behav 88(4–5):523–528

Milam KM, Stern JS et al (1980) Effect of lateral hypothalamic lesions on regulation of body weight and adiposity in rats. Am J Physiol 239(3):R337–R343

Miller MM, Tousignant P et al (1995) Effects of age and long-term ovariectomy on the estrogen-receptor containing subpopulations of beta-endorphin-immunoreactive neurons in the arcuate nucleus of female C57BL/6J mice. Neuroendocrinology 61(5):542–551

Minami T, Oomura Y et al (1990) 17 beta-estradiol depolarization of hypothalamic neurons is mediated by cyclic AMP. Brain Res 519(1–2):301–307

Moran TH (2009) Gut peptides in the control of food intake. Int J Obes (Lond) 33(Suppl 1):S7–S10

Moran TH, Norgren R et al (1990) Central and peripheral vagal transport of cholecystokinin binding sites occurs in afferent fibers. Brain Res 526(1):95–102

Moran TH, Ameglio PJ et al (1992) Blockade of type A, not type B, CCK receptors attenuates satiety actions of exogenous and endogenous CCK. Am J Physiol 262(1 Pt 2):R46–R50

Moran TH, Ameglio PJ et al (1993) Blockade of type A, but not type B, CCK receptors postpones satiety in rhesus monkeys. Am J Physiol 265:R620–R624

Morton GJ, Niswender KD et al (2003) Arcuate nucleus-specific leptin receptor gene therapy attenuates the obesity phenotype of Koletsky (fa(k)/fa(k)) rats. Endocrinology 144(5): 2016–2024

Morton GJ, Mystkowski P et al (2004) Increased hypothalamic melanin concentrating hormone gene expression during energy restriction involves a melanocortin-independent, estrogen-sensitive mechanism. Peptides 25(4):667–674

Murata Y, Robertson KM et al (2002) Effect of estrogen deficiency in the male: the ArKO mouse model. Mol Cell Endocrinol 193(1–2):7–12

Murray JF, Baker BI et al (2000) The influence of gonadal steroids on pre-pro melanin-concentrating hormone mRNA in female rats. J Neuroendocrinol 12(1):53–59
Musatov S, Chen W et al (2007) Silencing of estrogen receptor alpha in the ventromedial nucleus of hypothalamus leads to metabolic syndrome. Proc Natl Acad Sci USA 104(7):2501–2506
Muschamp JW, Hull EM (2007) Melanin concentrating hormone and estrogen receptor-alpha are coextensive but not coexpressed in cells of male rat hypothalamus. Neurosci Lett 427(3):123–126
Naftolin F, Horvath TL et al (1996) Aromatase immunoreactivity in axon terminals of the vertebrate brain. An immunocytochemical study on quail, rat, monkey and human tissues. Neuroendocrinology 63(2):149–155
Nakazato M, Murakami N et al (2001) A role for ghrelin in the central regulation of feeding. Nature 409(6817):194–198
Naleid AM, Grace MK et al (2005) Ghrelin induces feeding in the mesolimbic reward pathway between the ventral tegmental area and the nucleus accumbens. Peptides 26(11):2274–2279
Obici S (2009) Minireview: molecular targets for obesity therapy in the brain. Endocrinology 150(6):2512–2517
Ohlsson C, Hellberg N et al (2000) Obesity and disturbed lipoprotein profile in estrogen receptor-alpha-deficient male mice. Biochem Biophys Res Commun 278(3):640–645
Okura T, Koda M et al (2003) Relationships of resting energy expenditure with body fat distribution and abdominal fatness in Japanese population. J Physiol Anthropol Appl Human Sci 22(1):47–52
Olofsson LE, Pierce AA et al (2009) Functional requirement of AgRP and NPY neurons in ovarian cycle-dependent regulation of food intake. Proc Natl Acad Sci USA 106(37):15932–15937
Olson BR, Hoffman GE et al (1992) Cholecystokinin induces c-fos expression in hypothalamic oxytocinergic neurons projecting to the dorsal vagal complex. Brain Res 569(2):238–248
Osterlund M, Kuiper GG et al (1998) Differential distribution and regulation of estrogen receptor-alpha and -beta mRNA within the female rat brain. Brain Res Mol Brain Res 54(1): 175–180
Palmer K, Gray JM (1986) Central vs. peripheral effects of estrogen on food intake and lipoprotein lipase activity in ovariectomized rats. Physiol Behav 37(1):187–189
Park TH, Carr KD (1998) Neuroanatomical patterns of fos-like immunoreactivity induced by a palatable meal and meal-paired environment in saline- and naltrexone-treated rats. Brain Res 805(1–2):169–180
Pedram A, Razandi M et al (2009) Developmental phenotype of a membrane only estrogen receptor alpha (MOER) mouse. J Biol Chem 284(6):3488–3495
Pelletier G, Li S et al (2007) Oestrogenic regulation of pro-opiomelanocortin, neuropeptide Y and corticotrophin-releasing hormone mRNAs in mouse hypothalamus. J Neuroendocrinol 19(6):426–431
Peterson RS, Yarram L et al (2005) Aromatase is pre-synaptic and sexually dimorphic in the adult zebra finch brain. Proc Biol Sci 272(1576):2089–2096
Petrov T, Krukoff TL et al (1992) The hypothalamic paraventricular and lateral parabrachial nuclei receive collaterals from raphe nucleus neurons: a combined double retrograde and immunocytochemical study. J Comp Neurol 318(1):18–26
Peyron C, Petit JM et al (1998) Forebrain afferents to the rat dorsal raphe nucleus demonstrated by retrograde and anterograde tracing methods. Neuroscience 82(2):443–468
Pierroz DD, Ziotopoulou M et al (2002) Effects of acute and chronic administration of the melanocortin agonist MTII in mice with diet-induced obesity. Diabetes 51(5):1337–1345
Pissios P, Bradley RL et al (2006) Expanding the scales: the multiple roles of MCH in regulating energy balance and other biological functions. Endocr Rev 27(6):606–620
Qiu J, Bosch MA et al (2003) Rapid signaling of estrogen in hypothalamic neurons involves a novel G-protein-coupled estrogen receptor that activates protein kinase C. J Neurosci 23(29): 9529–9540
Qu D, Ludwig DS et al (1996) A role for melanin-concentrating hormone in the central regulation of feeding behaviour. Nature 380(6571):243–247

Reidelberger RD (1992) Abdominal vagal mediation of the satiety effects of exogenous and endogenous cholecystokinin in rats. Am J Physiol 263(6 Pt 2):R1354–R1358

Rinaman L, Verbalis JG et al (1993) Distribution and neurochemical phenotypes of caudal medullary neurons activated to express cFos following peripheral administration of cholecystokinin. J Comp Neurol 338(4):475–490

Rinaman L, Hoffman GE et al (1995) Cholecystokinin activates catecholaminergic neurons in the caudal medulla that innervate the paraventricular nucleus of the hypothalamus in rats. J Comp Neurol 360:246–256

Rinaman L, Baker EA et al (1998) Medullary c-Fos activation in rats after ingestion of a satiating meal. Am J Physiol 275:R262–R268

Rivera HM, Eckel LA (2005) The anorectic effect of fenfluramine is increased by estradiol treatment in ovariectomized rats. Physiol Behav 86(3):331–337

Rivera HM, Oberbeck DR et al (2009) Estradiol increases Pet-1 and serotonin transporter mRNA in the midbrain raphe nuclei of ovariectomized rats. Brain Res 1259:51–58

Rogers NH, Perfield JW II et al (2009) Reduced energy expenditure and increased inflammation are early events in the development of ovariectomy-induced obesity. Endocrinology 150(5):2161–2168

Roselli CE, Resko JA et al (2002) Hormonal influences on sexual partner preference in rams. Arch Sex Behav 31(1):43–49

Salamanca S, Uphouse L (1992) Estradiol modulation of the hyperphagia induced by the 5-HT1A agonist, 8-OH-DPAT. Pharmacol Biochem Behav 43(3):953–955

Santollo J, Eckel LA (2008) Estradiol decreases the orexigenic effect of neuropeptide Y, but not agouti-related protein, in ovariectomized rats. Behav Brain Res 191(2):173–177

Santollo J, Wiley MD et al (2007) Acute activation of ER alpha decreases food intake, meal size, and body weight in ovariectomized rats. Am J Physiol Regul Integr Comp Physiol 293(6):R2194–R2201

Schlenker EH, Hansen SN (2006) Sex-specific densities of estrogen receptors alpha and beta in the subnuclei of the nucleus tractus solitarius, hypoglossal nucleus and dorsal vagal motor nucleus weanling rats. Brain Res 1123(1):89–100

Schwartz MW, Porte D Jr (2005) Diabetes, obesity, and the brain. Science 307(5708):375–379

Schwartz MW, Woods SC et al (2000) Central nervous system control of food intake. Nature 404:661–671

Seeley RJ, Schwartz MW (1997) Regulation of energy balance: peripheral endocrine signals and hypothalamic neuropeptides. Curr Direct Psychol Sci 6:39–44

Seeley RJ, Woods SC (2003) Monitoring of stored and available fuel by the CNS: implications for obesity. Nat Rev Neurosci 4(11):901–909

Seeley RJ, van Dijk G et al (1996) The effect of intraventricular administration of leptin on food intake and body weight in the rat. Horm Metab Res 28:664–668

Shima N, Yamaguchi Y et al (2003) Distribution of estrogen receptor beta mRNA-containing cells in ovariectomized and estrogen-treated female rat brain. Anat Sci Int 78(2):85–97

Shimizu H, Shimomura Y et al (1997) Estrogen increases in vivo leptin production in rats and human subjects. J Endocrinol 154(2):285–292

Shintani M, Ogawa Y et al (2001) Ghrelin, an endogenous growth hormone secretagogue, is a novel orexigenic peptide that antagonizes leptin action through the activation of hypothalamic neuropeptide Y/Y1 receptor pathway. Diabetes 50(2):227–232

Shughrue PJ, Lane MV et al (1997) Comparative distribution of estrogen receptor-alpha and -beta mRNA in the rat central nervous system. J Comp Neurol 388(4):507–525

Simerly RB, Chang C et al (1990) Distribution of androgen and estrogen receptor mRNA-containing cells in the rat brain: an in situ hybridization study. J Comp Neurol 294(1):76–95

Simonian SX, Herbison AE (1997) Differential expression of estrogen receptor alpha and beta immunoreactivity by oxytocin neurons of rat paraventricular nucleus. J Neuroendocrinol 9(11):803–806

Slamberova R, Hnatczuk OC et al (2004) Expression of proopiomelanocortin and proenkephalin mRNA in sexually dimorphic brain regions are altered in adult male and female rats treated prenatally with morphine. J Pept Res 63(5):399–408

Smith GP (2000) The controls of eating: a shift from nutritional homeostasis to behavioral neuroscience. Nutrition 16:814–820
Sumner BE, Grant KE et al (1999) Effects of tamoxifen on serotonin transporter and 5-hydroxytryptamine(2A) receptor binding sites and mRNA levels in the brain of ovariectomized rats with or without acute estradiol replacement. Brain Res Mol Brain Res 73(1–2):119–128
Syed FA, Fraser DG et al (2007) Effects of loss of classical estrogen response element signaling on bone in male mice. Endocrinology 148(4):1902–1910
Tartaglia LA, Dembski M et al (1995) Identification and expression cloning of a leptin receptor, OB-R. Cell 83(7):1263–1271
Thammacharoen S, Lutz TA et al (2008) Hindbrain administration of estradiol inhibits feeding and activates estrogen receptor-alpha-expressing cells in the nucleus tractus solitarius of ovariectomized rats. Endocrinology 149(4):1609–1617
Thornton JE, Cheung CC et al (1997) Regulation of hypothalamic proopiomelanocortin mRNA by leptin in ob/ob mice. Endocrinology 138:5063–5067
Tritos NA, Segal-Lieberman G et al (2004) Estradiol-induced anorexia is independent of leptin and melanin-concentrating hormone. Obes Res 12(4):716–724
Tschöp M, Smiley DL et al (2000) Ghrelin induces adiposity in rodents. Nature 407(6806):908–913
Unger TJ, Calderon GA et al (2007) Selective deletion of Bdnf in the ventromedial and dorsomedial hypothalamus of adult mice results in hyperphagic behavior and obesity. J Neurosci 27(52):14265–14274
Uphouse L, Salamanca S et al (1991) Gender and estrous cycle differences in the response to the 5-HT1A agonist 8-OH-DPAT. Pharmacol Biochem Behav 40(4):901–906
van Dijk G, Thiele TE et al (1996) Central infusion of leptin and GLP-1 (7-36) amide differentially stimulate c-Fos-like immunoreactivity in the rat brain. Am J Physiol 271:R1096–R1100
Vasudevan N, Pfaff DW (2008) Non-genomic actions of estrogens and their interaction with genomic actions in the brain. Front Neuroendocrinol 29(2):238–257
Vaughan JM, Fischer WH et al (1989) Characterization of melanin-concentrating hormone from rat hypothalamus. Endocrinology 125(3):1660–1665
Voisin DL, Simonian SX et al (1997) Identification of estrogen receptor-containing neurons projecting to the rat supraoptic nucleus. Neuroscience 78(1):215–228
Wade GN, Zucker I (1970) Modulation of food intake and locomotor activity in female rats by diencephalic hormone implants. J Comp Physiol Psychol 72(2):328–336
Wallen WJ, Belanger MP et al (2001) Sex hormones and the selective estrogen receptor modulator tamoxifen modulate weekly body weights and food intakes in adolescent and adult rats. J Nutr 131(9):2351–2357
Wilkinson HA, Dahllund J et al (2002) Identification and characterization of a functionally distinct form of human estrogen receptor beta. Endocrinology 143(4):1558–1561
Willesen MG, Kristensen P et al (1999) Co-localization of growth hormone secretagogue receptor and NPY mRNA in the arcuate nucleus of the rat. Neuroendocrinology 70(5):306–316
Williams G, Bing C et al (2001) The hypothalamus and the control of energy homeostasis: different circuits, different purposes. Physiol Behav 74(4–5):683–701
Wise PM, Scarbrough K et al (1990) Diurnal pattern of proopiomelanocortin gene expression in the arcuate nucleus of proestrous, ovariectomized, and steroid-treated rats: a possible role in cyclic luteinizing hormone secretion. Mol Endocrinol 4(6):886–892
Woods SC, Schwartz MW et al (2000) Food intake and the regulation of body weight. Annu Rev Psychol 51:255–277
Wren AM, Seal LJ et al (2001a) Ghrelin enhances appetite and increases food intake in humans. J Clin Endocrinol Metab 86(12):5992
Wren AM, Small CJ et al (2001b) Ghrelin causes hyperphagia and obesity in rats. Diabetes 50(11):2540–2547
Wu MV, Manoli DS et al (2009) Estrogen masculinizes neural pathways and sex-specific behaviors. Cell 139(1):61–72
Wu-Peng S, Rosenbaum M et al (1999) Effects of exogenous gonadal steroids on leptin homeostasis in rats. Obes Res 7(6):586–592

Yeap BB (2009) Are declining testosterone levels a major risk factor for ill-health in aging men? Int J Impot Res 21(1):24–36

York DA, Bray GA (1972) Dependence of hypothalamic obesity on insulin, the pituitary and the adrenal gland. Endocrinology 90(4):885–894

Zhang Y, Proenca R et al (1994) Positional cloning of the mouse obese gene and its human homologue. Nature 372(6505):425–432

Zigman JM, Nakano Y et al (2005) Mice lacking ghrelin receptors resist the development of diet-induced obesity. J Clin Invest 115(12):3564–3572

Index

J. Russo (ed.), *Environment and Breast Cancer*, DOI 10.1007/978-1-4419-9896-5,

MIX
Papier aus verantwortungsvollen Quellen
Paper from responsible sources
FSC® C105338

If you have any concerns about our products,
you can contact us on
ProductSafety@springernature.com

In case Publisher is established outside the EU,
the EU authorized representative is:
Springer Nature Customer Service Center GmbH
Europaplatz 3, 69115 Heidelberg, Germany

Printed by Libri Plureos GmbH
in Hamburg, Germany